healthcare
OTHERWHERE

34th UIA/PHG International Seminar on Public Healthcare Facilities
Durban, South Africa. August 03-07, 2014
at UIA 2014 Durban Architecture Otherwhere

Proceedings
edited by Romano Del Nord

Conference organized by:

UIA International Union of Architects
UIA/PHG Public Health Group

Published by
TESIS Inter-University Research Centre
Systems and Technologies for Social and Healthcare Facilities
University of Florence
Italy

Scientific Editor:
Prof. Romano Del Nord
Director of TESIS Inter-University Research Centre
University of Florence

Session introductions (pp. 17, 63, 129) and volume layout:
Francesca Nesi
Arch. PhD
University of Florence

Published by

TESIS Inter-University Research Centre "Systems and Technologies for Social and Healthcare Facilities"

Department of Architecture DIDA
University of Florence

Via San Niccolò 93
info@tesis.unifi.it
+ 39 055 275 5348
Florence 50125
Italy

ISBN 978-88-907872-7-0
First Print 2015

The editors of the volume wish to thank Council for Scientific and Industrial Research (CSIR) in South Africa, especially Geoff Abbott and Peta de Jager for their support in collecting the papers and reports from the authors.

Cover photograph KwaZulu-Natal Research Unit for Tuberculosis and HIV (KRITH), Durban.

HHH Index

TESIS Inter-University Research Centre "Systems and Technologies for Social and Healthcare Facilities"
University of Florence, Italy

TESIS

Index

Foreword

by the Local Organising Committee

The occasion on the XXV International Union of Architects (UIA) World Congress in South Africa in 2014 provided an opportunity for members and friends of the UIA Public Health Group meeting (PHG) and GUPHA to meet and share experiences in a unique and vibrant setting between meetings held in Toronto, Canada in 2013 and in Dalian, China planned for 2015.

Unlike many of its precursors, the Durban PHG meeting was conceptualized as an integral part of the "main" UIA meeting and the UIA-PHG was formally recognized as a programme partner with an autonomous, dedicated, parallel track. This format allowed delegates the opportunity to enjoy the multitude of Congress activities, exhibitions and interactive events, and also for "other" Congress visitors to engage with the focused interests of the Public Health Group. The structure also resulted in the professional publication of academic papers of the proceedings of the UIA-PHG track through the general Congress outputs.

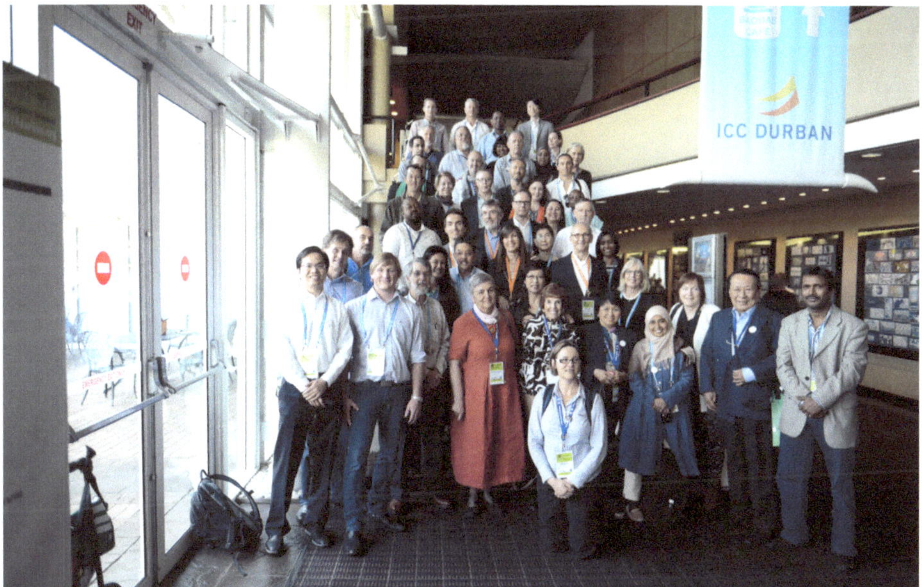

Participants attending the UIA Public Health Group Seminar held in Durban, South Africa, 03-07 August 2014.

This book is a compendium of activities and content related to the PHG at the 2014 Congress, which is in a long tradition of such dedicated healthcare architecture publications, including PHG proceedings, compiled under the leadership of Professor Romano Del Nord and his team at TESIS Inter-University Research Center Systems and Technologies for Social and Healthcare Facilities at the University of Florence, Italy.
The UIA meeting auspiciously coincided with the nomination of Cape Town in 2014 as World Design Capital, which prompted the local organizing committee to plan a field trip to a number of selected healthcare facilities in Cape Town (pg 181) in addition to a few in the host city of Durban (pg 187).

As well as traditional activities, such as a general UIA-PHG meeting chaired by Hans Eggen with the support of Janice Axon, the Congress saw the first International PHG Student Competition, with a number of fine entries and a prestigious jury (pg 189). This is already being followed by a second student competition, and, it is hoped, will become a regular event. Prize giving was undertaken at the annual dinner which was held in the unique, eclectic and local culturally inspired Ammazulu African Palace. Shortly after the conclusion of the Congress, the UIA-PHG established a Young Leader's Group, which seeks to ensure succession and continuity in the group through involving and inspiring emerging architects with an interest in this subspecialist field across nations and continents.

The local organizing committee need to pay respect to Warren Kerr, George Mann, David Allison, who provided leadership and encouragement throughout the organization. A number of important sponsors made the student competition and UIA-PHG exhibition stand possible, and these are acknowledged in text. We give thanks the many members and friends who paid service to UIA-PHG, on the peer review panel, who travelled great distances to Cape Town and Durban and participated in the pre-Congress and Congress activities.

Finally it is needed to thank the UIA 2014 Organising Committee, UIA 2014 Durban Scientific Committee and Review Panel especially the General Reporter, Dr Amira Osman and conference vendors who worked tirelessly to ensure that things ran smoothly.

We trust that this publication will provide treasured memories for those who visited Durban, consolation for those who couldn't make it and a valuable record of shared experiences. Enjoy!!

Geoff Abbott and Peta de Jager

Foreword

by the UIA Congress Organising Committee

The UIA 2014 World Congress, held from 3-7 August 2014 in Durban, South Africa, brought together architects, design and built environment professionals, pioneers in urban planning and thinking, activists, city makers, academics and researchers, students, government officials, decision makers and thought leaders, citizens and communities - to debate and discuss strategies for the design and delivery of more habitable, functional and beautiful cities.

UIA 2014 provided an opportunity for African architects to make their mark in the debate that perceives poverty eradication as a first unavoidable step in human progress. 2014 set out to explore how architects might play a pivotal role in addressing social inequalities. UIA Congress noted that Africa provides an abundance of opportunity – the ideologies of the last 100 years have done their time and failed, and the models aspired to in development are questionable. It posed the question: whether a lost respect and responsibility for our natural environment, commitment to our communities, and healthy social interaction could be rediscovered? This is a continent which has developed as others saw fit – now is the time for Africa to lead in anOTHER way forward…

The Congress theme OTHERWHERE and sub-themes of RESILIENCE, ECOLOGY and VALUES flowed from these desires: exploring OTHER ways of 'knowing' and 'doing', unlocking the multiple voices of Architecture. Congress organisers undertook to demonstrate that Architecture is as much spatial and formal as it is political, ideological, economical and theoretical – thus having the potential to influence thinking and policy. Having emerged from a century dominated by engineered, mechanised solutions and the marketing machinery of popular culture, the Durban Congress revisited the qualitative aspects of the world around us and, in so doing, brought attention to the perspective that, what we build is not only utilitarian but is, in fact, a humanitarian act; an investment in the environment and people through Architecture – reflecting people's aspirations, values and concerns. To enhance and support the academic aspects of the Congress, UIA 2014 involved a range of programme partners, who were instrumental in expanding the scope of the Congress. These partnerships aimed to use the event as a platform for furthering conversations on the Congress themes and pertinent built environment issues via collaborations planned to fit seamlessly into the main UIA 2014 event. The synergy between the between the event and the programme partners was acknowledged to be crucial to the development of the Congress programme and content.

Among programme partners was the Public Health Group of the UIA (UIA – PHG). The UIA - PHG is one of the working bodies of the UIA, the Union International des Architects or International Union of Architects which was founded in1955 and represents members and guest from all continents and a growing participation from more than 60 countries. Within the context of the UIA philosophy it is the vision of the UIA-PHG that world public health can profit by the dedication of architects to provide efficient, safe and aesthetic health care buildings and an environment that can contribute to a more rapid healing of the patients as well as an improvement in staff operations and satisfaction. To this end, UIA-PHG local organizing committee, saw Durban 2014 as a windfall opportunity to share its knowledge and experience – with an African flavor - not only within the group but also with other architects, engineers and consultants, health care managers and providers, health care organizations and governments, as well as to the general public who were present during the Congress as well as in the build-up to the event, as is its mission to do.

As programme partner, the UIA-PHG led a dedicated parallel track within the UIA Congress proceedings whilst still engaging with the overall Congress activities and debates. A pre-Congress tour to a variety of Cape Town and Durban healthcare facilities was arranged, which provided a useful window into wide disparities experienced African society. A healthcare focus international student competition – Healthcare OTHERWHERE – provided students from anywhere to engage with the special challenges and opportunities provided at Warwick Junction.

The UIA Congress received a total of 554 abstract submissions and 270 draft full papers, of which some 30 were healthcare related and identified for inclusion in the PHG track at the Congress. All congress submissions were subject to a rigorous two-tiered, double-blind peer review process before acceptance, inclusion and publication in the UIA Official Congress Programme, Book of Abstracts and Final Proceedings Book.

The UIA-PHG activities, together with the papers and presentations from the PHG track, are the focus of this publication, which combines the visual presentations presented at the Durban International Conference Centre and modified versions of the academic papers extracted from the full Congress proceedings.

The Multidisciplinary Approach in the Design of a Humanized Hospital

Romano Del Nord

romano.delnord@unifi.it
Professor, University of Florence, Director of TESIS Inter-University Research Centre,
Director of CSPE Professional Office, Italy

In the spirit of considering the printing and dissemination of the PHG Seminar Proceedings as an opportunity to disseminate updated knowledge and information useful for supporting the culture of hospital designers in operational terms, the editor of this volume, as a side event to the seminar, wished to offer a contribution to the increasingly topical debate on the criteria, methods and tools in order to steer hospital design towards the humanization of spaces for care. These contributions derive from the results of research conducted on behalf of the Ministry of Health in Italy.

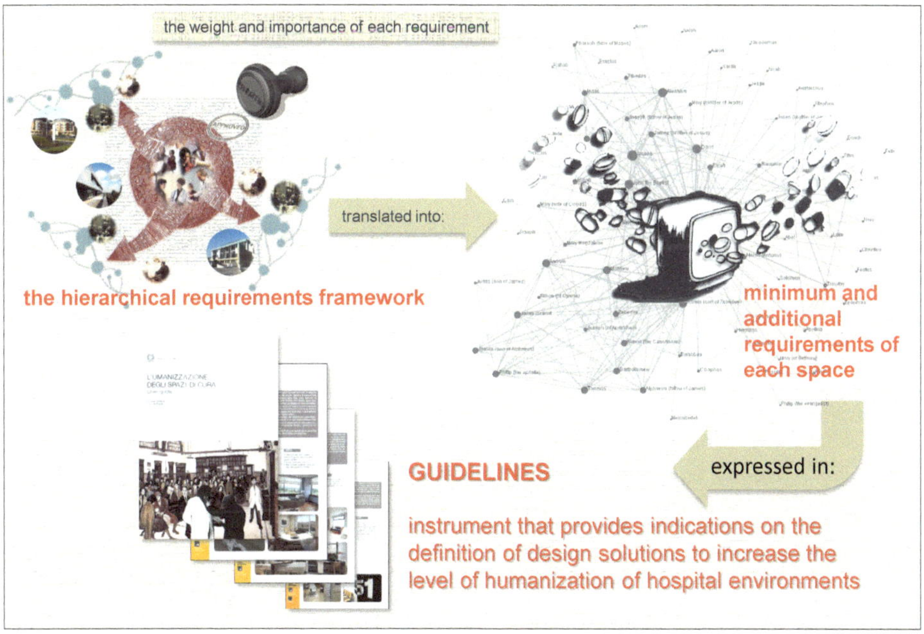

Figure 1. The guidelines for the design of humanized hospital environments.

The irrepressible intrusiveness of biomedical technologies in therapeutic processes, now more than ever, is leading to full and shared awareness that how the hospital space is used is heavily influenced by the physical and emotional impact of the facility on the users and that the arrangement of the space can play a complementary role to that of the treatments provided within.

This affirms the vision that conceives of the hospital environment as a healing environment, namely therapeutic in itself. In short, the hospital increasingly becomes the constructed expression of a society's degree of civilization and of its culture of hospitalization which modern environmental psychology is transforming into a science with mechanisms that link the dynamics of treatment to the emotional and perceptual centrality of the patient.

Of the tasks assigned to the designer, the one increasingly considered to be strategic concerns the ability to prevent conditions of environmental stress inside the hospital facility also operating through the psychological-environmental component. To pursue this objective it is necessary to act on user behaviour patterns which on the one hand are conditioned by the morphological-spatial configurations of the areas and on the other by the perceptive and sensory stimuli of the environment: a patient in uncomfortable or pathologically critical conditions reacts in relation to the explicit or implicit messages transmitted by the space.

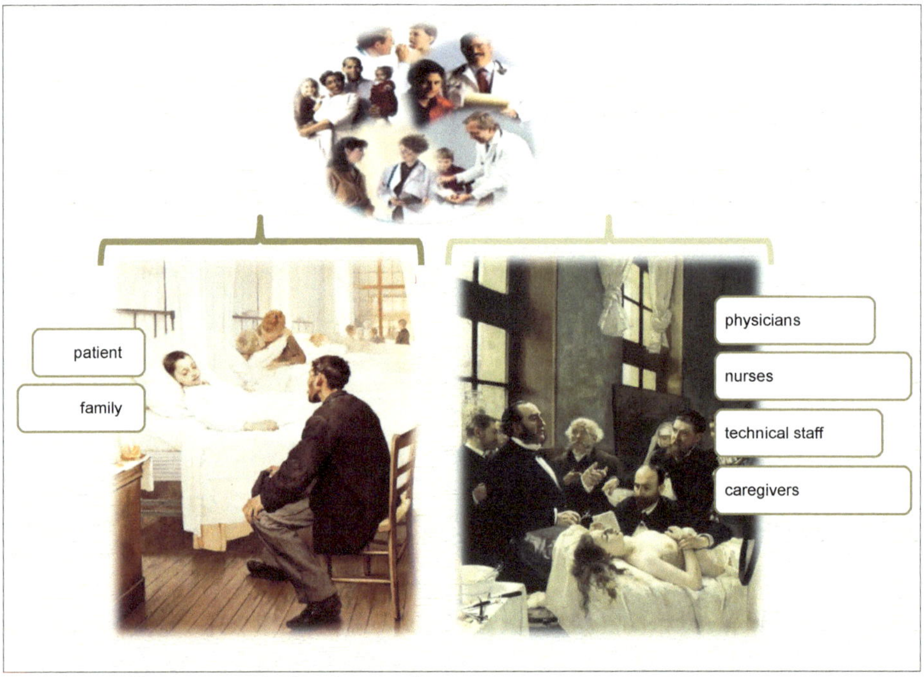

Figure 2. Profile of users involved in the research.

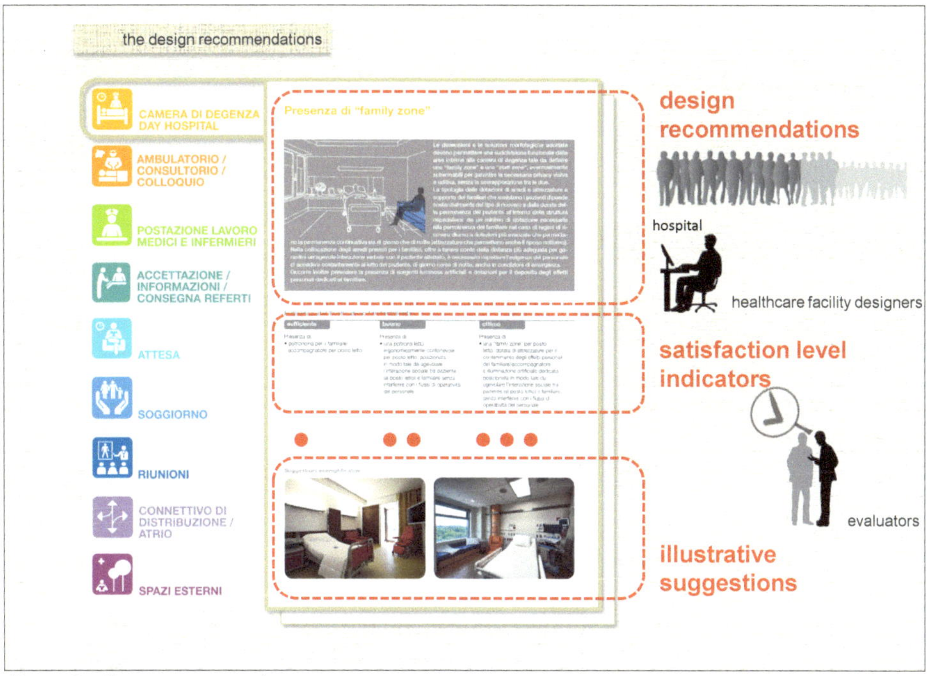

Figure 3. Design recommendations.

It follows that there is a need to focus on as many of the aspects as possible that affect sensory perception and to translate them into the correct design of the different hospital areas. In operational terms this translates into closer collaboration between psycho-social and design sciences: collaboration which is undoubtedly extremely useful but difficult to put into practice in the sense that the languages adopted by the different disciplines are difficult to interpret and translate across sectors.

It is therefore necessary for designers, on the one hand, to question the meaning of the expression "requirement" linked to psychological phenomena; and for environmental psychologists, on the other, to know how to convey their information so that it can be used effectively in the process of formulating design-related decisions.
What is not acceptable, however, is for the facilities become the testing ground of a esthetic and formal languages detached from the complexity of the services to be provided and inconsiderate of the principles of human dignity which, insofar as service facilities for the community, must be guaranteed for ordinary citizens. A condition that could be satisfied by using design approaches based on the "real" principles of multidisciplinarity and deriving from the acquired conviction that the "physical space" for treatment can perform an effective therapeutic action if conceived so that the principles of human/space conflict are attenuated, stress-inducing phenomena are reduced and perceptual/sensory phenomena are correctly assessed.

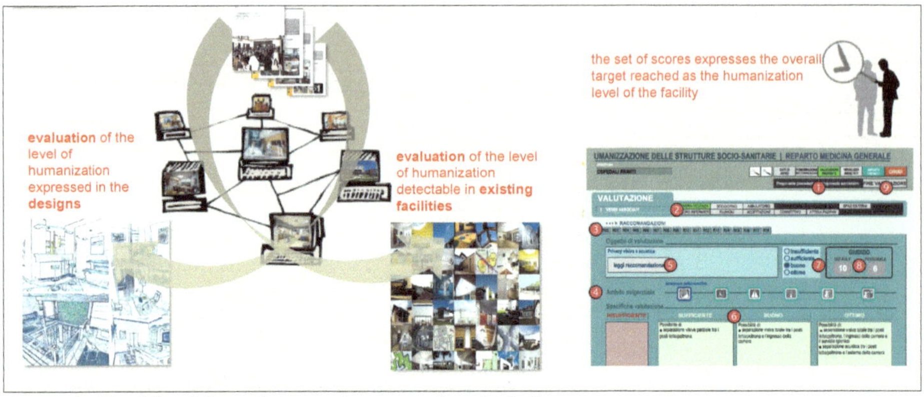

Figure 4. The IT tool for evaluation, objective and method of use.

Faced with such a scenario, the critical point for designers and decision makers is to identify the logics and methods, namely how, through suitable design and decisions-making strategies, it is possible to create the environmental conditions to promote health and restore it when it is compromised.

The promotion of health action (macro level), as we know, is carried out in two main directions which can be identified as generation and maintenance. Generation can be associated with actions to correct factors that create stress and bad health in built environments (corrective action of land reclamation); the creation of new environments free of factors known to be negative (prevention action);and the implementation and reinforcement of salutogenic factors (actions to induce the causes of good health). The action to restore health (micro level) is that which directly calls on the involvement of the health facilities system as a whole and more specifically affects hospital design models.

In the broad and complex operational sphere of actions to improve the health of people the role of the designer assumes special importance. The latter, in fact, as the inventor and author of habitat transformations, is concerned with crucial decisions about the physical and environmental qualities which are determinants for the onset of pathogenic phenomenon or the improvement of health and wellness conditions.

The designer not only acts on health determinants, which are physical by nature, but also on social determinants (how people's behaviour can be influenced by acting on the space). In fact, the ultimate aim of the design action does not so much lie in the object itself but rather on the effect it produces in social terms. In this sense it is projected into a meta-design perspective. For all these reasons the new design strategies must take inspiration from a more up-to-date way of understanding and interpreting "health", "disease", "treatment", and "wellbeing".

Taking these assumptions as a starting point the Interuniversity Centre for Research TESIS of the University of Florence and the DAD Department of Turin Polytechnic have developed – on behalf of the Italian Ministry of Health – a research project

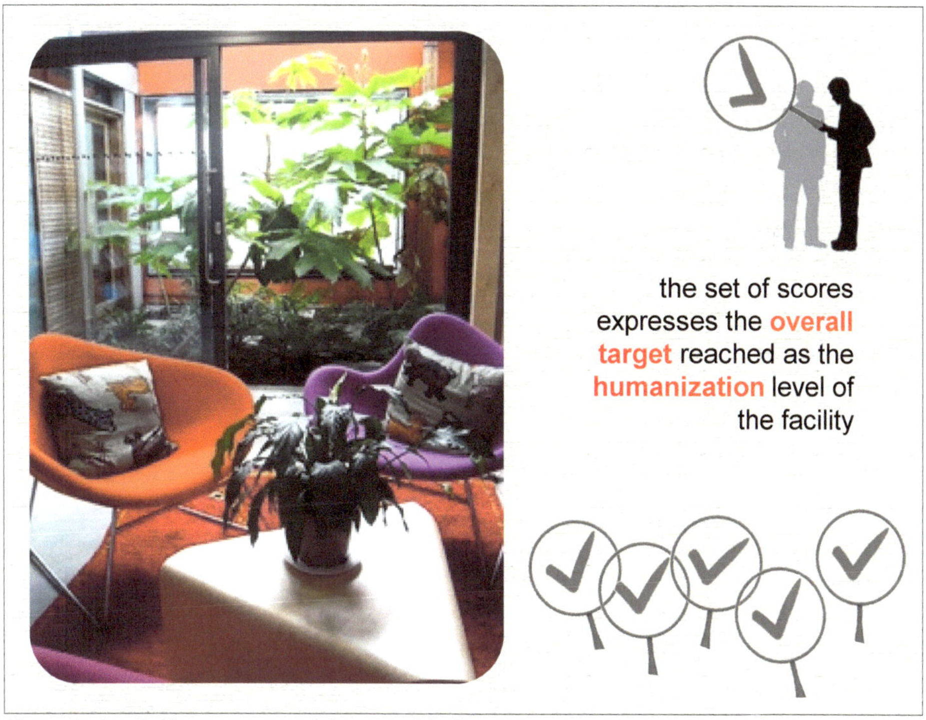

Figure 5. Level of humanization of designs and facilities.

aimed at defining the principles and criteria for the "Humanization of spaces for care" (Figure 1).
To give the research the marked value of an interdisciplinary approach and operational pragmatism, the working group involved researchers and professors qualified in hospital design, environmental psychology, medical statistics, sociology and medicine, as well as medical and nursing personnel, facility managers and professors of the health disciplines most concerned.
Collaboration with research institutions that have been operating abroad for some time on the same topics developing positively tested proposals turned out to be particularly profitable.

Starting with the assumption that the objective of humanizing healthcare facilities has already been widely absorbed and shared by the culture of users and decision-makers and the awareness that the state of developments and propositions has already reached a level of universally shared convergences, the task of researchers has been to organically systematize what, moreover, can already be verified in the highest quality designs and works, with stimulating feedback in the post-occupancy evaluations. The primary purpose has thus become that of offering a valid contribution to the dissemination of knowledge and information useful to those who systematically or occasionally operate in the area of designing socio-healthcare facilities and in particular spaces used for treating sick people where the fragile condition of the patient collides with a frequent lack of comfort, hospitality and psychological and physical well-being that could instead help to speed up the recovery process.

During development the research adopted the methodology of the performance design approach with particular attention given to the perceptual and sensory aspects that, in this case, best connote the specific characteristics of the requirements framework. The surveys carried out in the field have helped to corroborate the results of the desk-based research and to support the construction of the importance hierarchy attributed by users to the aspects that most affect the perception of humanization (Figure 2).

The system of the guidelines produced obviously refers to the humanization components that concern the quality of the spaces perceived in the different human-environment interaction methods. Nevertheless, in the full conviction that the objectives of the effective humanization of the hospital facilities primarily affect forms of interpersonal interaction, it was considered appropriate to contextualize the issue of communication between the different users of the system so that the implications can be focused on in terms of the spatial requirements.

For easier application possibilities the "design recommendations" – which represent the guiding tool available to the operators concerned – have been structured "by functional area" and have been enhanced with photographic suggestions which are not meant to influence the designers or decision-makers but to point out how certain requirements have been met in recently produced works (Figure 3). In some cases the levels of service required are higher than the current average, both in terms of the benefits expressed and the economic implications. However it should not be forgotten that, especially in hospital facilities, the initial investments costs represent a lower value than that of the overall management costs of just two years of life and that the impact of the perceived benefit by the user also has economic implications, particularly if referred to the work conditions and burn-out of the medical and nursing staff.
The last part of the research, concerning the model for assessing the level of humanization of designs and facilities (Figure 4-5), in any case points out how the target to be taken as a reference to steer the humanization requirements can be decided freely, case by case, by the head of the implementation programme, thereby making the tool flexible, open and susceptible to ongoing and gradual updates.

Planning, Design and Construction Improvement Processes

Session introduction

Research plays a key role in the process of improving the construction of healthcare facilities as it renews the areas of investigation and provides the framework for action that allows the precise application of strategies defined for the construction of buildings.

The importance of research on the healing environment and evidence-based design is documented through a large body of publications that have essentially been published in North America, Europe and Australia. The challenge for healthcare construction researchers and developers is to see how the information and theories on hospital design developed over the past 20 years can be adapted to the different needs of developing countries, with limitations due to scarce resources and cultural and political differences. The challenge for researchers is to understand how the research results can be applied to different contexts and what necessary adjustments and changes need to be made to practical models in use.

The need to optimize the economic resources available meant that the studies were developed to improve the efficiency of staff involved in the care process. Field research has shown that the involvement of patients' families and friends is a factor that helps to ease the work of the staff and positively contributes to the care process. The use of a real-scale mock-up has shown that it is possible to intervene on the layout of the building to improve efficiency in the care of patients.

The rapid changes in technology and healthcare practices related to them mean it is inevitable for researchers to reflect on the possibility of making the healthcare building as flexible as possible and capable of accommodating the changes imposed by the evolution of care.

In this context the open building approach offers a valid theoretical framework from different points of view as it allows action to be taken at different scales of the project, from urban development to detail: devising the city reorganization plans, drafting guidelines, and designing a hospice or analysis laboratories within the university hospital.

System Separation in Healthcare Architecture
From Tradition to Innovation of the Hospital Laboratory

Hans Eggen

H.Eggen@ittenbrechbuehl.ch
M.Sc. ETH SIA, Senior Partner, Itten + Brechbühl AG, Bern, Switzerland

Why is system separation needed? Life cycle economies with complete separation of the 3 building systems combined with an updating of medical technical equipment as tertiary system is nowhere more relevant than in the hospital laboratory. Primary system for 100 years / Secondary 20 years / Tertiary for 5 years of life expectancy.

How was it introduced for the treatment building at the University Hospital in Berne? An architect's competition for the primary system alone, separated from a later competition for the secondary system. My former company was the winning team. This treatment building contains the emergency department, x-ray, the surgical department, the intensive care and also the laboratory. The aspect of grey zones as undefined empty areas within the layout for later use will be explained.

What was the development of hospital laboratories during the last 40 years? The process from decentralisation to centralisation, then to concentration - achieved. Introduction of 80% automation of all laboratory services - implemented. A socialisation among different specialists - introduced. New technologies - continuously introduced. Miniaturisation as a next step is already in preparation and ongoing implementation.

How could the turnaround be achieved technically?
- The open plan and the anticipated layout has to prove its flexibility
- Dimensions between floor and ceiling are important
- Introduction of different types of water and water evacuation
- Individual HVAC for special units to be introduced later where required
- The still free grey zones may be used for coming innovative further ideas

Why system separation? – A conclusion

Keywords: *System separation, life cycle economies, new technologies in use for laboratories.*

INTRODUCTION

The Hospital Laboratory is as a specific type of the different existing typologies. It is not a lab for teaching purposes where every room is identical (Figure 1), nor a lab for pure scientific research like Synchrotron (Figure 2). It is not a laboratory intended to make a product like vaccines on an isolated island in North Germany (Figure 3). The hospital laboratory only serves the requirements of the patients in the hospital.

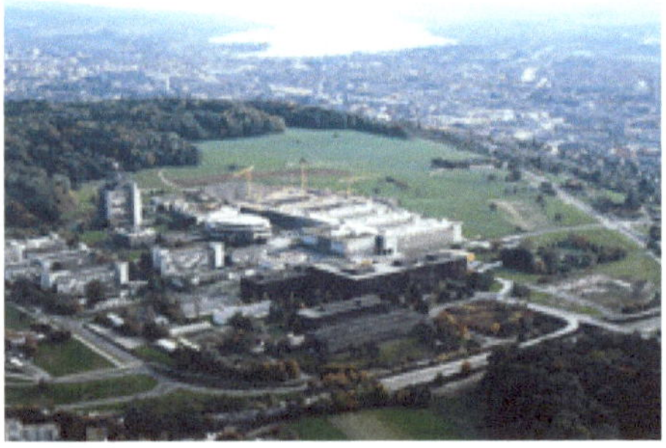

Figure 1. Laboratories for teaching purpose, Technical University of Zürich.

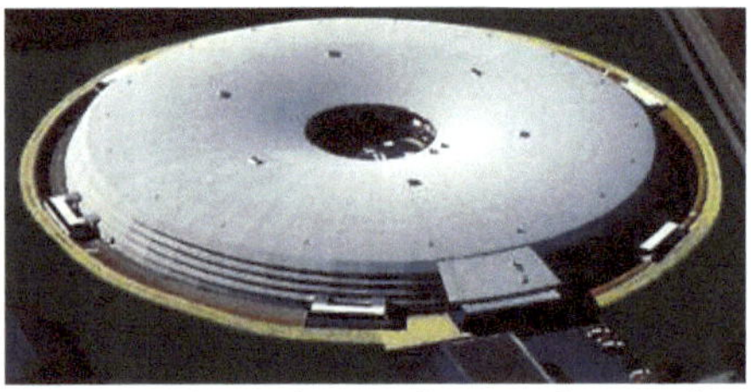

Figure 2. The Synchrotron for scientific research.

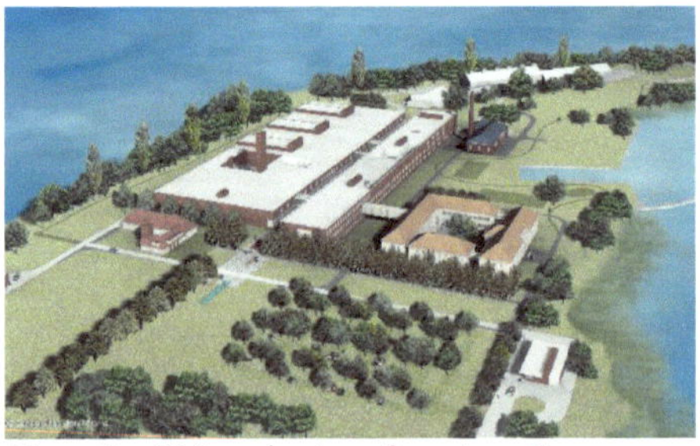

Figure 3. FLI production of vaccines, Germany.

WHY IS SYSTEM SEPARATION NEEDED FOR A HOSPITAL LABORATORY?

It is a relatively small facility and fully integrated in the treatment process. It is clear however that at the university hospital such a laboratory takes the lead in many different activities and is therefore changing continuously. Whatever will be developed in medical science will mark its footprint from the very beginning in the laboratory, already with adequate equipment together with a specific process to produce and certify the results. How should such a treatment building be conceived in order to be efficient today but easily adaptable for all the coming requirements in the future, if nobody can imagine it. System separation in healthcare architecture with the laboratory is a typical example.

This is the overall site of the University Hospital in Bern (Figure 4). The primary system came out of a first conceptual Architects completion in 1998 with the idea of building an empty structure, while a second competition for the next phase, for the secondary system could be launched. A building of 100 m by 100 m is very deep. The idea with these light shafts looks good on the plan but you can imagine that it will only serve the upper floors. Further down, artificial light has to be introduced. The advantage of the deep plan is that it can produce very efficient treatment units.

HOW WAS SYSTEM SEPARATION INTRODUCED FOR THIS BUILDING?

What you can see here is the primary system, consisting of floor slabs, columns and the facade. It was actually

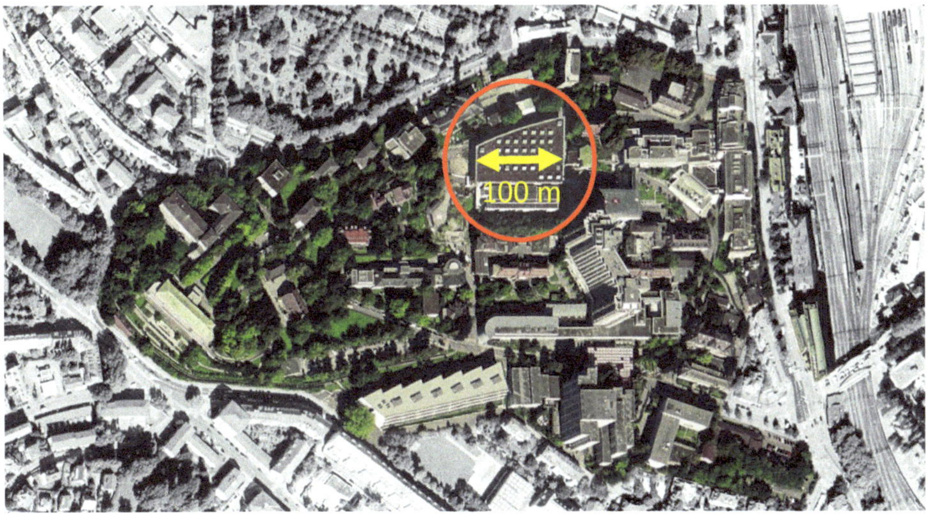

Figure 4. Site of the University Hospital in Bern.

built like this as a pure primary system when we started our competition for the secondary system. The life cycle of this primary system is expected to reach 100 years, while the inner separation walls and the equipment will change at shorter cycles.Here is the primary system as a plan (Figure 5).

The secondary system consists of the separation walls and the technical installations to each room. Finally there is the tertiary system with the equipment and the corresponding conduits. Here the view on the top level of this treatment block is precisely into the same space designated for the laboratory with the secondary system under construction (Figure 6).

For the laboratory, we originally had no separation walls as you can see here at the opening of the laboratory. There was however a large step until the tertiary system for the laboratory was fully equipped and put into operation (Figure 7). From that moment, the equipment on the workbenches started to change very fast.

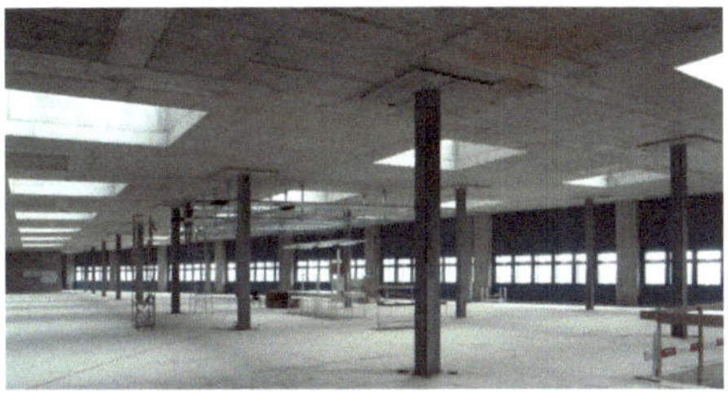

Figure 5. The primary system.

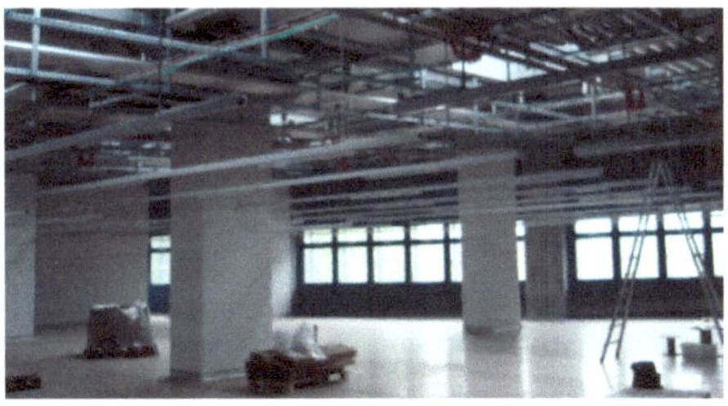

Figure 6. The secondary system.

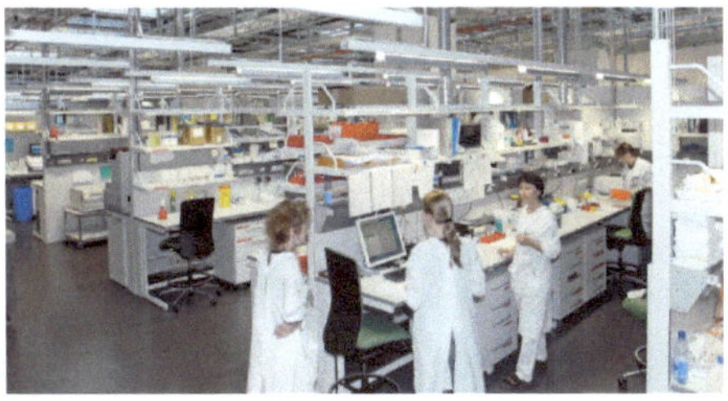

Figure 7. The tertiary system.

THE DEVELOPMENT OF THE HOSPITAL LABORATORY

The process started 40 years ago from a decentralised pavilion hospital finished in 1973 (Figure 8). The centralised treatment building contained all laboratories on one floor only (Figure 9). Today however, the laboratory is even more concentrated in "one open room" only.

Already in 1973 the modular layout was conceived similarly for each individual laboratory discipline (Figure 10), adopting also a typology of laboratory furniture. Water was available on each laboratory desk (Figure 11). Staff however were kept mentally strictly separated within each individual discipline. The main disciplines were laboratory for haematology and the central chemical laboratory. I realise now that from that moment, rapid development brought a large number of new medical specialities to Switzerland from all over the world. Medical knowledge, you may call it the disciplines, has multiplied over a few years. For each new discipline, an adequate new laboratory space had to be integrated. The space was available because the technical development was even faster, with reference to miniaturisation of the equipment and the beginning of automation.

WHY IS TODAY'S LABORATORY SO DIFFERENT?

In 2005, when the first phase of the INO was inaugurated, the laboratory was concentrated on the top floor in this corner and remained here also after the second phase had been added in 2013 (Figure 12).

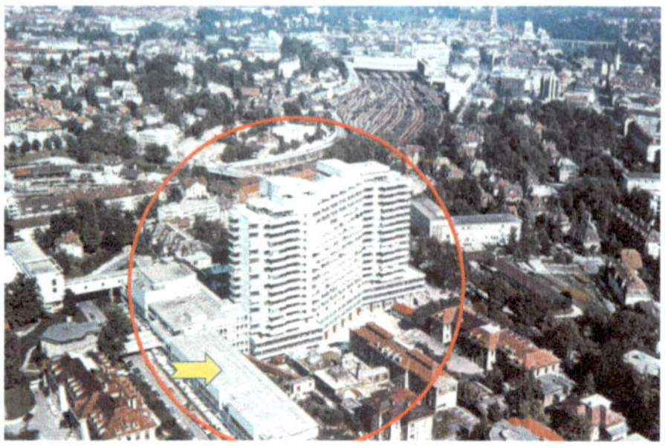

Figure 8. Centralised university hospital with a centralised treatment building, 1973.

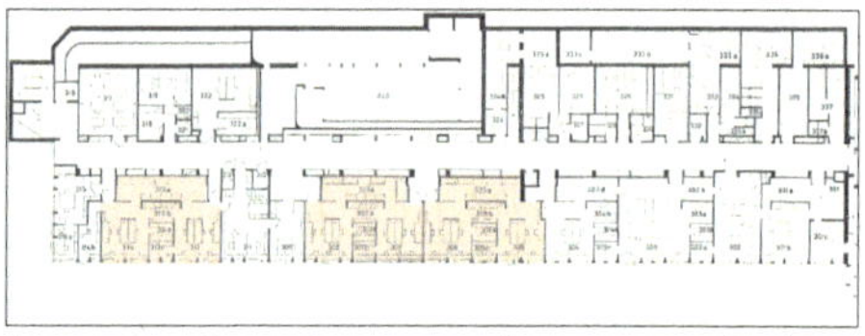

Figure 9. Centralisation on the site in one building on one floor only.

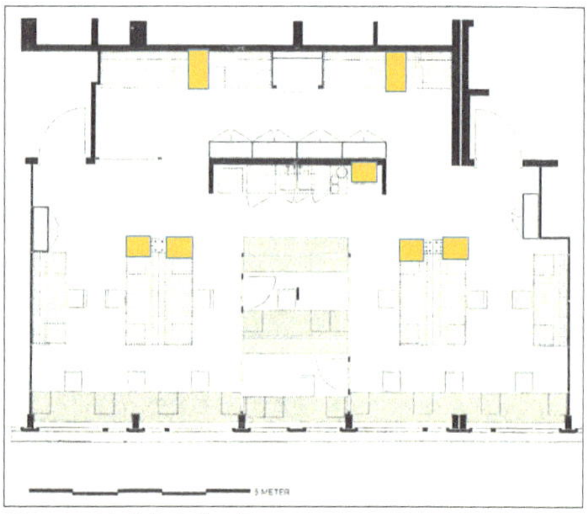

Figure 10. Modular layout.

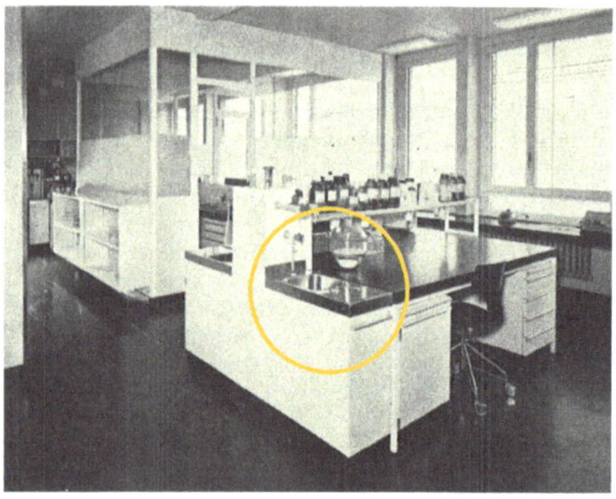

Figure 11. Modular furniture.

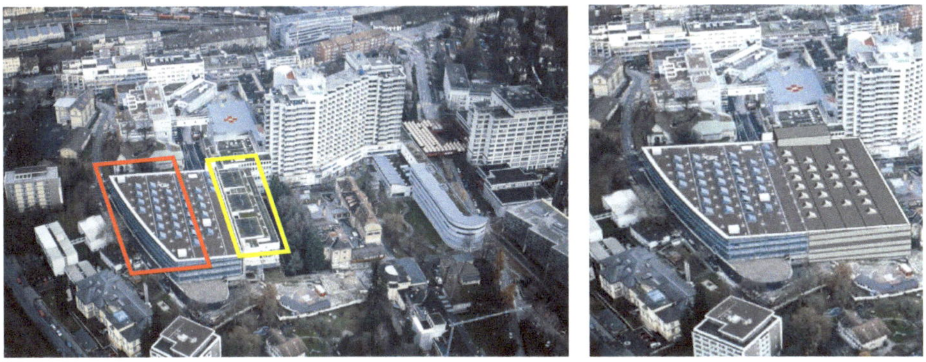

Figure 12. INO laboratories in 2005 (left) and in 2013 (right).

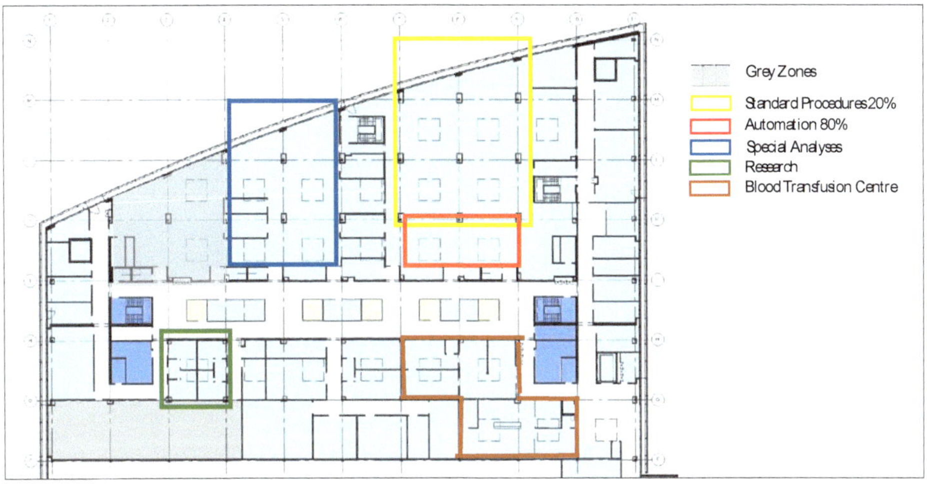

Figure 13. INO laboratories floor.

From centralisation in 1973, with separated disciplines in units, towards an open plan and concentration in one room, is a large step but logical for an adaptable structure. Only the standardised procedures of the laboratory services are placed here. The blood transfusion centre has been developed on the same floor in adjacent rooms. Results are produced by machines, the auto analysers, at the moment 80% out of 100%. The remaining "empty rest" of the whole laboratory space is allocated generally for special analyses and research and is still not yet consumed by the continuous development which leads to the most important statement: such "grey zones" were distributed over all floors of the treatment building. Areas kept empty and fully reserved for real future development. The grey zones are becoming more and more valuable every day and have not been fully used until today (Figure 13).

The standard procedures of the chemical analysis: reception of material; labelling; triage; sample preparation. From here,

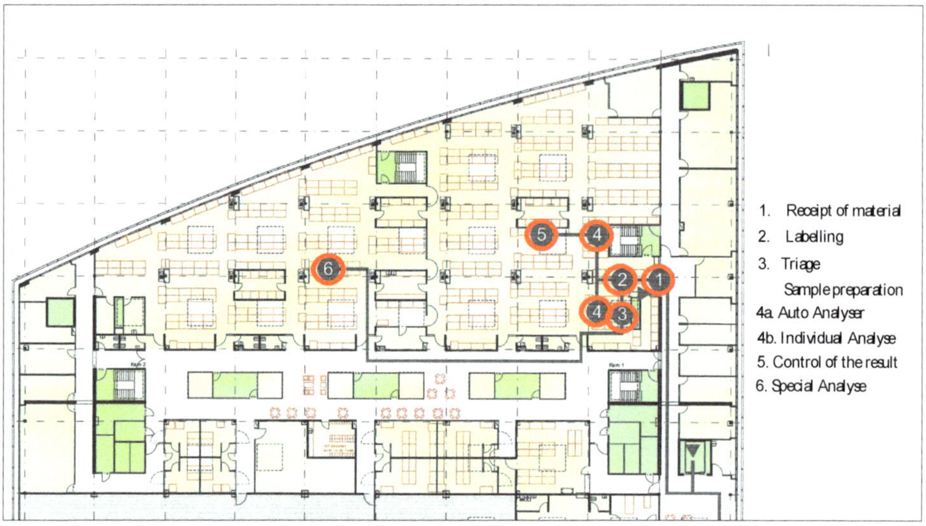

Figure 14. INO, general laboratory process.

the sample goes either through the auto analyser, or an individual analyser, or even a special analyser. There are many more standardised and certified procedures within this laboratory (Figure 14).

Concerning the internal communication, we intended to use this double corridor with all the roof lights creating an atmosphere of detention (Figure 15).

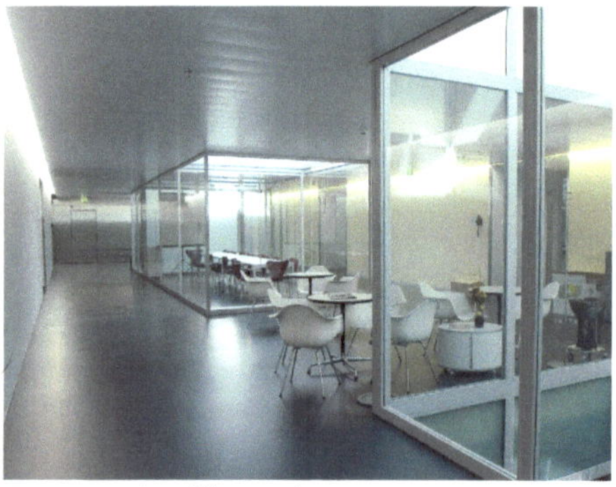

Figure 15. Double corridor.

ZONES WITHIN THE LABORATORY REQUIRING SYSTEM SEPARATION

Research

The cubicles reserved for research are placed on the other side of the middle corridor, fully separated from the standard procedures. Each room has an individual access and a HVAC system with negative pressure to avoid any doubts of cross infection. It can be used for a specific research purpose and without any standard procedure (Figure 16).

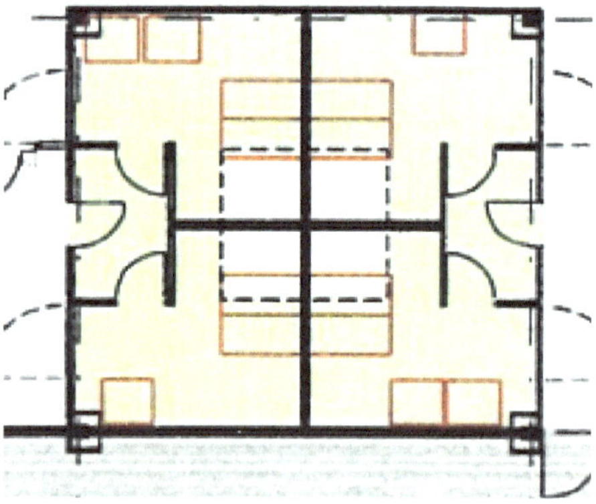

Figure 16. Research fully isolated.

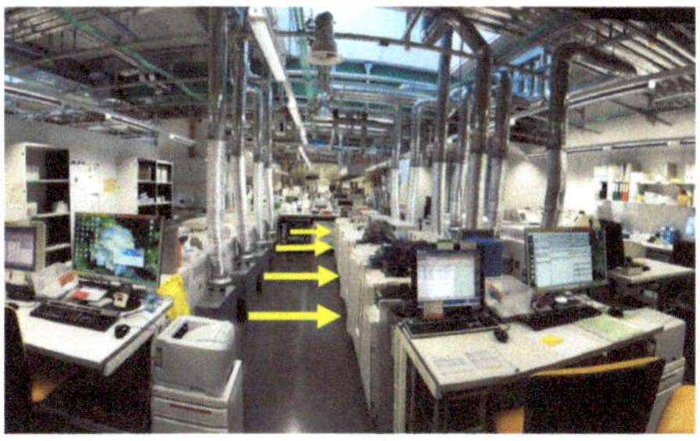

Figure 17. Special zones within the laboratory.

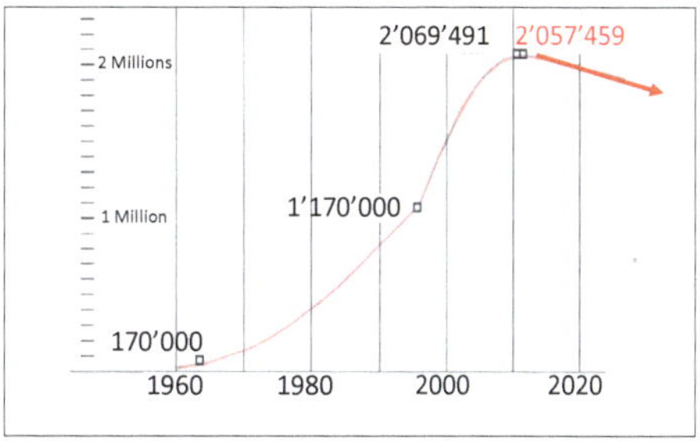

Figure 18. Number of chemical analyses.

Full Automation

Within this small area, 80% of all the chemical laboratory analysis is performed with auto analysers. These machines were selected at the last possible moment and arrived only 3 months before the opening of the laboratory. We had not seen them before and were surprised by the dimensions, of approximately 18 m by 7 m. Everyone was astonished to see that it could be installed within the flexible layout without any major problems.

Here is a wide angle view from the front part. All parts of the machines are linked together on the right hand side as well as on the left hand side in a similar row (Figure 17).

The development of the number of chemical analyses

1964: 170.000
1996: 1.170.000
2011: 2.089.491
2012: 2.057.491 (this shows a reduction for the first time already in 2012)

A reduction of 1-2 % annually is now anticipated due to cost reduction in relation with the DRG system. Even if the machines could produce more results, nobody wants more information than is absolutely necessary. In other words, empty work benches could be used for other purposes in the future (Figure 18).

Masses spectrograph

First of all, we the architects had to cope with new requirements, since the machines work with vacuum, which requires: absolute constant temperatures; absolute constant humidity.
In the original zoning plan, we had anticipated (not yet built) some island cubicles with special conditions. At this time, we had no idea if it would be needed in the future but we knew that this could happen. Last year, the architects suddenly had to identify necessary allocations for 5 of these special machines, introduce the cubicles with such HVAC conditions and connect the machines. It is definitively the beginning of a new chain of research programmes in health care with the aim of serving patients. It could be realised without asking for a complete new building within the same floor space and be handled with the same number of staff because system separation and an open plan could make it possible (Figure 19).

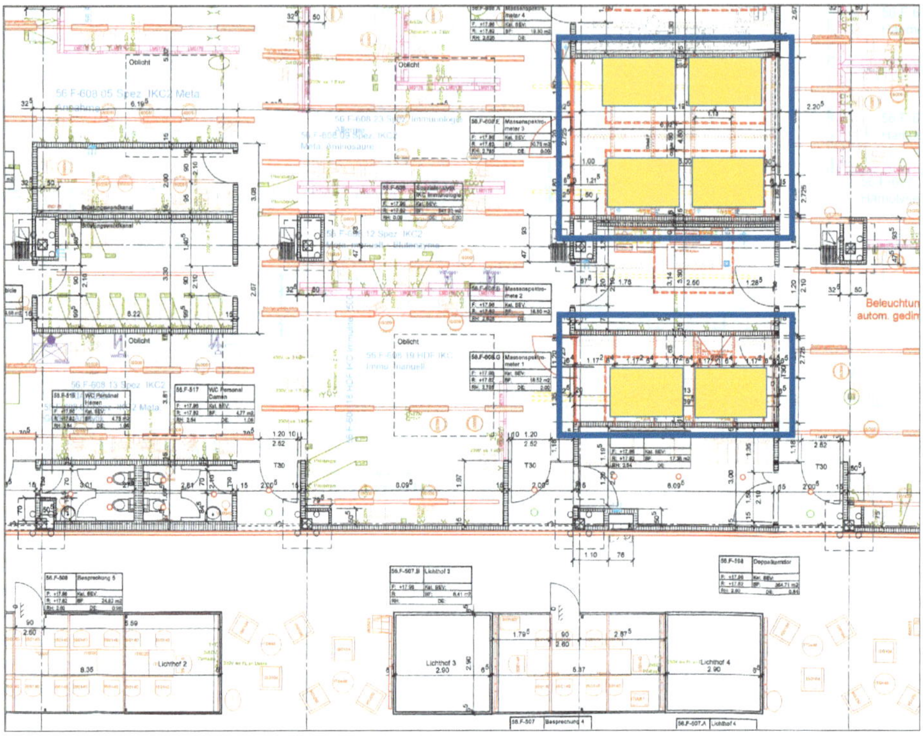

Figure 19. Masses spectrography localization.

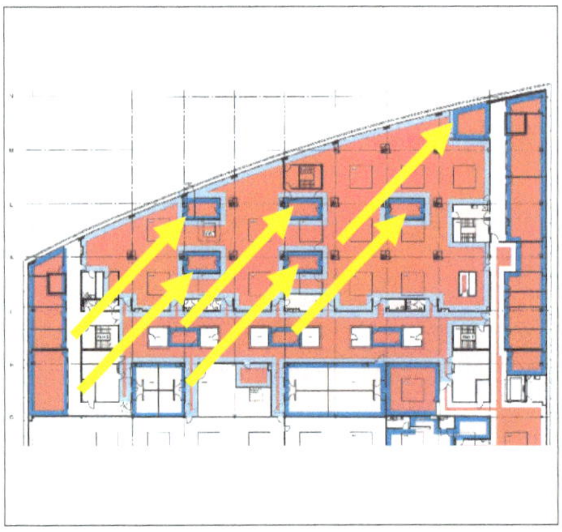

Figure 20. Special zones within the laboratory.

CONCLUSIONS

System separation is of great value. For a new piece of equipment (with a new process), a location can be found within the existing building, installed, and put into operation (overnight) and used by the same number of staff. Many more examples could be found to prove such statements, especially in the hospital laboratory department. The laboratory is a wonderful place of work for male and female staff, all concentrating their efforts for the benefit of patients.

Smart Staff: Reducing Cost of Staff by Patient and Family Involvement, Effective Expertise Level and Efficient Architectural Layout

Bas Molenaar

basarch@planet.nl
Prof., EGM Architects, Dordrecht, The Netherlands

The cost of medical staff runs up to 70% of the total cost of healthcare and is increasing to the extent that healthcare becomes unaffordable. The complexity of procedures due to safety requirements does not make the work easier. The skills needed on the different levels of care require adequate training and results in diverse salary scales for medical staff. The second mayor issue is the aging of the working population. In the Netherlands the payment grows with the age of the worker on the assumption that the skill level is growing at the same speed. Research on ways to reduce staff is required to keep healthcare affordable.

Salutogenesis

The responsibility for a person's health shows an increasing focus on maintaining a healthy status instead of curing when medical problems occur. The salutogenic paradigm falls within the larger paradigm of positive psychology and is a preventative model as opposed to being a disease model.

Slowly evidence is gathered that indicate that people and systems that develop the ability to implement the salutogenic way of living will live longer and perceive a good health, enjoy a better quality of life and mental wellbeing.

In the Netherlands this also applies for the care, from elderly care to psychiatry and mentally disabled persons. They are stimulated to stay as long as possible in their own home, supported by friends and family and - when needed by professional medical care.

Design

In the design of a ward of hospital self-control of temperature, sun blinds and fresh air by opening the window can stimulate the activity of the patient. Also the free choice of food, music and art helps the patient to get control on its environment and day schedule.

Family

The help of family and friends for tasks that are not medical helps nurses to focus on their medical tasks. The presence of family constitutes an important source of psychological stability for the patient, as well as a source of support

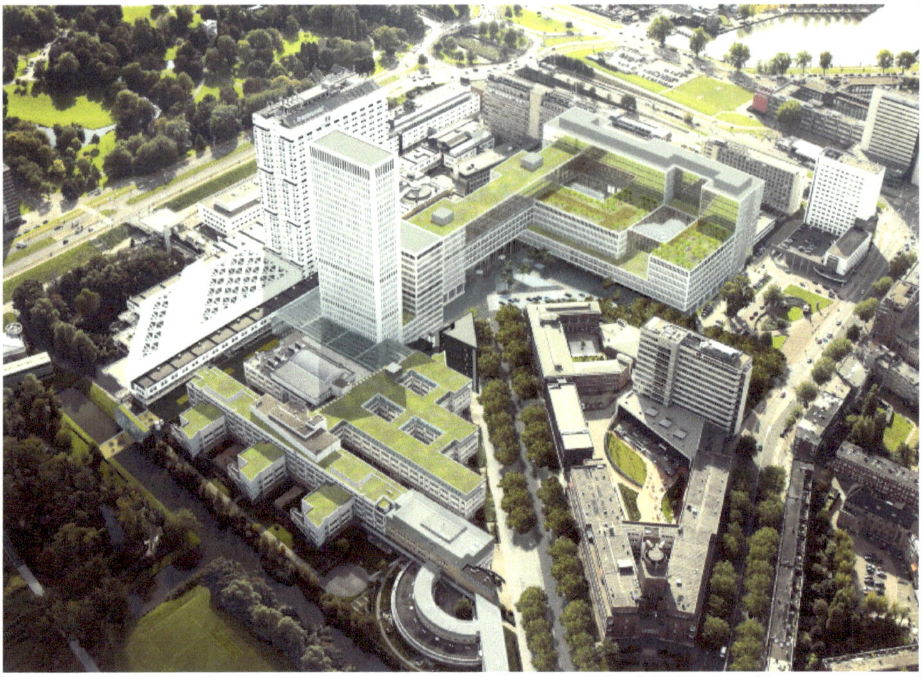

Figure 1. Erasmus Medical Center, the recent studies on the new wards of the Erasmus University Hospital in Rotterdam illustrate the most recent trend in design and layout.

for better recovery, since it helps him to maintain a contact with his house and his friends. Family can direct the patient in order to participate in self-care activities and effectively face any complications of his illness.

STAFF EFFECTIVENESS

Planning of the right level of skill according to the healthcare status of the patient can affect the cost of medical staff in a positive way. Build examples in Singapore, the Rhön-Klinikum hospitals in Germany and commonly in Scandinavia show step back facilities to adjust the level of care to the patient needs at lower cost. In the Dutch hospitals specializes nurses can partly take over the work of medical specialists and doctors when trained and audited on the right level. Rehabilitation hospitals with less expensive medical infrastructure can take care of patient who need less intensive medical care that can be provided by medical staff of lower skill and according lower salary.

WARD LAYOUT

The new Erasmus ward that is still in its construction phase is based on 100% private patient rooms (Figure 2). They bring the risk of cross infection down; provide ultimate privacy that is comfortable for the patient as well as improving the communication between medical staff and patient and all rooms have place for overnight stay of family. The wards will comprise of 469 medium care

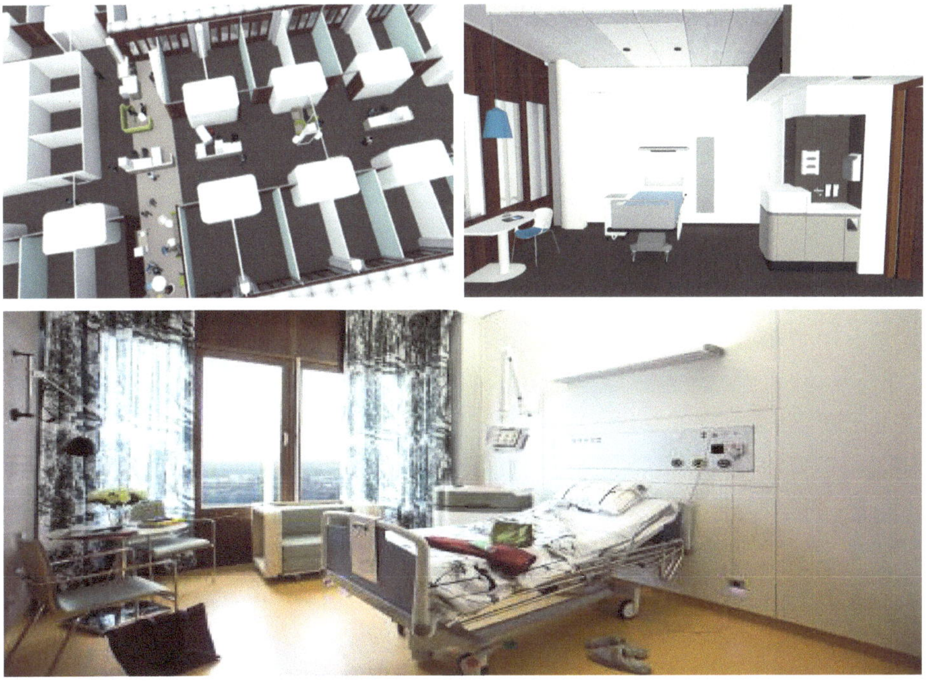

Figure 2. EMC: 100 % private patient rooms.

beds, 56 intensive care beds and 80 places for day-care treatment. The uniform layout of the ward enables grouping patients according to their need of specialized care. Each ward is divided in units of an average of 8 beds, connected with shared facilities in between.

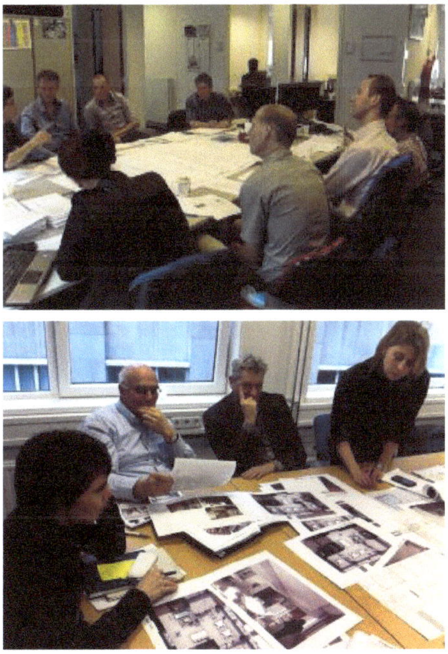

Figure 3. Evaluation of designs at every step.

The location of medical supplies in decentralized stations is essential to provide effective medical care. Also decentralized docking stations replace the rigid nursing station because patient information is accessible thru wireless connected devices. The area between the rooms is much broader than a standard corridor and allows small local storage of medical supplies, decentralized nursing stations and room for patients and visitors. This implicates a new type of central space,

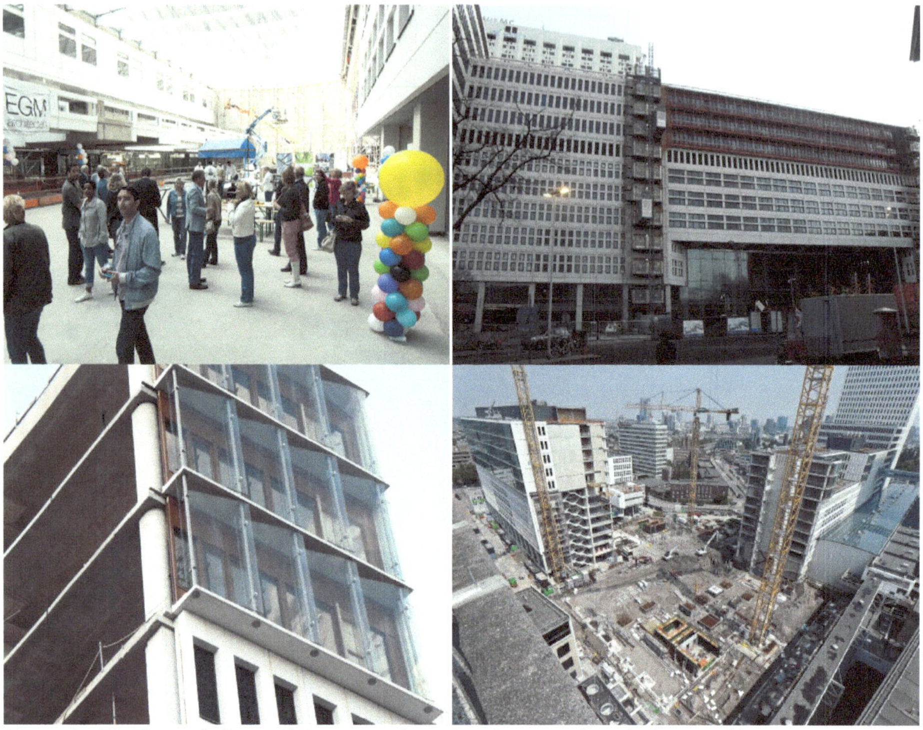

Figure 4. The design challenge of Erasmus MC was based on providing the best possible care on a university medical level.

with friendly furniture, daylight and pleasant lighting shared by nurses, patients and visitors. This will be quite a change compared to the current wards, and nurses are now being trained to take the best advantage of this new lay-out. A mock-up room will be set up this summer, while the complete building will be operational in 2017. Continuous evaluation will help to improve the working methods and help to allow nurses to deliver effective and patient friendly care (Figure 3).

Universal model or adaptable model

The layout of the ward of the Erasmus MC is on the level of a university hospital with high standards. The same principles of adequate staff skill, family support and an environment that stimulates an active role of the patient can also be used for simple wards with limited space and budget.

Conclusions

It is very hard to find research data on this topic, mainly because there are too many issues that influence cost. The wards of the Erasmus MC have been designed to get the best possible care for patient. As the project is still under construction the impact of the design on cost will have to be evaluated later (Figure 4).

Air, Surfaces and Hospital Associated Infection (HAI): An Interdisciplinary Empirical Approach towards Architectural Design Validation, a Health Care Design Initiative

Jako Nice

jnice@csir.co.za
Built Environment, Architectural Engineering, CSIR, South Africa

Architectural design validation is not an unfamiliar notion; however the subjective nature of our field evokes much contention. Health care design presents a much more tangible possibility through inter disciplinary research for validation. A collaborative approach using epidemiology, microbiology, medical and engineering fields presents evidence for an empirical architectural validation model.

Scientific evidence has firmly established the causal relationship between microbes and disease. Furthermore, science has established causal associations between certain environmental conditions and proliferation of certain disease causing micro-organisms. Microbiologist, epidemiologist, doctors and engineers have developed models and methodologies to define infection rates and occurrences. When one correlates this with the cost per capita as was done in the United States, the financial burden of HAI weighs heavily on national healthcare budgets.

This abstract attempts to present a new design construct, a microbial design construct for architecture. A theory grounded on interdisciplinary observation on the causal nature of, air quality and risk, surface type and space, microbial 'fallout' and persistence.

People, users are infected and affected by indoor environments daily; therefore a microbial architectural model of design for the built environment could address these pertinent challenges with empirical authority.

The literature presents indicators for indoor environment quality and microbial conditions, in considering the diverse fields of research, striking correlation relationships are found.
It recognises the potential for developing a microbial model for Architectural design that can serve as empirical design validation.

Keywords: *Architecture, microbial, HAI (Hospital Associated Infection), interdisciplinary.*

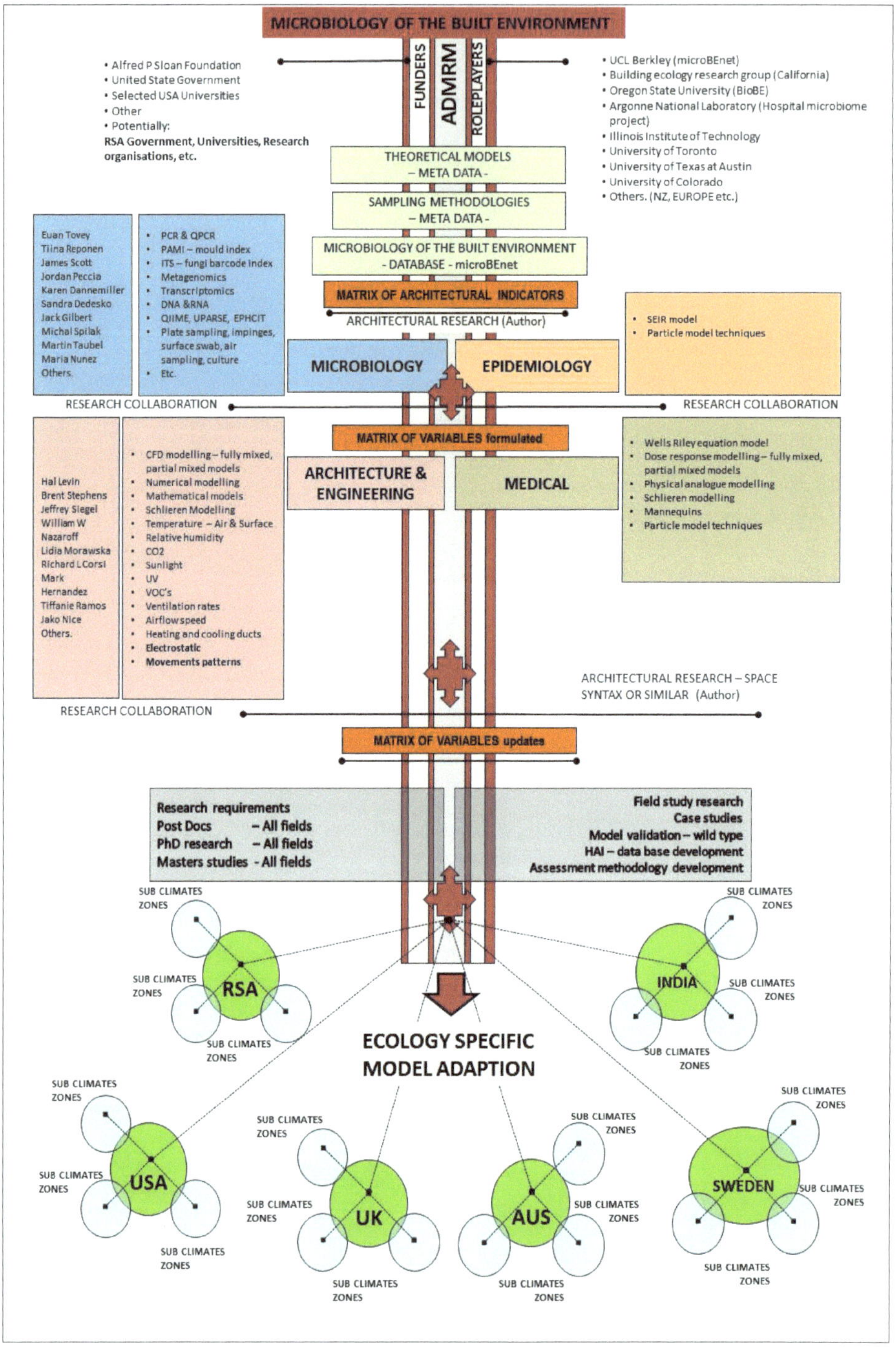

Methodology.

User LED Design: Redevelopment of the Christchurch Hospital, New Zealand

Jane Carthey[1], Roger Carthey[2]

jcarthey@gmail.com, rcarthey@thinc.com.au
[1]Australian Health Design Council, Australia
[2]Thinc Health, Australia

Building the new Christchurch Hospital is part of an overall Canterbury-focused strategy of delivering 'the right care, in the right place, to the right person, at the right time'. In 2010 and 2011, major earthquakes hastened implementation of the project. In mid-2013, design consultants were appointed to work with clinical user groups to design a new building that includes: additional operating theatres; ~360 inpatient beds; purpose-designed space for children; an expanded intensive care unit, and an emergency department.

Initiated prior to appointment of the design consultants, and now running in parallel with the project, the Canterbury District Health Board (CDHB) set up a 'Design Lab' to enable clinicians, engineers, architects and user groups to work together to rethink how health services are provided.

Derived from the principles of rapid prototyping similar to those promoted by design 'thinktanks' such as IDEO, the Design Lab concept was brought to the project by a US architectural firm in response to the CDHB CEO's interest in lean, and process design from other non-healthcare related industries. On the Christchurch project, this interest has been further developed to focus on patient safety and the patient experience.

This paper examines the interaction between the Design Lab process, the 'user-led design philosophy', and its impact on the traditional role of the healthcare architect working within a normal time and fee-constrained project delivery environment. In particular, it will examine the broader implications for the project including sequencing of various parts of the design, and the impact of often 'naïve' user led design input on the delivery program and budget. It will describe the negotiation of this environment by the project team and will evaluate the success of this approach to the design of a new, major hospital in an urban New Zealand setting.

Keywords: *healthcare design, user-led design, lean process design, prototyping, project delivery.*

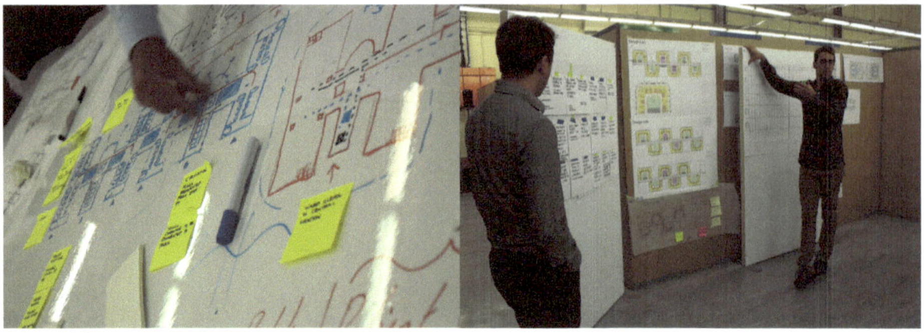

Design lab.

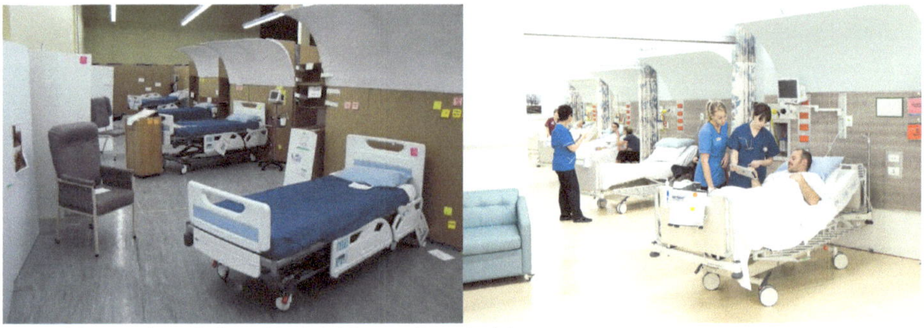

Low fidelity mock up (left) and high fidelity mock up (right).

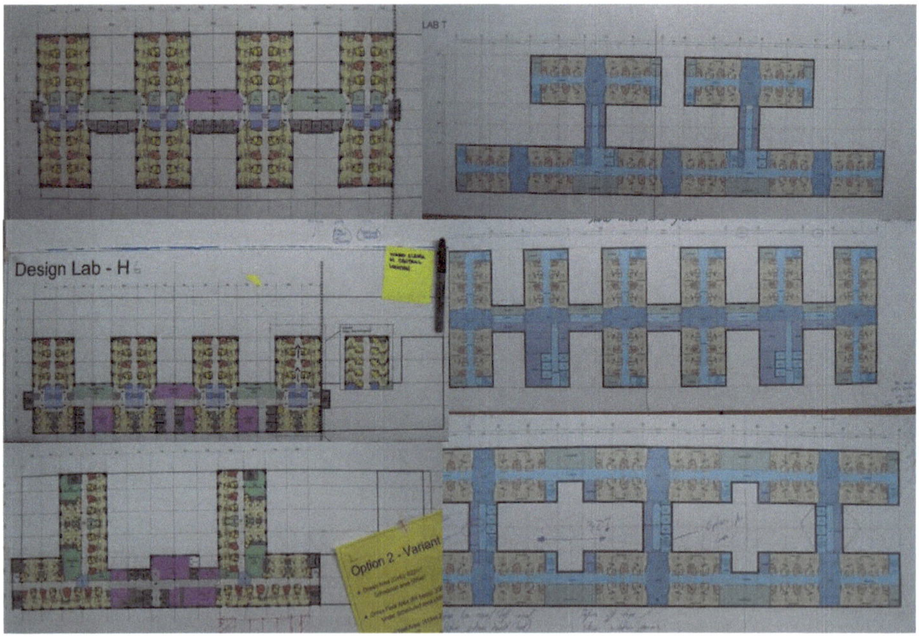

Ward configuration assessments.

Transformation of a Hospital Building to a Hospice: Open Building as Strategy for Process and Product - An Example from the Netherlands

Karel Dekker

karel@decco.net
Karel Dekker, KD/Consultants, The Hague, The Netherlands

This paper presents a case study describing a five year search for a new building for a Hospice, and the transformation planning, design and construction of an existing hospital building (polyclinic) into a Hospice of 1200 m² using Open Building as strategy for process and product.
The paper describes the state of the art of the Rent-Buy principles used in the Netherlands. Applying this principle in this case resulted in the client renting a renovated base building (primary system) for 30-40 years and acting as owner for the secondary system.
A new principle is that the tenant (the Hospice) is financing improvement of the primary system. The net present value calculations for decreased rent compared with these investments shows a positive balance for the client. The budget system is based on a strict distinction of the primary, secondary and tertiary systems.
A competitive tendering (bidding) process was used for choosing a contractor as part of the design team. A distinction in tendering (bidding) was also made for the primary system (base building) and the secondary system (fit-out or infill). This corresponded to a technical separation between primary and secondary systems, in which all installation technology belongs to the secondary system (infill). To increase the capacity of the primary system for future changes, buffer spaces were created for future expansion. Gyproc's CableStud were used for flexible wire management to good effect. Decentralized HVAC systems were used, offering maximum flexibility in future transformation of spaces.
The paper concludes with an evaluation of the process and product innovations used in the Hospice project, and makes recommendations for improving decision-making for flexibility in healthcare facilities.

***Keywords:** open building, hospital building, rent-buy, hospice, health care.*

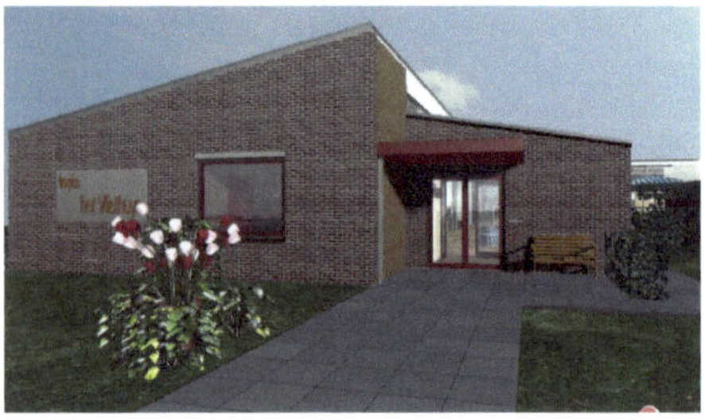

Hospice design September 2012. The transformation planning, design and construction of an existing hospital building (polyclinic) into a Hospice of 1200 m² using Open Building as strategy for process and product.

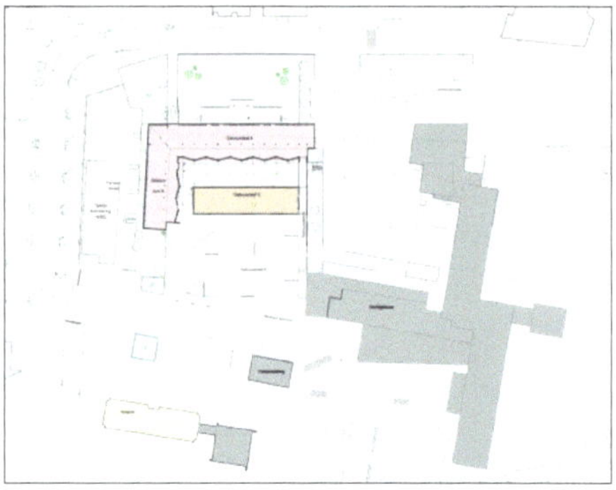

Hospital area.

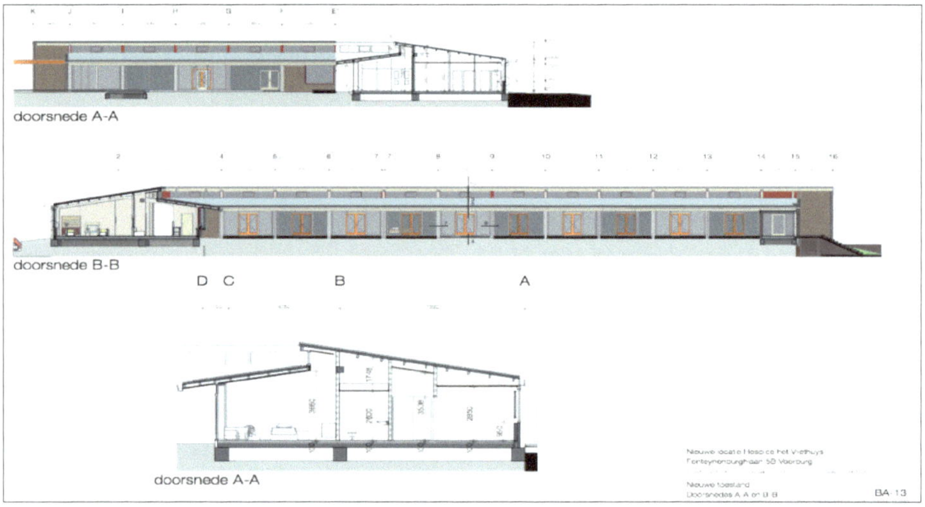

Hospital sections.

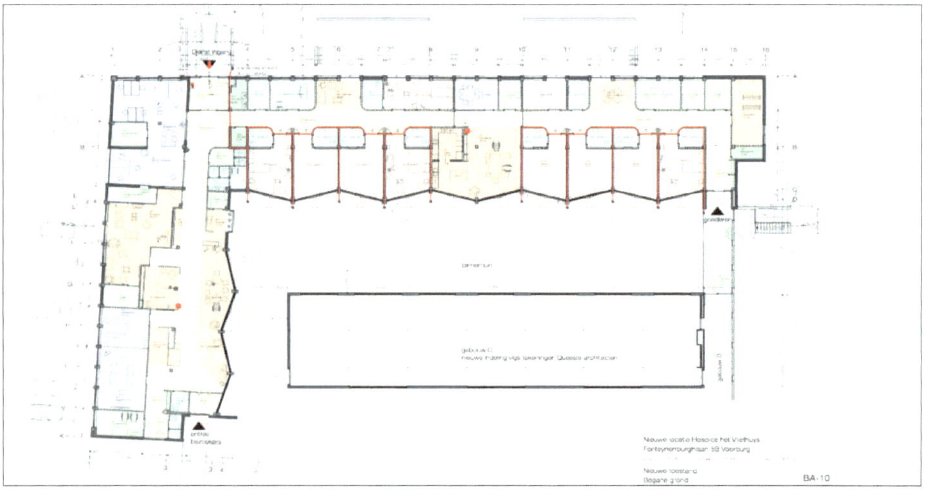

First design infill.

Healthcare Facilities Designed for Flexibility: The Challenge of Culture Change in a Large US Public Agency

Stephen Kendall[1], Thom Kurmel[2], Karel Dekker[3], John Becker[4]

[1]Emeritus Professor of Architecture, Ball State University, Muncie, Indiana
[2]TDK Consulting, LLC, Lorton, Virginia
[3]KD Consulting, Voorburg, The Netherlands
[4]Director of Facilities, Defense Health Agency, Washington DC

The US Department of Defense Health Agency (DHA) has an international network of healthcare facilities to serve personnel serving in the armed forces. The DHA has a budget approximating $3 billion per year for the acquisition of new facilities and the maintenance and upgrading of existing facilities. Recently, the DHA – driven by a US government-wide mandate - has made a commitment to a policy of sustainable facilities. DHA leadership recognized that a key element of a sustainable asset portfolio is that the facilities must be flexible – planned for the likelihood of expansion, contraction, alteration or change of function or a combination of these – and thus capable of meeting the challenges of changing missions, patient demographics, medical practices, and medical technology. This paper discusses the work being done to introduce flexibility as a high level principle in the DHA policies, practices and criteria. The paper discusses the recommendations being made to implement flexibility by the insertion of flexibility requirements in the key guidance documents used by architects and engineers in designing new and renovating existing DHA facilities. Because many of these are recommended to be mandatory (not simply incentives), their adoption is expected to require a change in the culture of DHA and in the entire decision-making chain for the acquisition and management of DHA healthcare facilities. This paper reports on the recommended flexibility requirements and the culture change required for their full implementation.

Keywords: *Healthcare facilities, flexibility, whole-life performance, sustainability, open building.*

Introduction

This paper reports on the second of two research contracts with the National Institute of Building Sciences one of whose clients - the United States Department of Defense Health Agency (DHA) – asked for a.) Recommendations on introducing flexibility as a high level principle in their policy documents; b.) Assistance in writing flexibility requirements in acquiring healthcare facilities; and c.) Recommendations for tracking how their facilities transform over time for the purpose of assessing the merits of mandated flexibility requirements.

DHA's goal is to assure the long-term value of their facilities portfolio and to assure the wise investment of approximately $3 billion per year expended in acquiring new and maintaining and renovating existing facilities worldwide.

The recommendations recognize that the DHA has already adopted measures that lead positively toward a more flexible portfolio. The effort reported on here has therefore been aimed at several things:
a. defining the term flexibility as having both technical and decision-making dimensions;
b. clarification of current developments within the DHA and in the building industry at large toward flexibility, with particular reference to newly adopted patterns of decision-making;
c. formulating and describing these developments in a larger conceptual framework (Open Building);
d. making recommendations of mandatory flexibility requirements in the acquisition and management of the DHA facilities portfolio with the goal of high performance under conditions of change in medical practices, demographics and building technology.

Fundamental Principle for Achieving Flexibility

Acquisition of assets expected to have a long use-value can only come out of decision-making processes based on a recognition that the built environment is never finished, and that continuous transformation must be recognized and planned for. Use-value itself is not only a technical term when associated with health care facilities: the concepts of use and value exist in a social body that understands that the value of the physical environment is not a static phenomenon but is evolving on the time axis.

Flexibility – like sustainability - is fundamental to a facilities life-cycle (whole-building life) agenda. Even though flexibility is not an industry standard, it should be a DHA requirement, like LEED and building codes, and should appear in all design guidance documents, cutting across lines of authority and decision-making.

Background

Too often, the term flexibility is used to describe only technical performance or physical characteristics, such as added floor-to-floor height; or standardization of spaces to enable multiple uses of the same space; and so on. While technical solutions can be helpful to assure long-lasting (flexible and sustainable) assets, our studies demonstrate that technical matters alone are insufficient to achieving a flexible building stock, and sometimes actually thwart long-term utility of facilities if poorly employed. If clients retain decision-making patterns that result in physical facilities that lack the capacity to adapt, improved technical solutions offered by product manufacturers, architects and engineers will prove to be insufficient remedies.

Even before commissioning is complete, healthcare facilities are being adjusted and continue to be transformed in small and large ways, over many years, because of changing priorities, practices and policies. The concept of "continuum of care" therefore applies not only to people whose health these facilities are designed to recover and enhance, but to facilities themselves. This suggests that the current focus on near-term planning, budgeting, funding, design, construction, commissioning and outfitting of facilities must be supplanted by a longer view of continuous transformation. This long view must be supported by scenario planning and cost modeling and by data collection necessary for evaluating the return on investment of flexibility strategies. "Facilities maintenance" may not be an adequate concept or term of reference for the realities facing MHS assets. More "open ended" and "continuous improvement" attitudes and methods of accounting and management are needed, if the DHA expects its facilities to be sustainable and to provide continuous world-class operational and physical performance.

To support the flexibility principle outlined above, the Phase I Flexibility report recommended adoption of a serial decision-making model for managing uncertainty and change. Adoption of this model will enable greater transparency and more effective and rapid corrective policy and acquisition measures. This model is based on the principle of decoupling parts of a facility having long term utility from the parts having shorter-term utility (System Separation). This model is partly in use in the DHA with the Initial Outfitting and Transition contract (IO&T) as a separate acquisition activity, and with the use of "incremental funding waivers" in fast-track projects, allowing, for example, funding for an early "foundation package" before design of the rest of the building in detail is completed. The model is conventional in the commercial real estate markets in the United States and internationally.

The serial model has three "system levels":

- *Primary System* (Base Building - an "open building:" structure, skin and primary mechanical, electrical and plumbing systems);
- *Secondary System* (Fit-out – all components and spaces directly supporting functionality, including the parts of the overall mechanical, electrical and plumbing systems specific to a given program of functions);
- *Tertiary System* (Furnishings, fixtures and equipment – short-term investments such as equipment, furnishings, consumables).

The principle understanding embodied in this decision-making sequence (for new construction and for comprehensive reactivation of existing facilities) is that all facts and requirements cannot be known at once - at the beginning of a many-decades-long process from decision-to-build/renovate, through appropriations, commissioning, move-in and later adaptation to new requirements. Decisions are inescapably made sequentially during initial acquisition and then continuously over the life of the facility. How could it be otherwise?

Design decision-making for facilities should be decoupled based on the expected lifecycle (use-value) of the system "level" concerned. That is, the tertiary system can change without excessive disruption of the secondary system; and the secondary system (representing evolving DHA mission, functional and space requirements) can change with minimal disruption of the primary system, an investment designed to be useful over a long period of time.

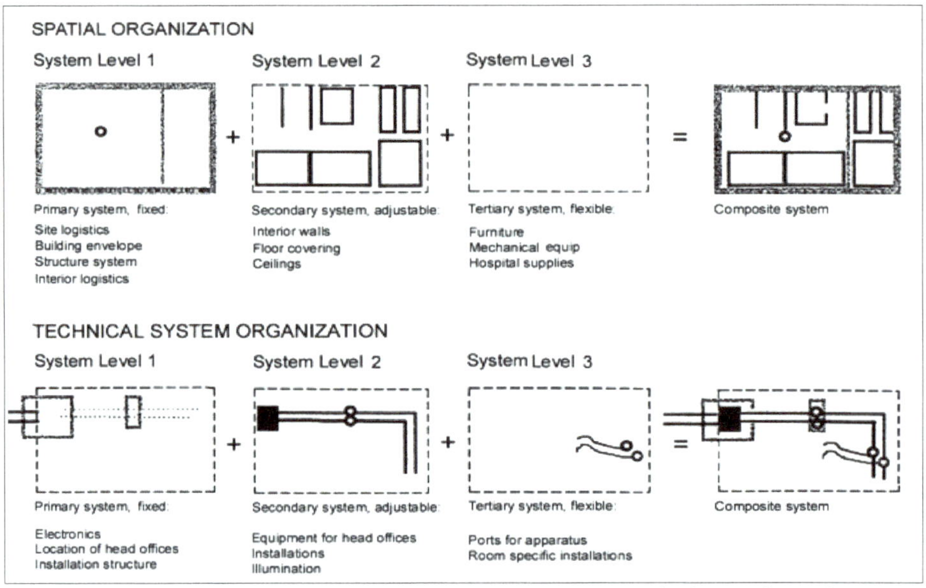

Figure 1. (source: Office of Properties and Buildings, Canton Bern, Switzerland). Translating the principle in Figure 1 into an acquisition-sequencing model, the recommended sequence (bottom sequence Figure 2 below) is actually an evolution from the recently implemented separation of IO&T (Initial Outfitting and Transition) contracts (as shown in the middle diagram in Figure 2).

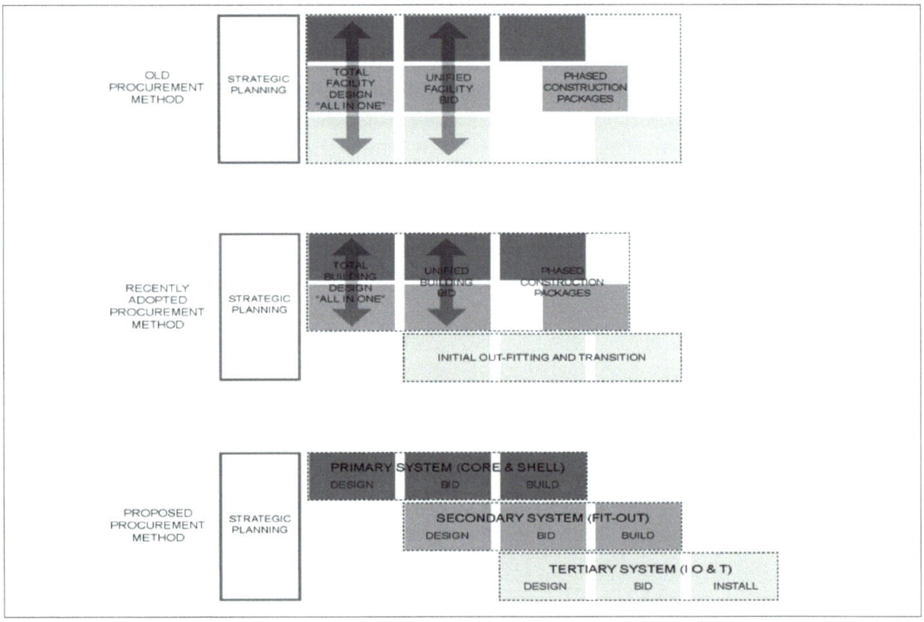

Figure 2. Evolution from a parallel to a serial decision-making process. The "old" procurement model may be suitable for simple projects. But the greater the project size and complexity, the longer the critical path to realization is, and the greater the chance that the investment will undergo significant transformation later, the more important decoupling and sequencing of decisions becomes.

ANALYZING DHA DOCUMENTS IN PREPARATION FOR WRITING NEW FLEXIBILITY REQUIREMENTS

Two DHA documents were analyzed in preparation for making recommendations for flexibility requirements. First was the UFC 4-510-01 (Uniform Facilities Criteria for Medical Facilities). Hundreds of pages long, it is periodically updated and has been the principle vehicle by which facility design requirements are promulgated. The second was the World Class Facilities Check-list, a public access website which undergoes continuous updating. UFC 4-510-01 requirements were analyzed and an assessment made as to how pertinent existing requirements are to flexibility. An Excel chart was used to:

1) Indicate relevance of existing requirements to flexibility by assigning them numbers 1, 2 and 3: 1 means no relevance; 2 means moderate relevance and 3 means high relevance;
2) Introduce the distinction between Primary, Secondary and Tertiary systems, and with an "X" depict the relevance of the UFC paragraph to one or more of these levels.

This analysis led to recommendations to augment the text of current UFC Flexibility Requirements.

ANALYZING THE UFC DESIGN SUBMITTALS

The Design Submittals contained in the UFC 4-510-01 are instrumental because they instruct architects and engineers in the preparation of drawings and specifications at each mandated design submission: Conceptual, Schematic, Design Development and so on. Because implementing flexibility necessities that architects and engineers explicitly demonstrate how they are complying with the requirements, and the client must monitor compliance, the Design Submittal requirements are – and will be – an essential instrument in implementing flexibility.

Because a direct relationship exists between the thirteen recommended UFC flexibility requirements (discussed later) and the UFC Appendix C Design Submittals requirements, it is important to make an explicit link between these as well.

If flexibility is to be implemented successfully across the DHA portfolio, the Design Submittals required of architects and engineers must be periodically assessed and revised. The client (DHA) must develop the methods, skills and culture to update these requirements as experience is gained and maintain vigilance of compliance over time.

The work of adjusting the Design Submittals was not part of the research contract and is therefore not reported on in this paper but is recommended for further study. However, the full analysis on the basis of which such development can be done was included in the final report.

THIRTEEN RECOMMENDED AMENDMENTS AND ADDITIONS TO THE FLEXIBILITY REQUIREMENTS IN THE WORLD CLASS CHECK LIST

A comprehensive examination of the World Class Facilities checklist revealed several flexibility requirements, indicated in ***bold/italic*** in the full list of recom-

mendations below:
- Site Capacity;
- ***Building Expansion Flexibility;***
- ***Geometry of the Structural System***
- ***Natural Light;***
- Floor-to-Floor Height Requirement;
- Loading Capacity of Floors;
- Minimal Internal Structural Walls;
- Flexible Facades;
- Separate Systems;
- Layout and MEP flexibility for the Secondary System;
- Opportunity for Vertical Mechanical Equipment in the Future;
- ***Multifunctional Use of Rooms;***
- Capacity for Variable Inpatient Bedroom Sizes.

Based on extensive review of best practices in the industry worldwide, and following the principles enunciated in the official report, the existing requirements were augmented and additional requirements were added, as listed above. All of these were provided in the final report, following the World Class Facilities Check-List format.

LINKING FLEXIBILITY TO PRINCIPLES OF RESILIENCY AND ADAPTATION TO CLIMATE CHANGE

We were also asked to link flexibility to the principles of resiliency. Discussions with leading experts and by reviewing recent literature lead to the following assessment. Both resiliency – the ability to withstand and recover from extreme natural and human-caused events – and capacity to adapt to climate change relate strongly to flexibility. While the causes of facility change differ (evolving functional and satisfaction factors over time drive the need for flexibility) the required facility performance common to all has to do with reducing the ripple effects of change in one part of a facility to all parts of that facility or installation.

In decision-making for flexibility, an economic and political (social/organizational/behavioral) assessment is required to evaluate the efficacy and return on investment of implementing a given flexibility strategy from a portfolio of candidate strategies. The same assessment is needed in preparing a facility for resiliency and capacity to adapt to climate change. That is, if flexibility is achieved, resilience and capacity to adapt to climate change are easier to achieve. That said, some of the recommended flexibility strategies are demonstrably more relevant in achieving resiliency and climate change adaptability than others. A thorough analysis of and elaboration of these points of convergence is needed.

LINKING FLEXIBILITY AND SUSTAINABLE BUILDINGS – MOVING BEYOND TECHNIQUE

Up to now, the discourse on high performance and sustainable buildings - in published technical reports, academic and industry conferences, in client organizations and among service providers - has been largely devoid of a fundamental rethinking of decision-making patterns. The discourse has focused on technique, not control (who decides what, when). Discussion about technique is preferred because of its presumed objectivity and purported grounding in technical rationality.

Discussions about control, on the other hand, inevitably encounter questions of the distribution of control (no single person can control everything), for which there are no "right" answers that can be justified by technical rationality. The literature also calls this "task partitioning." Organizations steeped in the culture of technical rationality, but who also must inescapably operate in complex patterns of distributed control, do not have good theory on which to establish policy and practices linking technique and control: thus the avoidance of systematic restructuring of decision-making. This difficulty is particularly evident in a large governmental organization such as the DHA which have grown larger over time and which accumulate patterns of decision making with few opportunities for a thorough overhaul.

Based on the above observation, a high-level tenet is important to include in the introduction section of the newly published UFC 1-200-01 (Uniform Facilities Criteria High Performance and Sustainable Building Requirements). In the interim, these principles can be implemented in the medical facilities infrastructure by including them in the UFC 4-510-01and in the World Class Checklist.

Conclusions: Adjustments in the Client Organizational Culture

To successfully implant a flexible (and high performance and sustainable) facility methodology as a normal way of doing business, DHA must develop the needed expertise and tools, as well as clear requirements to monitor and enforce a key principle: facility changes should have minimal consequences for the primary processes of the facility in adjacent areas, or above or below the affected floor area of the facility. This principle is relevant for new construction and for the reactivation or renovation of existing buildings.

Therefore, building elements and spaces with an expected long life should be strictly and explicitly decoupled from building elements and spaces with shorter expected use lives. This decoupling must be implemented in all phases including the planning, budgeting, design and construction (and renovation) processes.

The reason for decoupling is to assure that the change of a building element with a short life (e.g. an element serving a specific function) does not require disruption or change (or only minimal change quickly accomplished) of an element with an expected long life (i.e. an element or configuration that supports many building functions). For example, changing a wall with an expected short life should not require demolishing the structure; changing an electrical outlet should not require demolishing the wall it follows.

Within each of the three "systems levels" (Primary, Secondary, Tertiary), it is possible to find "fixed" and "variable" parts. For instance, the façade is assigned to the primary system. But within the "façade" category, some parts may need to be replaced or upgraded more frequently than other parts (e.g. windows may need to be replaced before the entire building cladding comes due for replacement; in that case, the building envelope as such is "fixed" and the windows are "variable"). There is no precise or scientific basis for decoupling or for deciding what should have a long asset life and what should have a short (or shorter) useful life. Part of the reasoning is certainly technical. But an equally if not more important set of criteria has to do with what could be called "interests." Decentralized interests may not be as easily discernable in a top-down organization such as DHA or other large, centralized organizations, as compared to large private healthcare systems with many geographically disbursed, semi-autonomous facilities such as, for example, Sutter, St. Joseph or Ascension Health Care Systems.

What is common across these cases is that a hierarchy of interests exists. At the highest level are interests in the long-term survival and maintenance of the asset base. In the case of the DHA, it is the US Congress. They are in the game for the very long haul. On the other end of the hierarchy of interests are the doctors and other caregivers. They are the direct service providers and are ethically and professionally committed to offering the best care with the best medicine, technology and personnel. A model may explain, in which system levels are paired with "interests":

- *Primary System*: Central Organization (Agency, Governing Board);
- *Secondary System*: Local Healthcare Facility Management Group;
- *Tertiary System:* Doctors and Nurses.

Needless to say, this practice of linking physical systems with "interests" has become conventional best practice in the bulk of commercial property development in much of the world and is increasingly found in other use types such as laboratories, institutional and multi-family residential properties. This model, when adopted for use in DHA facilities, will enable not only a positive return on investment, but also a more effective and fluid transfer of knowledge, experience and innovation between the private sector and the DHA, despite inevitable and important differences.

Rhizomatic Healthscapes

Alan Mee[1], Eric Wright[2], Phil Astley[3]

[1]School of Architecture and Landscape, University College Dublin, Ireland
[2]Department of Architecture, University of Johannesburg, and BOOM architects, South Africa
[3]UCL Bartlett School of Construction & Project Management, London, England

This paper deals with organisational and working models for spatially chaotic, informal and/or unplanned city settlements where there is low access to public health services and services in general, workforce, technologies and space that enable service transformations through which they are delivered. These situations require new approaches to planning and design processes.
The Rhizomatic theory and methodologies covered in this presentation are developing on the ground in the current 'aformal terrain' studio underway right now in johannesburg. This studio is the beginning of an intended long term engaged process with the UJ, UCL and the community of Denver informal settlement.

This studio model investigates co-productive and collaborative methods of working within and beyond architectural scales, employing 3 main concepts; Spatial justice; Humane settlements; Scenario planning.

These processes aim to facilitate dialogues within highly uncertain strategic and spatial environments.

The term and the use of 'rhizomatic healthscapes' extends the philosophical approaches of Deleuze and Guattari, in that it describes this research problem as one that allows for multiple connections between 'semiotic chains and organsiations of power where the informal, unplanned or aformal settlement is an 'inter-being' of culture.

On this basis methodologies require continual mapping of growth and change.

The paper essentially distends along 3 main trajectories. This presentation takes the form of these:

1. Emergent Theories - linkages of rhizome theory to unexplored territory within spatial theory;
2. Two Healthscape Sites - comparison of 2 previously unrelated sites (joburg/dublin) in doing so a particular understanding of 'rhizome' is deepened, tested, expanded by specific choices;
3. Approaches and Methods - identify and introduce a new set of tools for spatial disciplines (practitioners) working within 'creative spatial sciences.

Emergent Theories

In current global conditions the political, social and environmental effects of the rampant production of space lead to reactionary movements such as insurgent urbanism (Davis 2013) which seek, under pressures of poor governance and constrained civic capacity, to address emerging manifestations of spatial chaos.

...cities are what we might call a "mess"... Urban data isn't simply discovered, it is invented, manipulated and crafted; and cities aren't 'solved', they are created through the actions, motivations and decisions of their citizens... Uzman Haque in praise of messy cities.

Given these conditions, it is suggested in this paper that a new focus on healthcare can become more spatial and public, leading to a rhizomatic renewal of community identity as well as of the spatial, public and health landscape.

While allowing for the local economies of design, considering appropriate responses to rapid spatial change can include those from the broader creative spatial sciences (urban design, spatial planning), with arguably deeper consideration of assemblages and critical urbanism, as well as a broader geographical set of scales.

This broadening of scales refers to the north-south divide investigating complex relationships observed between social movements cutting across social and historical boundaries, with a focus on 'urban learning assemblages'.

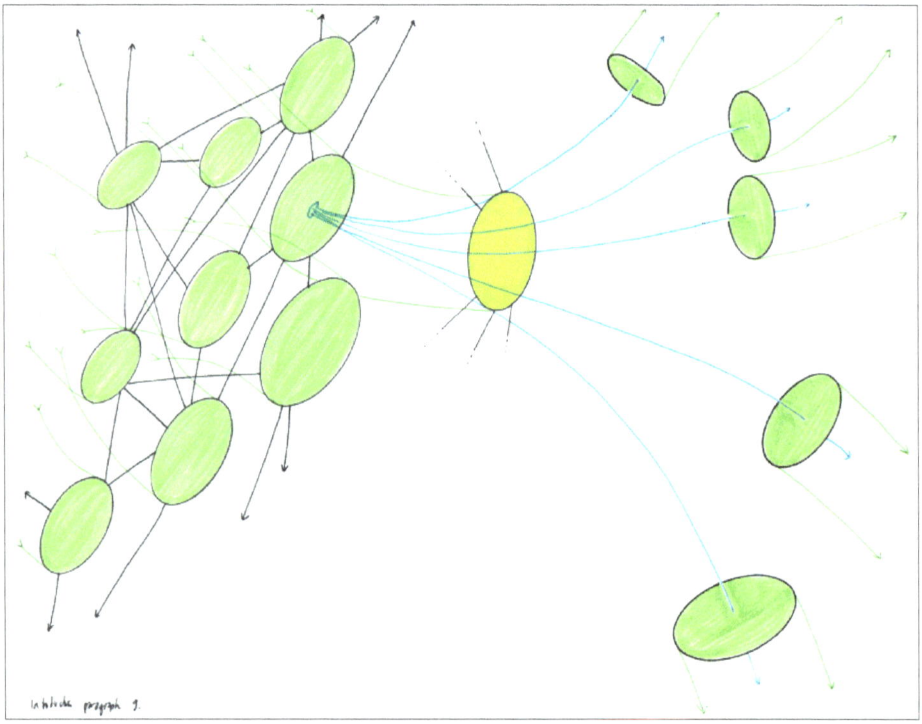

Figure 1. Drawing of 1000 plataues © Marc Ngui.

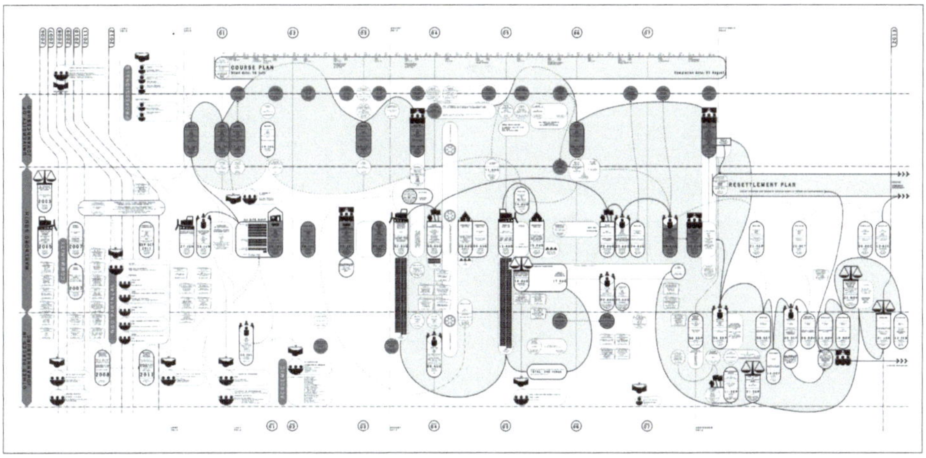

Figure 2. Processes of Engagement Map, Informal Studio Marlboro South © BOOM architects.

Recent discourse on spatial planning, with reference to Deleuze and Guattari's 'normative political vision, that aims at a condition of radical freedom for humans beyond the state and capitalism'.
Purcell describes their definition of a rhizome as 'a form for the act of mutual augmentation through connection', and further as 'an acentered, non-hierarchical network of entities in which each member has the potential to communicate horizontally with any other'. Figure 2 aims to demonstrate these acentered, non-heirarchical interactions and connections.

In the paper it is argued that in any system comprising a dense web of interdependent factors 'one can break into the system and intervene at any point in an attempt to shift its direction, disrupt its current trajectory and improve its performance.'
By this an ecological framework is proposed:
- the clinical micro system (the space where the care, intervention, treatment takes place);
- the meso-system (a system of systems eg between the specialist hospital and the neighbourhood);
- the exo-system (the link to the professional schools, the workforce);
- the macro system (values/politics) ie the whole healthscape as an armature.

Identifying and collecting data for each system level and related elements (non-physical technology to physical) will elicit a new 'mindset' that can support success in collaborative relationships.

From this intention system resilience is promoted across and between microsystems in the face of informal, unpredictable changes in providers and individuals.

The application of scenario planning as an 'open design approach', identifying possibilities through dialogue to inform planning across healthscapes was identified by Astley an others in preceding work. This approach would untie care activities (service delivery) from the building fabric and enable operational change in the system.

Scenario planning undertaken with trans-disciplinary teams at a strategic and operational level would set out design systems enabled by infrastructural and physical possibility. The scope from strategic to operational encompasses the systems theory at varying scales. Reference to earlier 4 scales, micro, meso, exo, and maxo (Figure 3).
In our current iteration of this immersive, participative planning and design process this is referred to as co-produced communty action planning' (Figure 4).

In these processes the aim is, through collaborative discussion, to improve the resilience of the microsystem whilst the physical infrastructure and space can be improved. By this the dynamic arrangements and ecologies of the setting are respected, repaired and improved.

To summarise, emergent theories in the paper identifies:

- non fixed health provision;
- new models of health care practice;
- connections of emerging ecological theory around 'health' as a wider role-wellbeing and spatial justice.

TWO HEALTHSCAPE SITES

Sandyford in Dublin unplanned, (Figure 5) and Marlboro South informal, (Figure 6) in Johannesburg.

Unplanned referring to forms and ecologies outside or in contrast to the intended/expected and informal referring to scenarios within, and despite of inadequate provision from governance.

Although very different in the many respects, the two sites do share some characteristics:

Both can be considered. Peripheral edge cities – as unplanned and unequal developments, each could be seen as 'bounded' physically, socially, spatially.

Having poor or non-existent public realm provision, poor public health provision, and 'unusual' land ownership scenarios, eg. totally privatised, no/few owner occupiers, etc. Seen as 'spatial products', that is, 'emerging manifestations of spatial chaos.'

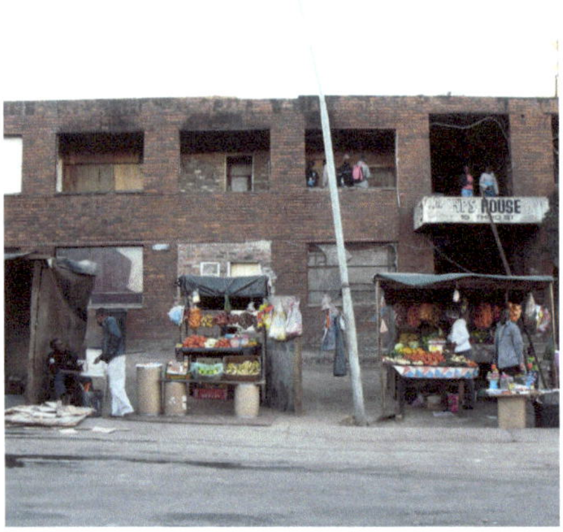

Figure 3. Microsystems level. © Alex Opper.

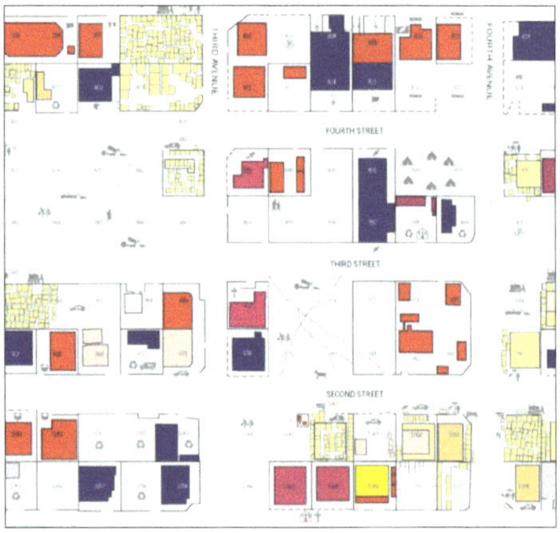

Figure 4. Land-use map, Marlboro South, 26'10 south Architects based on mapping by UJ, 2012 ©.

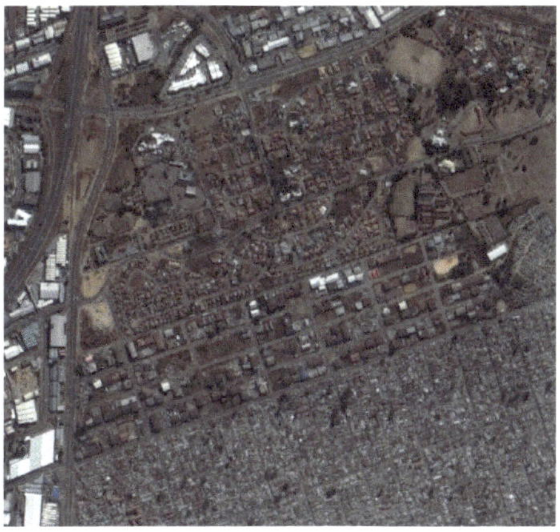

Figure 5. Marlboro South.

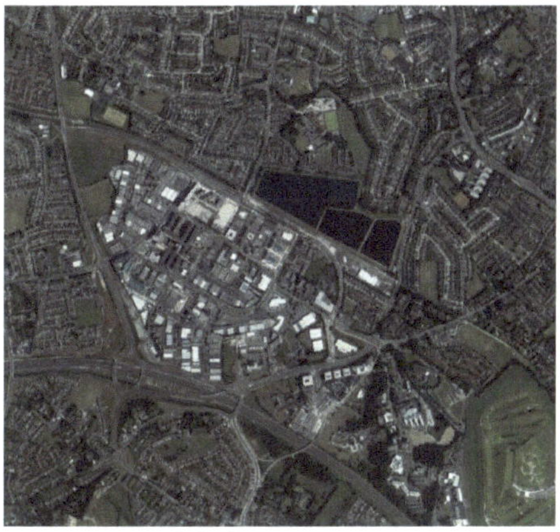

Figure 6. Sandyford in south Dublin.

One 'microsite' in each city is looked at - investigating possible provision of appropriate rhizomatic healthscapes.
It is not intended that the two locations chosen here are seen as comparable sites in relation to historical, cultural, or other location specific aspects, but more as two separate places, subject to some similar forces, especially related to rapid urbanization, globalization, but also potential for self-organisation.

At this point in the developing research and working methodologies this comparison informs readings of emerging spatial theory and towards more appropriate methodologies and tools.

Sandyford in south Dublin, and the 'former Sandyford Industrial Estate', evolved in the 1980's towards a more mixed use site including retail, and lastly emerging after 2000 as an unplanned, sharply contrasting (in terms of density) unfinished commercial and residential development, effectively stalled since the end of the economic boom in 2008.
Sandyford has a population of 2,600 approx., spread over one square kilometer, so a quite low overall with just a few high density apartment blocks, alongside unfinished/abandoned developments.

Even though very high levels of self-reported health occur, it is a new neighbourhood with almost no public health provision, real public amenities, or walkable areas. It also houses one of the few private hospitals/clinics in the country, which attracts patients from all over the island, but is not an option for local low-income residents. Sandyford relies on this privately run hospital to serve the area, with the support of the Local Authority there is a lack of public primary care centre (PCC) facilities in the neighbourhood
The situation is compounded by the fact that public realm provision, including parks, public open space and playgrounds are all low or missing, and there is a roads dominated spatial character in general.

The presence of a private hospital as the dominating health provision in the area is an indicator of fixed and obdurate health provision (Figure 7).

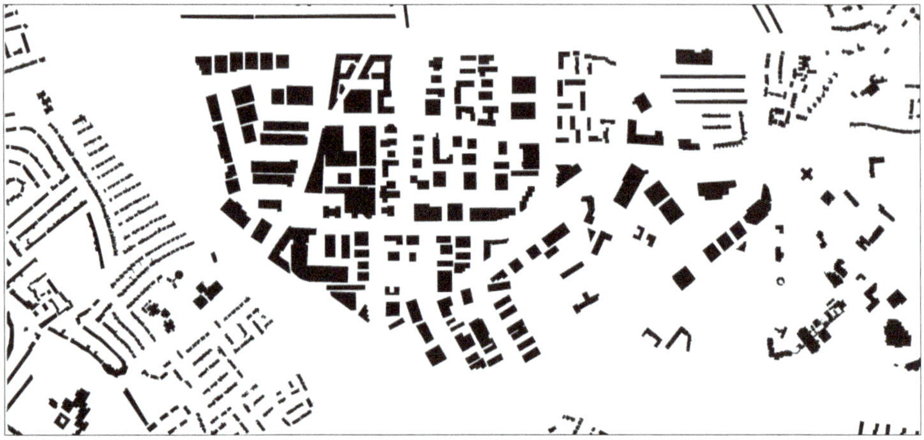

Figure 7. Figure ground Sandyford © Alan Mee.

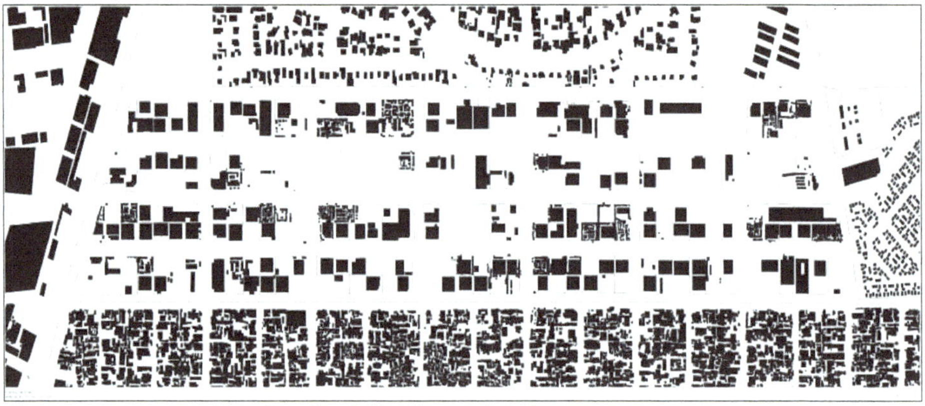

Figure 8. Figure ground Marlboro South © 26'10 south Architects.

Marlboro South in extreme contrast to Sandyford acts as a temporary accommodation zone for the displaced residents of the Alexandra Township to the north of the city centre (here the word temporary sits in stasis as many residents have been finding or constructing shelter here since as early as 1996). With a population of approximately 4,000 people, this site comprises a 2km long informal settlement of low-rise buildings, with a severe lack of public services. An enumeration of the area undertaken by SDI (Slum Dwellers International South African Alliance) revealed that many residents are on very low incomes. Many sites were never occupied and many of the warehouses that were built, were either vacated or abandoned in the 1980's. Some stats form the MS2012 studio - Only 21% of the sites still function as intended. Many of the remaining structures are standing empty.

Some areas, consisting of open land between structures, are used as (illegal) dumping sites or parking lots. Some buildings are used as crèche's, clinics or churches. 18.8% of the area is used as formal (0.02%) or informal (18.78%) housing.

APPROACHES AND METHODS

It could be argued that value systems in both areas sometimes bear resemblances: the need, desires and aspirations; to drive a new car, for example, or have satellite tv, can override the need for basic infrastructure like water supply (Marlboro South) or public footpaths (Sandyford). The general edge city morphologies also demonstrate some surprisingly similar patterns in both places: big box sheds, motorways, informal/ mixed density settlements. The following 'Framework for Dialogue' (Figure 9) intends to stimulate official responses to issues of health, spatial justice and quality in unplanned urban environments. Earlier reference was made to the Processes of Engagement Map as a record of the work in Marlboro South. The basis of the studio was to provide a defined service of an overarching supporting process of development driven by residents themselves, and aided by NGOs and CBOs.
Within this meta-programme a 'nested' healthscape design process is suggested, including products and responses to informal and spatially chaotic scenarios.

The following 'tools' and 'systems' are proposed:
- a 'Framework for Dialogue';
effecting open building (system separation) intelligences;
- overturning 'unmappings', systems beyond state;
- seeking rhizomatic or assemblage groupings.

These will be covered in more detail in the Figures 10-12.

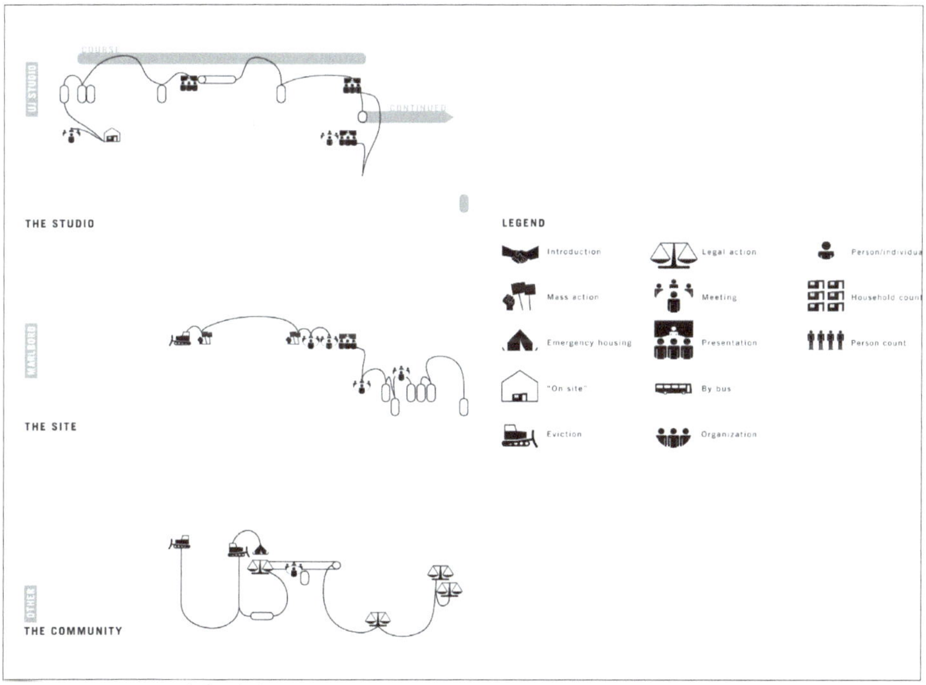

Figure 9. Framework for dialogue.

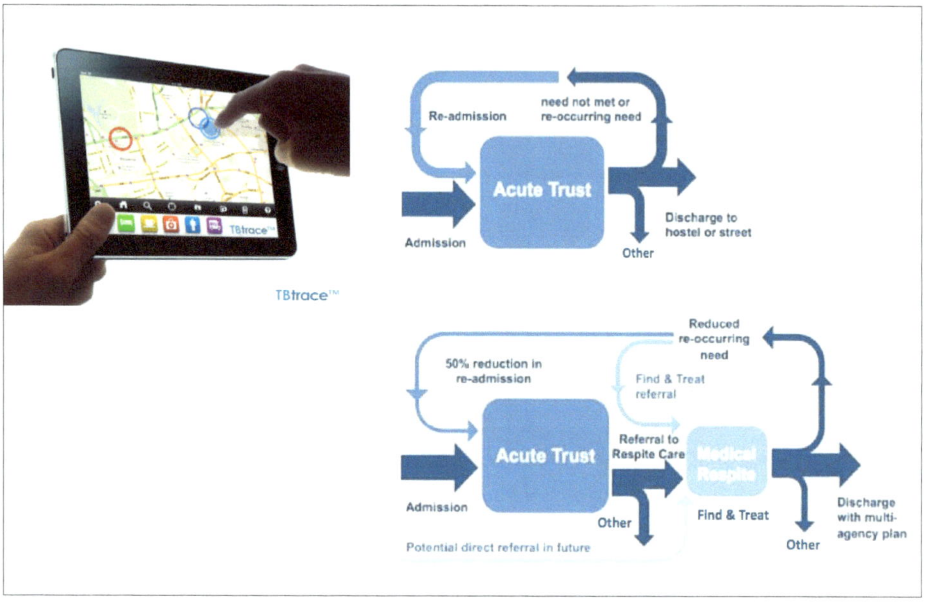

Figure 10. UCLH/UCL remote monitoring, screening and video organised therapies. Photograph source: TB 'Find and Treat'. Medical Respite Centre scheme. Diagrams source: Pathway Medical Respite Centre A new model of specialist intermediate care for homeless people. May 2012.

THE 'FRAMEWORK FOR DIALOGUE'

Scenario planning is proposed as a tool to facilitate multi-disciplinary dialogues. My colleague Phil Astley has worked with a multi-disciplinary clinical team on a research-led health interventions in the London Pathway project for the diagnosis and provision of TB services for informally housed and individually homeless.

The aim of the project was to articulate and prepare for the development of health space for respite care. Space would be supported by an innovative mobile imagining, 'Find and Treat', interventions as well as the use of oral medicine management and internet treatment by TB specialists with both client and health provider 'at large' in the meso and exo system.

1 - Existing model, existing feedback loop of unmet needs causing repeat admission and increased attendance in acute services;

2 - The pathway model, proposed medical respite centre reduces unmet need lowering repeat admission by approx 50% and minimising re-attendance in acute services, with increased discharge into appropriate accommodation with multi-agency planing.

The spatial aspect of this work (through the framework of dialogue shown in Figure 11) is the growing recognition that successful interventions need to be about more than dealing with illness, but to provide social and well being support linked to housing and employment initiatives.

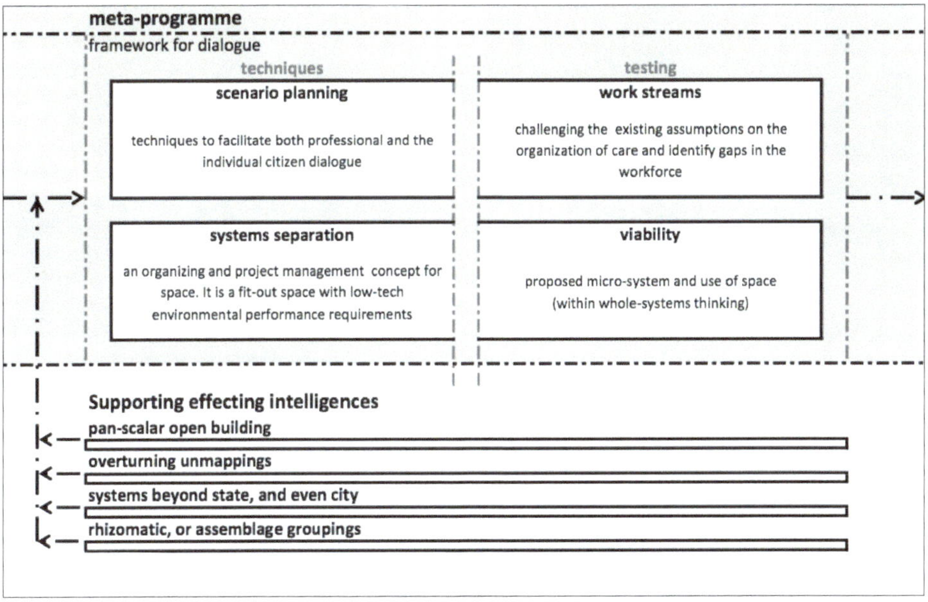

Figure 11. Framework of dialogue.

The aim is to provide improved care for physical ill health problems, while also working to address mental health and substance misuse issues. The main organisational aspects of this integrated approach are:

- Scenario planning, as the technique to facilitate both professional and the individual citizen dialogue;
- Workstreams, to challenge the existing assumptions on the organization of care and identify gaps in the workforce;
- Systems separation, as an organizing and project management concept for space. It is a fit-out space with low-tech environmental performance requirements (eg ventilation);
- Viability, of the proposed micro-system and use of space (within whole-systems thinking).

These framework flows incorporate the following emergent tools, approaches and methods: Really a conclusion for this presentation:

1. Pan-scalar open building

Effecting open building intelligences that utilize systems separation techniques involves a 'pan-scalar' opportunity, that is, within buildings, but also beyond, outside, or at a scale which includes broader communities, both digital and actual, and for temporary as well as permanent uses.

2. Overturning Unmappings

The importance of mapping overlapping social indicators and health inequalities is acknowledged in this paper.

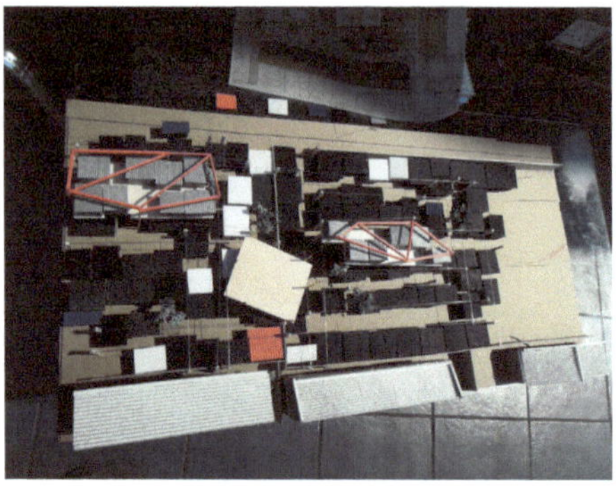

Figure 12. Pan-scalar open building; overturning unmappings. Model by UJ student Jaco Jonker.

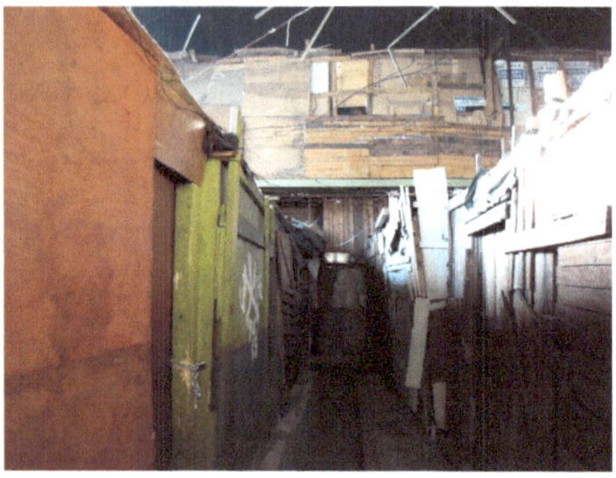

Figure 13. Systems beyond state: rhizomatic, or assemblage groupings.

In this respect, lack in provision of amenities, rights, and space are often hidden in the absence of clear understandings of land ownership, zoning and other power dynamics.

Revealing these aspects of the built environment to local residents through graphical and other mappings or 'unmappings' of inappropriately accepted readings of these places can be a way to open dialogue on possibilities for healthscapes and spaces to emerge from collaborative discussion.

3 - Systems beyond State

In political geography, certain state centered African development has been described as a 'monstrous hybrid' in an argument which favours cities 'and their city-regions' over states in attempts to eradicate poverty. In this sense systems beyond state, and even beyond city, could become effective.

4 - Rhizomatic, or Assemblage Groupings

In a rhizomatic healthscape, the health provision network would organize itself. An assemblage urbanism would allow for self-organisation of systems of provision and care, as assemblage groupings.

This paper has analysed the critical spatial, health, systems and open building theory and literature, before outlining a definition of 'Rhizomatic Healthscapes'. Which is defined as non-fixed health provision which minimises obduracy (inflexibility) and extending it to design scales around and above architecture.

Design Research and the Globalization of Healthcare Environments

Mardelle McCuskey Shepley, Yilin Song

mshepley@arch.tamu.edu
Texas A&M University, Texas

Objectives. Global healthcare practice has expanded in the past 20 years. At the same time the incorporation of research into the design process has gained prominence as best practice among architects. The authors of this study investigated the status of design research in a variety of international settings. We intended to answer the question, "how pervasive is healthcare design research outside of the United States?"
Method. The authors reviewed the international literature on the design of healthcare facilities. Over 500 international studies and conference proceedings were incorporated in this literature review. A team of five research assistants searched multiple databases comparing approximately 16 keywords to geographic location. Some of those keywords included: evidence-based design, salutogenic design, design research, and healthcare environment. Additional articles were gathered by contacting prominent researchers and asking for their personal assessment of local health design research studies.
Results. While there are design researchers in most parts of the world, the majority of studies 1) focus on the needs of populations in developed countries and 2) generate guidelines that have significant cost and cultural implications that prohibit their implementation in developing countries. Additionally, the body of literature discussing the role of culture in healthcare environments is extremely limited.
Conclusion. Design researchers must address the cultural implications of their studies. Additionally, we need to expand our research objectives to address healthcare design in countries that have not been previously considered.

***Keywords**: evidence-based design, design research, proxemics, culture.*

Introduction

Global healthcare practice has expanded over the past 20 years. Simultaneously, the incorporation of research into the design process has gained prominence as best practice among architects. These two trends are interlinked; one of the outcomes of design research is providing information about indigenous user needs.

Using research to support international practice is a means of providing more appropriate environments for individuals whose culture is unfamiliar to the designer.

Thorne (1993) suggests that Western medicine has been embraced as the only appropriate medicine in much of the world. However, Verderber (2003) argues that traditional care may play a more important factor in the future.

Furnham and Smith (1988) suggest that the seemingly disparate worldviews of East and West are reconcilable and may be manifested in the high-tech/high touch philosophy of many healthcare facilities. "Given the profound effects of culture and spirituality on one's identity and subsequent behaviors, it stands to reason that a physical environment that supports cultural and spiritual beliefs would contribute positively to one's health and recovery" (Kopec & Han 2008, p. 116).

One of the primary considerations for international healthcare design is culturally-based spatial behavior. The associated research area is called proxemics. The expression proxemic behavior, coined by Edward Hall in 1963, is "the study of microspace as a system of biocommunication" (p. 1022). Related to human topology, choriology (the study of organized space), and chaology (the study of boundaries) (Hall 1963), the study of proxemics was popular during the 1970s, but little research was conducted since.

In light of the need to provide research to designers, the authors of this study aimed to investigate the availability of design research across international settings.

We intended to answer the question, "how pervasive is healthcare design research outside of the US?"

EVIDENCE-BASED DESIGN (EBD)

EBD is the process associated with the use of research to inform the design process. While the use of design research has been gaining momentum over the last several decades, the notion of EBD was initiated in North America and Europe in the 1980s. Similar to evidence-based medicine, the purpose of EBD is to use research to inform professional practice. This is particularly critical in the creation of healthcare facilities. EBD can be used to expand our awareness of cultural needs, and inform design decisions (Shepley 2011).

Unfortunately, many of the recommendations stemming from EBD involve increased construction costs. Research tends to be directed at specific design solutions, such as private rooms, and sometimes loses its focus on the original intention (e.g., infection control), inhibiting the pursuit of less expensive options. In countries with sufficient resources, we argue that, while capital costs increase with EBD, maintenance costs will decrease and a return on investment (ROI) will be forthcoming. In many developing countries, regardless of the truth of this ROI, funds are simply not available to support certain design recommendations. EBD may be "expensive, demanding costly materials; hospitality-style rooms and lobbies, and large expanse of lush gardens that are costly to maintain" (Pati n.d.). In response to this circumstance, Sherif (1999) discusses strategies that should be used in developing countries. These approaches include the reduction of built area, uses of simple but appropriate construction systems, modular design, implementation of daylighting and ventilation, specification of heavy-duty materials and efficient HVAC systems.

Pati (n.d.) also points out that cultural, legal and financial limitations impact the flexibility of design decision-making and that no single solution fits all cases. "EBD should be viewed as a process to optimize performance within cost, legal, cultural and operational boundaries" (Pati n.d.). He notes, for example, that safety is not a binary concept of safe versus unsafe, rather it is an indicator of the degree of risk a culture will take based on socio-economic resources.

This paper attempts to summarize the available literature. This is an optimistic endeavor and we are likely overlooking critical publications. One of the purposes of the authors, however, is to incite a response on the part of the readership informing us of our oversights and enabling us to have a broader understanding of the status of health design research.

Methodology

In order to examine the role of EBD in the global development of healthcare environments, the authors reviewed the international literature on the design of healthcare facilities. Over 500 studies and conference proceedings were incorporated in this literature review and filtered according to their global applicability. We obtained many of the articles by contacting prominent researchers and asking for their personal assessment of local health design research studies. These researchers were located in China, Egypt, Germany, India, Iran, Israel, Singapore, and other countries. A team of five research assistants searched multiple databases comparing the following keywords to geographic location: "evidence-based design," "design research," "healthcare environment," "spatial behavior," "proxemics," "design culture," "salutogenic design", and related terms. Greater keyword success was achieved by searching for specific countries or regions (e.g., China, Iran, Israel, and Sweden) in lieu of the term "international." Other keywords were terms associated with EBD. For example, Planetree, an approach to patient care that incorporates the physical environment and patient centered care, share similar objectives with proponents of design research. Planetree includes an international certification program, the recipients of which are located in the Brazil, Canada, Netherlands, and United States (Planetree 2012).

The literature review team members and external experts were multi-national in composition and included individuals who were either native speakers or had reading knowledge of English, Farsi, French, German, Hebrew, Italian, Mandarin, Portuguese, and Spanish. Countries were included in which publications or abstracts appeared in those languages.

The references were consolidated into tables according to keywords and country of origin as a means of organizing the disparate material. The objective was to determine the degree to which designers throughout the world are incorporating EBD in the creation of healthcare buildings. The topics ranged from the design of rooms to full blown urban environments. The methodologies varied from qualitative research on health behaviors to quantitative research on the environment and infection.

As research focusing specifically on health design was limited in many countries, the summary included international design literature of all kinds, if the outcomes could be interpreted as potentially applicable to healing environments. For example, most publications on culturally-based responses to the environment were considered to be useful to the design of healthcare settings. The primary purpose of this project was to garner a sense of the role research plays in design from an international perspective.

Results

A primary finding of this literature review is that rigorous research is minimal outside of North America, Europe and Australia. In many regions publications are limited to project descriptions. Such case studies and reviews of international projects may describe the use of EBD principles in the programming, and design of projects.

Several venues include both research and case studies such as the journals World Health Design and Healthcare Design and books such as Sustainable Healthcare Architecture (Guenther & Vittori 2008) and Therapeutic landscapes: An Evidence-based Approach to Designing Healing Gardens and Restorative Outdoor Spaces (Cooper Marcus & Sachs 2013).

Websites, such as Healthier Places, published by Architecture and Design Scotland, provide references and case studies that are also useful resources.
While acknowledging the contributions of case studies and project descriptions, the authors of this paper focused on design research. Design research is an essential tool contributing to the highest quality healthcare environments. The following is a map of the outcomes of this literature review, organized by geographic region. These regions include, the African continent, Asia and Eurasia, Australasia, Continental Europe and Nordic countries, Latin America, Middle East, and the United Kingdom (UK) (Figure 1).

Discussion

The results of this study demonstrate that there is insufficient research on environments in developing nations. Three conclusions are clear:

- more research on the design of healthcare facilities is needed in many regions in the world;

- there are too few studies on cultural differences in environmental preference across nations, races and ethnicities; the outcomes of studies done in one country might not be culturally appropriate for another. As a result proposed environmental interventions may contribute more to stress than healing. In evaluations of new and old hospitals, staff and patients did not have higher satisfaction with new buildings (Abbas 2012);

- there are too few studies on healthcare environments in economically challenged countries; the studies in other, more fiscally stable countries may recommend environmental interventions that are not achievable.

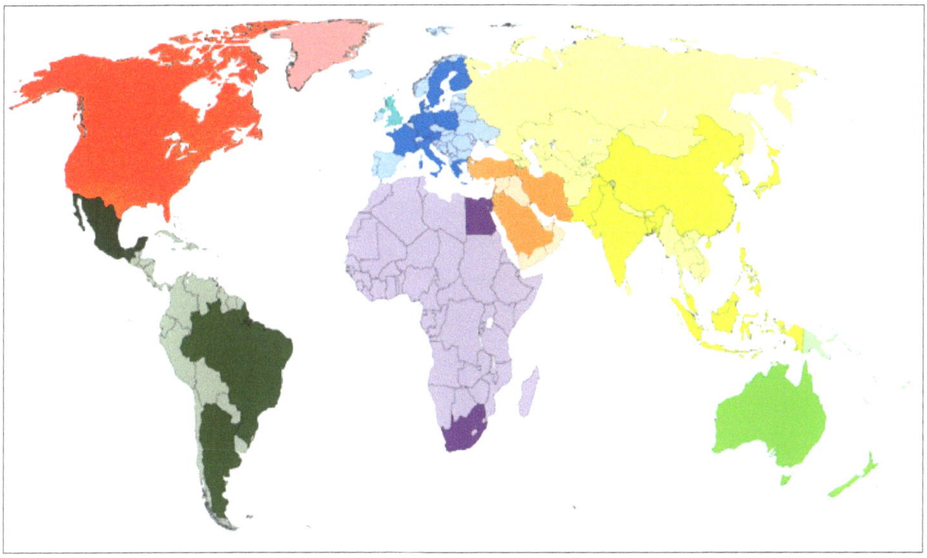

Figure 1. World map designating the geographic regions used in this paper. The countries for which we did not uncover literature are indicated by lighter tones.

CULTURAL CONTEXT

In the absence of research, non-local designers must be more aware of the cultural needs of the populations for whom they are serving. When informed by research, healthcare architects can more adequately address indigenous needs in two ways: 1) they can support healthcare staff who in turn care for patients, or 2) they can address the needs of patients directly (Shepley, 2011). In order to do this, however, they must increase their cultural understanding.

There are no particular models for increasing the competency of architects. However, Campinha-Bacote's (2002) proposed schemata for culturally competent health service providers a potential framework (Figure 2). Campinha-Bacote's model includes the attributes of knowledge, skill, awareness, desire and encounters. The role of knowledge can be readily interpreted as design research/EBD. Research can contribute to guidelines for effective and supportive healthcare environments. The use of research should work in tandem with partnering with local firms and studying the indigenous architecture.

ECONOMIC CONTEXT

The economic circumstances of a country have an enormous impact on the healthcare environment infrastructure. The total healthcare expenditures, which tend to parallel the prevalence of research, clearly demonstrate the need for research in the developing world. The highest healthcare and research expenditures per capita takes place in North American, European and Western Pacific countries where life expectancy is highest and infant mortality is lowest (WHO 2013).

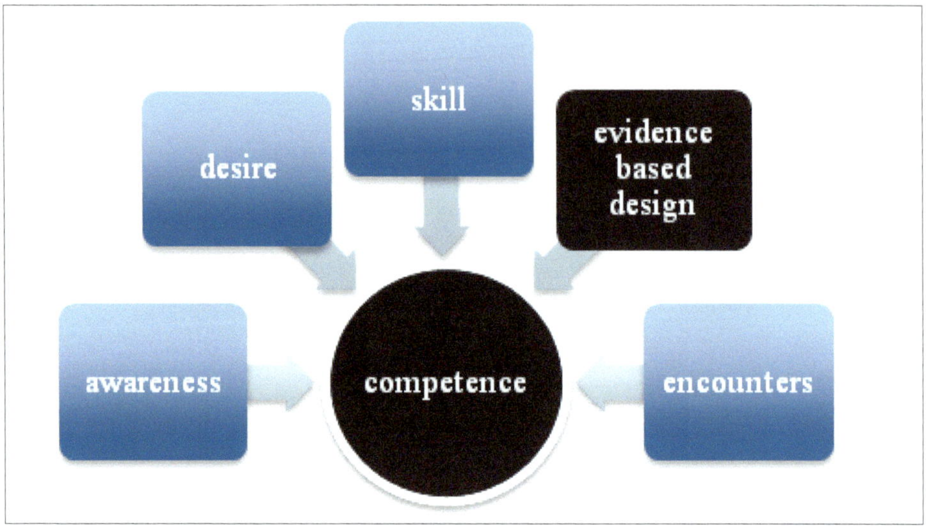

Figure 2. Cultural competent health facility design and research based on the Campinha-Bacote model (2002) and Shepley (2011).

Designers in Southeast Asia, Africa and Central America are likely to focus on meeting the basic requirements of the indigent populations and design research is perceived as a luxury. This underlines the need of researchers outside of these countries to seek funding in their country of origin and collaborate with researchers within these countries. In supporting those countries, research priorities should be emphasized and the tools used in developed countries altered for this application (Abbas 2012). Design research must be focused on specific design objectives (e.g., infection control) rather than specific solutions (e.g., private patient rooms), the latter of which is only practical in regions with greater resources.

CONCLUSIONS

The intention of this paper was to summarize the state-of-the-art in international design research and practice and address the issues of cultural competency and economic viability in developing countries. Progress toward creating the most appropriate healthcare environments is a global endeavor requiring the contribution of all designers and researchers intent on improving global quality of life.

ACKNOWLEDGMENTS

This paper is an abridged version of a manuscript, which was accepted for publication on April 26, 2014 in the Journal of Health Environments Research & Design (HERD). The full version in HERD includes detailed citations and references, and an expanded body of text.

The authors would like to acknowledge the contributions of Xiaohan Gao, Victoria Garcia, Farzad Golestanirad, Naomi Sachs, and Mario Salinas to both papers.

REFERENCES

Abbas, MY., 2012. 'Children, youth & environments (CYE): Lessons for developing countries?', *Procedia - Social and Behavioral Sciences*, vol. 38, pp. 15-22.

Campinha-Bacote, J., 2002. 'The process of cultural competence in the delivery of healthcare services: A model of care', *Journal of Transcultural Nursing*, vol. 13, no. 3, pp. 181-184.

Cooper Marcus, C & Sachs, NA., 2013. *Therapeutic landscapes: An evidence-based approach to designing healing gardens and restorative outdoor spaces*, John Wiley & Sons, Hoboken, New Jersey.

Furnham, A & Smith, C., 1988. 'Choosing alternative medicine: A comparison of the beliefs of patients visiting a general practitioner and a homoeopath', *Social Science and Medicine*, vol. 26, no. 7, pp. 685-689.

Guenther, R & Vittori, G., 2008. *Sustainable healthcare architecture*, John Wiley & Sons, Hoboken, New Jersey.

Hall, ET., 1963. 'A system for the notation of proxemic behavior', *American Anthropologist*, vol. 65, no. 5, pp. 1003-1026.

Kopec, D & Han, L., 2008. 'Islam and the healthcare environment: Designing patient rooms', *Health Environments Research & Design Journal*, vol. 1, no. 4, pp. 111-121.

Pati, D., n.d. *Evidence based design during financial turmoil*, Viewed 8 February 2014, <http://www.Healthdesign.org/sites/default/files/news/ Evidence%20Based%20Design%20during%20Financial%20Turmoil.pdf>.

Planetree, 2012. Hospital Israelita Albert Einstein: Humanizing healthcare in Sao Paulo, Brazil, in *Planetree Case Studies*, viewed 16 November 2012, <http://planetree.org/?page_id=314>.

Shepley, M., 2011. 'Using evidence-based design to support different cultures in healthcare environments', in *ACSA 2011 Fall Proceedings*, Washington, DC, pp. 153-160.

Sherif, AH., 1999. 'Hospitals of developing countries: Design and construction economics', *Journal of Architectural Engineering*, vol. 5, no. 3, pp. 74-81.

Thorne, S., 1993. 'Health belief systems in perspective', *Journal of Advanced Nursing*, vol. 18, no. 12, pp. 1931-1941.

Verderber, S., 2003. 'Architecture for health- 2050: An international perspective', *The Journal of Architecture*, vol. 8, no. 3, pp. 281-302.

World Health Organization (WHO), 2013. *World Health Statistics 2013*, viewed 8 February 2014, <http://www.who.int/gho/publications/world_health_statistics/EN_WHS2013_Full.pdf>.

Design Issues for Healthcare Buildings

Session introduction

The design of buildings dedicated to healthcare is an extremely complex professional and research field. Work in this particular design sector requires ongoing study and results can be achieved over a period of decades; there are cases where designers have devoted their entire careers to this area of research. The complexity is due to the fact that in addition to the scientific and technical skills of architecture affecting the design and construction process it is necessary to have a proper understanding of all sociological and psychological factors underlying the use of architecture for healthcare. From their birth until old age environments for care and health promotion play a decisive role in the well-being of the people and this is why it is necessary to adopt all the design solutions that increase the positive perception of the environment.

The design of birthing environments has been addressed since antiquity. One of the priorities in this design area is to create an environment in which the mother feels at ease in a familiar-looking and domestic space. On the other hand this consideration of the psychological sphere of perception must be accompanied by a careful study of the measures that ensure the safety of the mother and baby.

Similarly even in paediatric hospitals it is necessary to adopt all the design solutions that allow children to face the treatment and hospitalization period in the best mood possible by decreasing the difficult stress conditions related to illness and treatment. Creating environments where children can spend time in hospital with the possibility of playing games and engaging in recreational activities goes hand in hand with knowledge of new technologies for creating interactive and friendly environments.

Even the design of environments for the elderly requires a careful analysis of the aging population; the environment must meet the needs of people faced with spending a period of time there providing the best quality of life possible. It should also take into account the need to adapt the urban spaces of the city to people who have reduced mobility thus preventing the creation of areas isolated from the rest of the community.

Even the design of environments devoted to mental health care requires a careful interdisciplinary analysis of the needs of patients and the families of the personnel involved in the care process. The environments must be able to help people with mental health problems to feel part of the community, and function so that these places are perceived as familiar. Architecture can support the process of the deinstitutionalization of environments dedicated to mental health care and can make a positive contribution in overcoming the stigma and prejudice linked to the disease.

Moshe Zarhy
A Life for Health Facilities

Peter R. Pawlik

Peter R. Pawlik
Dr. AKG of Germany, Berlin, Germany

Moshe Zarhy, born in 1923 in Jerusalem, counts among the second generation of architects, who have contributed decisively to shaping the face of today's modern state of Israel. By his functional, aesthetical and unadorned style he can be seen in direct succession to the founding fathers of Israeli architecture, who - in the twenties and thirties of the twentieth century - laid the foundation for the settlement of Palestine.
In his life as an architect he has achieved supreme international recognition. Numerous national as well as international distinctions were conferred upon him. One field of work, however, has been of particular interest to Moshe Zarhy since the beginning of his activities: Health facilities. It is in this field that he has achieved mastery by a multitude of outstanding and ground-breaking hospitals.
He has been involved in the International Union of Architects' (UIA) since the mid-sixties. As a voting member of the Public Health Working Group, Zarhy has represented the Israeli National Section in all UIA Congresses since 1969. He was UIA Council Member during the years 1990-1993, was elected UIA vice President Region II for the terms of 1993-1996-1999, and has served as Director of the UIA Work Programme "Architecture for Science and Hi-Tech Facilities" since 1999. Moshe Zarhy has been elected as FAIA - Fellow of the American Institute of Architects.

This lecture will give an insight into his substantial work, including his influence on the work of the UIA.

Introduction

Moshe Zarhy was graduated from the Technion - Israel Institute of Technology, Haifa in 1945 and concluded post-graduate studies at the Ecole d'Urbanisme in Paris in 1949-1950. He has been practicing since 1950.
Moshe Zarhy is the Founder of Zarhy Architects. He was joined at the firm by his son, architect David Zarhy and architect Anat Patrycha Zarhy in 1978. They currently run the firm. The firm is active in all areas of architectural planning; public institutions, housing projects, urban planning, private homes, education buildings, hotels and commercial buildings, sports facilities and IDF (Israel Defense Forces) projects. Special emphasis has been put on planning and

developing Medical Centers, Health Facilities, Science and High-Tech facilities. Moshe Zarhys' main projects are the Sheba Medical Center in Tel Aviv with 700 beds; the Meir Medical Center in Kfar Saba with 620 beds; about 4,200 dwelling units at 11 different locations; the ATIDIM Industrial Park in Tel Aviv and several Hi-Tech Projects, as Iscar Industries in Upper Galilee and the Weizmann Institute of Science in Rehovot.
During 60 years of professional experience, Moshe Zarhy has provided comprehensive architectural services for numerous major building projects. He is the author of many professional papers. His projects have been widely documented in the international professional press.

Born in 1923, Moshe Zarhy was, strictly speaking, not among the founding generation of what was to become Israel, but he grew up in the environment moulded by 'the Big Three', the architects Dov Karmi, Zeev Rechter and Arieh Sharon, popularly known as The Three Animals. Moshe Zarhy has known all of them personally. The strong European influence on architecture in this region is probably due to the origins as well as the education of many immigrants. This can be briefly exemplified by the backgrounds of the three above-mentioned architects. Karmi (1905-1962), born in Odessa/Ukraine, took up studies in Art and Design in Jerusalem before deciding to study architecture in Ghent/Belgium. Rechter (1899-1960), equally of Ukrainian origin, came to Palestine in 1919 and first worked in different offices before establishing himself as a self-employed architect. In 1926 he went to Rome for a year and came into touch with Russian constructivism. He gained further European experience from 1929 to 1933 in Paris. Arieh Sharon (1900-1984), of Polish origin, emigrated to Palestine in 1920 and first worked as an apiculturist in a kibbutz, but also contributed to planning the main building. The kibbutz community sent him to Germany for a year, where he met Walter Gropius in Weimar and was imparted the new, ground-breaking education of architects.
One of the fellow students of Moshe Zarhy at that time was Yaakov Rechter, son of the famous architect Zeev Rechter. Zeev Rechter had three children, beside Yaakov two daughters: Aviva and Tuti. By Yaakov Moshe got to know the Rechter family and fell in love with Aviva. They married in 1944 and had 3 children, Yael (1948), David (1951) and Rivi (1954).
Since 1945, Moshe worked for Zeev Rechter with a break for postgraduate studies in Paris (1949-1950).

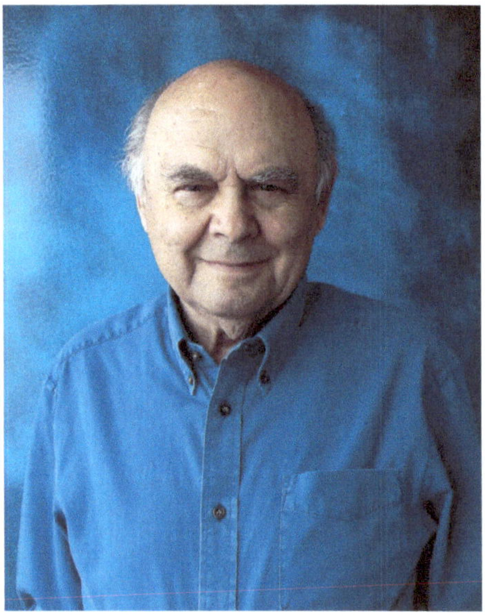

Figure 1. Portrait of Moshe Zarhy 2011.

Meir Medical Center in Kfar Shaba

His first work for a hospital project started in 1945 for the nurses' school in the Meir Medical Center in Kfar Shaba. The design of the hospital is based on plans submitted to an architectural competition in 1947, which won first prize. The hos-pital was planned as a T.B. hospital based on an explicit programme for a specialized hospital for lung diseases. Later it was transformed into a general hospital. New wings to house medical services were added and it developed into a medical center, consisting of the various facilities to provide comprehensive medical care.

The building consists of three main blocks. The ward block, the largest one, contains 10 typical medical wards, 40 beds each, in five typical floors.

The disposition of the main ward block and the basic composition of the whole edifice were based on the requirement to have southern orientation for all patients' rooms. Crossventilation was made possible by leaving spaces along the corridor, facing the northern wall of the building. The final master plan from Zarhy Architects is from the year 2010 (Figure 2-3).

Sheba Medical Center, Tel Hashomer, Ramat Gan

The general composition of the hospital buildings is arranged about a main east-west axis (the spine) which is also the axis of the wards, with secondary axes (the ribs) of the health and maintenance services. The ground floor of the building containing the wards serves as a link

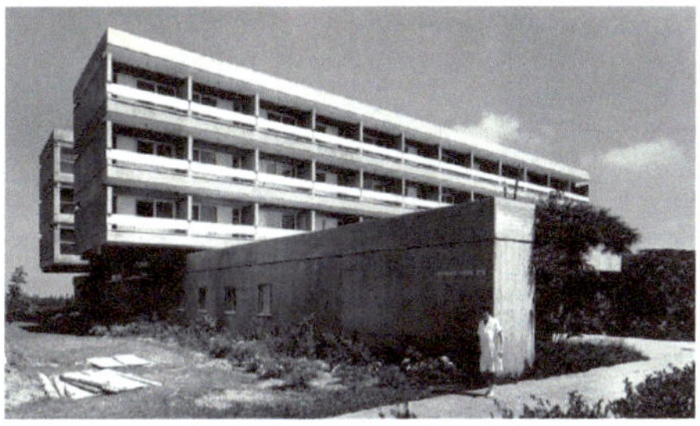

Figure 2. School of Nurses, Kfar Shaba, 1952.

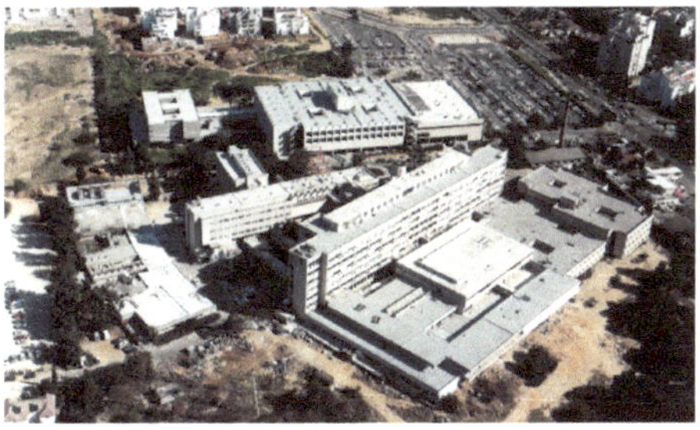

Figure 3. Meir Medical Center Kfar Shaba, 1952-2010.

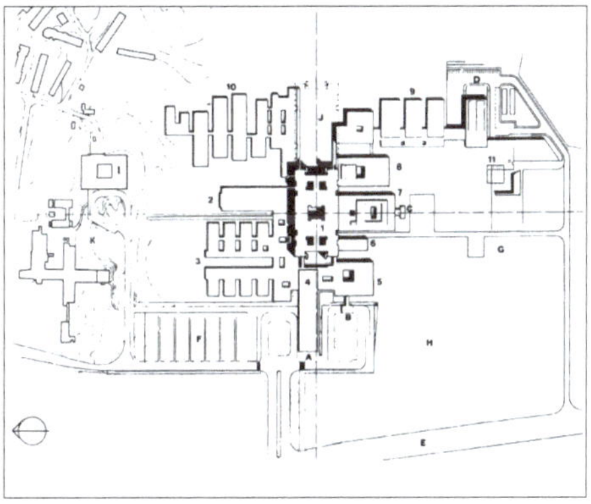

Figure 4. Sheba Medical Center – Site Plan.

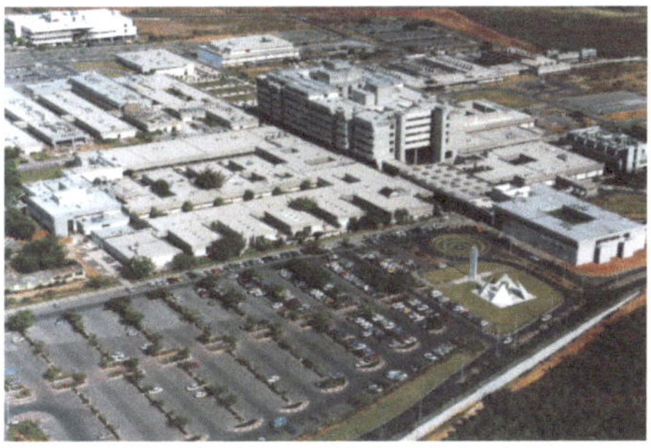

Figure 5. Bird's view of Sheba Medical Center.

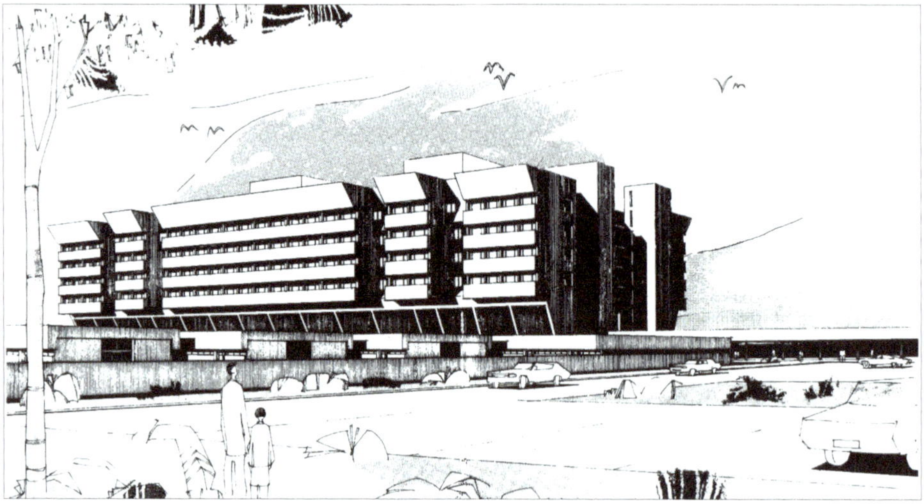

Figure 6. The ward's block of Sheba Medical Center, 1967-2010.

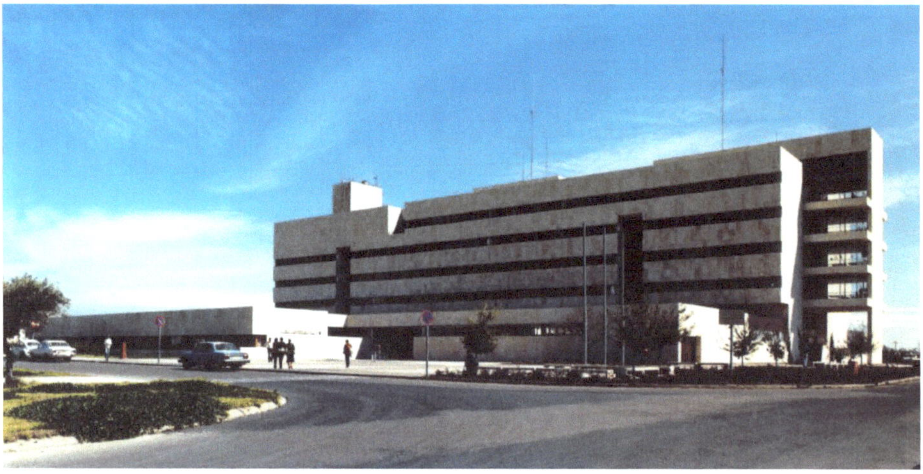

Figure 7. The Safed Governmental Hospital, 1962-1973.

between the entrance and its adjoining facilities, the casualty and admittance section and the different health service wings.

This scheme permits the complex to be planned so that each wing can be enlarged separately if necessary, with the added possibility of enlarging the whole complex (Figure 4-6).

The Safed Government Hospital, Safed, Upper Galilee

The master plan enables a large general hospital to be built in stages. In the first stage there was built close to 250 general beds with the possibility of rationally increasing the size to 500 beds, including beds for chronic diseases and psychiatry. All the medical and technical services are planned so that they can be expanded considerably with minimum interference to the running of the hospital.

The new building is situated on a site of 112.000 sq. m. on one of the ridges of the mountains of the town's outskirts. Although the steep slopes gave rise to problems in the hospital's design, the site was ideal from the point of view of location, climate and view. The crucial architectural problem was to relate the scale of this very large building with the more intimate one of the town of Safed. Advantage was taken of the site to suitably scale down the building by conceiving it as a superstructure, containing the wards, resting on a base of two floors, which blend into the site. Medical and technical service areas are located in the lower part of the building (Figure 7-8).

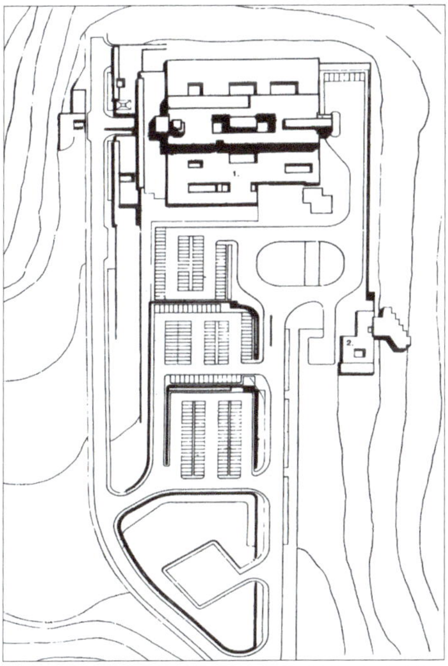

Figure 8. The Safed Governmental Hospital, Masterplan.

MOSHE ZARHY RESIDENCE, RAMAT HASHARON

An architect's attitude is clearly expressed when he builds a house for himself. His own residence in Ramat Hasharon, a three-storey concrete masonry building with an angular single-storey extension feature timeless modernity. It was built in 1953 (Figure 9).

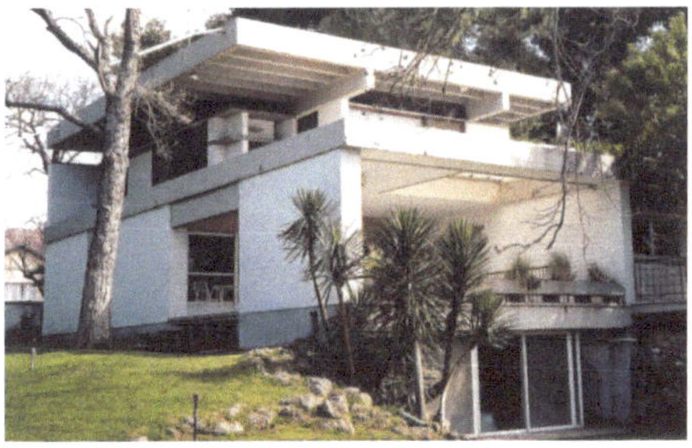

Figure 9. Moshe Zarhy Residence, Ramat Hasharon, 1953.

ARLOZOROV 150, TEL AVIV

The building's new program includes a mix of uses; Zarhy Architectural office is located on the first floor, while the residential units are above it. The main concept and programmatic organization were drawn from the unique existing reference Arlozorov street section, where Ficus trees are planted along unique and dense architectural sequence. In the new design, a small urban plaza was created, eliminating the clear separation between the building and the street. The new plaza is also used as a divider between the office main entrance on the right, and the residential main entrance to the left. The location of the office on the first floor, under the banyan trees, strengthens contact with pedestrians and allows them a glimpse into the backstage of architecture as a main event. The project was finished in 2011 (Figure 10).

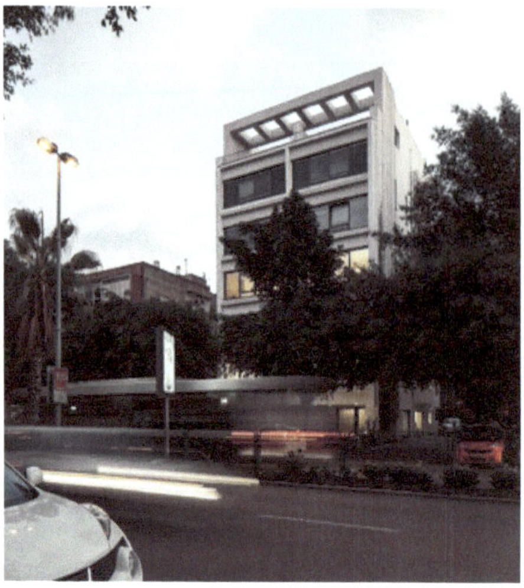

Figure 10. Arlozorov Street: office and residence of Moshe Zarhy, 2011.

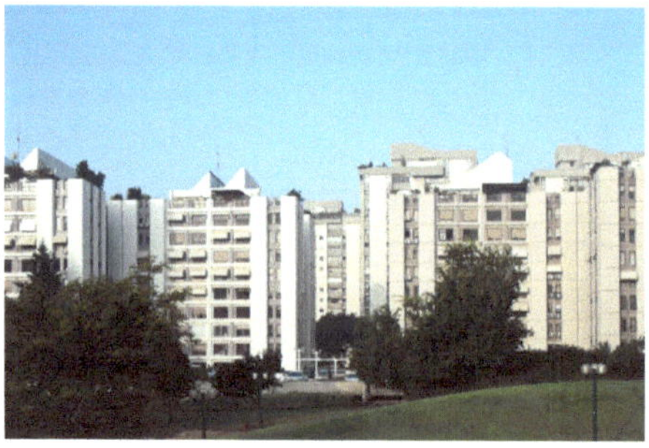

Figure 11. Six residential blocks (350 units) in Ramat Aviv, 1991.

HOUSING ESTATES

Rather than satisfying the individual residential needs of wealthy clients, however, Israel depended on creating living quarters in great numbers for a continually growing population. It is above all in the foundation of new towns that rationality, planning with suitable materials and industrial prefabrication were necessary to provide affordable housing for all.

Together with the Israeli concrete industry Moshe Zarhy had developed the Modul Beton Israel Building System in the early 1960s. In 11 different places in Israel, new neighborhoods with 4.600 dwelling units were created, 1956-1994 (Figure 11-12).

SYNAGOGUE AND JEWISH MEMORIAL, MOSCOW/ RUSSIA

The building is located in the Poklonnaya Hill park in the heart of Moscow. Situated in the midst of an urban park, this symbol was created for the Jewish people of Moscow who fought with the Russians during the Second World War.

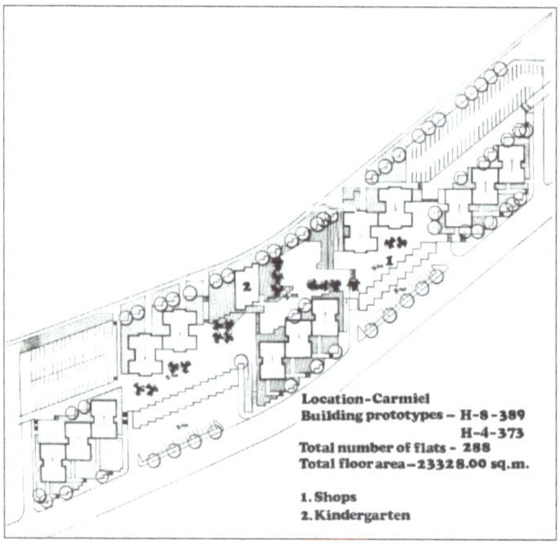

Figure 12. Site plan of location Carmiel.

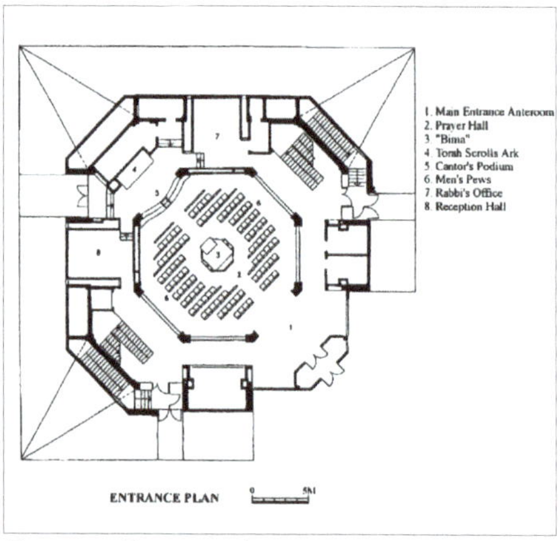

Figure 13. Entrance plan.

The architects refrained from introducing direct symbolism into the design, thereby allowing each visitor to have a different interpretation of the subject memorialized and encouraging a distinctly intimate experience (Figure 13-14).

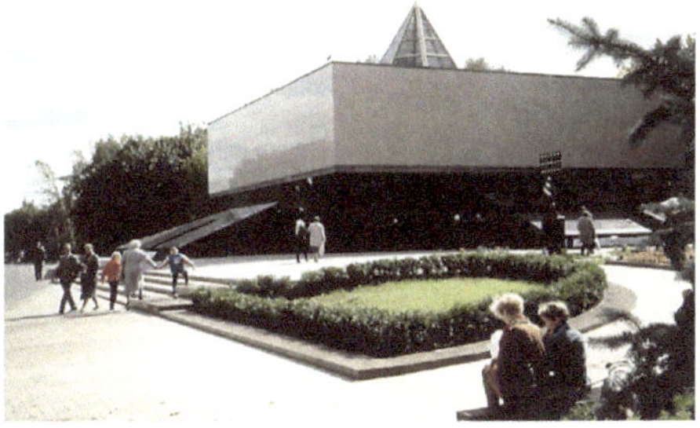

Figure 14. Synagogue and Jewish Memorial, Moscow 1993-98.

SWIMMING POOL, TECHNICON HAIFA

The building is located at the Technicon – Israel Institute of Technology – campus in Haifa. Designing an indoor Olympic swimming pool requires bridging large spans. In this case, the structural solution enhanced the architecture – the covering is made of a series of precast concrete elements, each in the form of a three-hinged arch. This solution created an elegant, slender, and fluent structure (Figure 15).

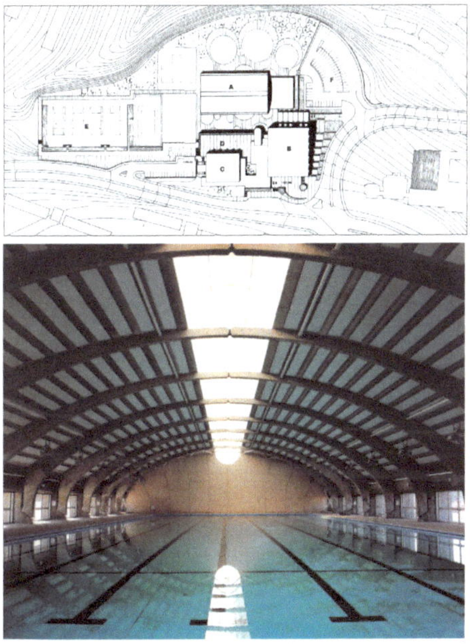

Figure 15. Sports Center and Swimming Pool, Haifa 1979-80.

ISCAR INDUSTRIES, UPPER GALILEE

Tefen, the site of Iscar's campus, is a mountainous rural area in the Galilee, in northern Israel. The buildings define an open and central garden with a ring service road surrounding the site and servicing the buildings via a multi-purpose yard. The buildings are articulated as simple, horizontal, rectangular volumes made of precast concrete elements. They function as open systems enhancing flexibility and change, while generating a formal aesthetic language attained from the gestalt effect of the campus' configuration (Figure 16-17).

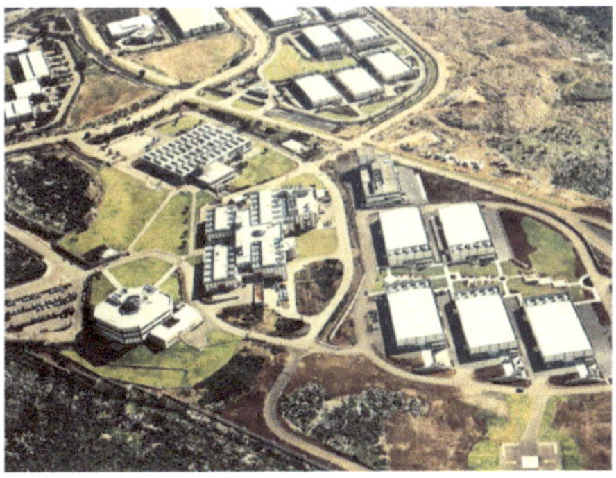

Figure 16. Iscar Industries 1985-2000.

ATIDIM, INDUSTRIAL PARK FOR SCIENCE-BASED INDUSTRIES, TEL AVIV

The complex is comprised of buildings specially designed for high-tech based industries. The building is part of this

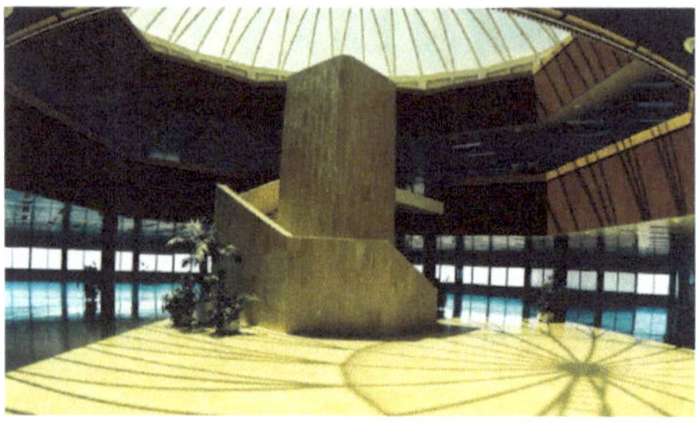

Figure 17. Main entrance.

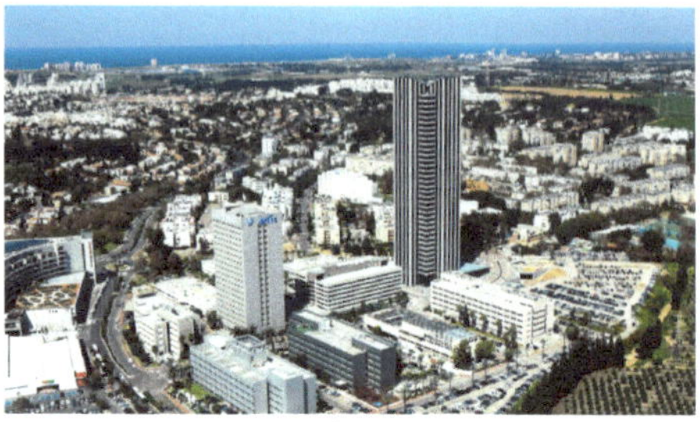

Figure 18. ATIDIM, Tel Aviv 2000-2011.

complex, whose master plan was devised by Zarhy Architects in the 70's. Its design philosophy established a new paradigm for high-tech campuses in an urban environment and has triggered major development in its adjacent areas and created Tel Aviv's main employment quarter, mixing workplaces, leisure and retail. The solution of Zarhy Architects creates maximal envelope in relation to floor area: the building is conceived of as two intersecting volumes creating a flexible floor plan that allows for either a division into several companies or unification for a single corporation. Architecturally, the elevations of the two volumes are articulated differently, one horizontally and the other vertically, helping to lighten the building's mass. It was developed a unique technology that treats both the glass and the stone cladding as a curtain wall. This sophisticated system reinvents the use of stone as a cladding material (Figure 18).

CONCLUSIONS

At his ninetieth birthday in November 2013, Moshe Zarhy could look back on his outstanding life as an architect. He has planned and built about 20 health facilities, several residential projects with about 4.500 units, private homes, several industrial, Hi-Tech and cultural projects. He had great influence into the work of the UIA and especially the Public Health Group. Between 1970 and 2006 Moshe Zarhy held about 40 lectures worldwide, mainly about healthcare and Hi-Tech-facilities.

The book "Health Facilities in Israel", published in 2014, gives an insight into the remarkable life and work of Moshe Zarhy.

The Story of Birth

Fani Vavili[1], Argyri Chalkia[2]

faniva@arch.auth.gr, argychal@arch.auth.gr
[1]Architect, MA, PhD, Professor, Aristotle University of Thessaloniki, Greece
[2]Architecture Student, Aristotle University of Thessaloniki, Greece

This paper investigates the relation between childbirth and space. Given the current movement of giving birth at home in many developed countries, it is interesting to examine under which conditions it takes place and what is the role of architecture. The space of delivery in all periods is studied, starting from Greek mythology. In fact, place is investigated at the birth of the god Zeus and which was, in antiquity, the perception of birth practices and space. Ancient figurines and paintings enhance the data for the space of delivery. Also, the study refers to obstetrics and the movement from birth at home to the maternity wards, as a result of medical progress. After that, the return to home birth is studied, because of the requirements of pregnant women for natural delivery, while water births are mentioned, as a new space element in the delivery process. Finally, current attempts for a new approach are investigated, in combination with current architectural concepts for childbirth (birth centres, delivery rooms like at home in maternity wards). The aim is to understand the relationship between architecture and childbirth and to highlight the significance of space in such an important moment of human life. In addition, it intends to sensitize the architects in order to design, with respect and care, the birth spaces, where the first contact of the fetus with the new world takes place.

Keywords: *architecture of child birth, health care design and obstetrics, mythology and childbirth, birth practices and space.*

"A mother's womb is the optimum environment for development; there the foetus… It is lulled by body movement and the rhythm of mother's heartbeat. It would be hard indeed to find a better initial space in the world." Sehosian 2003

Introduction

One may wonder: why 'the story of birth'? In fact, this paper is directly related to architecture and its offering to people. Architecture places the human existence at the centre of its design's interest and always aims to create sustainable conditions for people. So, architecture would not be absent from the most important time in a human's life, birth.
It is important to consider that, in all periods, childbirth evolved in a space, whether it was outdoors or a specified enclosed space. So, space and its organi-

zation, the atmosphere, the equipment and the materials, which are all involved in the delivery, are architecture.

Through the centuries and following the advance of medicine and construction, societies tried to create safe spaces for giving birth. Then, the architect started to design space for the moment of childbirth, sometimes consciously, sometimes not. Though a historical overview, the change of birth space is studied, starting from the house to hospital maternity wards (obstetrics), and finally present discussions of a return to home birth.

The main question is, in all cases, how the architects can interfere in such an important moment of human existence and how positively they can influence the moment of birth.

Childbirth in Myths

According to Hesiod's Theogony, which is the first attempt to record beliefs about the creation of the world, Rea gave birth to Zeus in the absence of her husband Cronus and in full secrecy. She wanted to avoid Zeus being swallowed by his father, as happened to the rest of his children (Giannis, 2010). Based on the mythology, the birth of the god Zeus took place in a cave at the top of Mount Psiloritis, in Crete (Figure 1). The leader of the Greek Olympian Gods was born in a place that nature offers, an enclosed space, without natural lighting. This darkness of the cave resembles the womb, which hosts the miracle of human life.

In ancient Greek mythology, Hera and Eileithyia are characterized as the goddesses of childbirth (Wikipedia, 2014). According to the goddesses, the birth was an act of regeneration and it had to

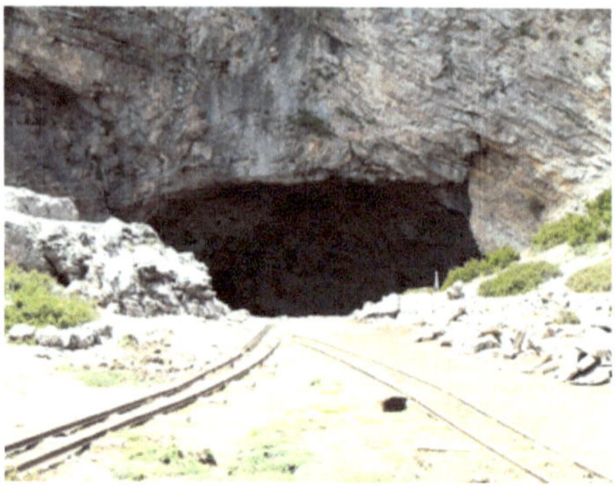

Figure 1. "Cave of Zeus", Mount Ida, Crete. Source: Wikipedia.

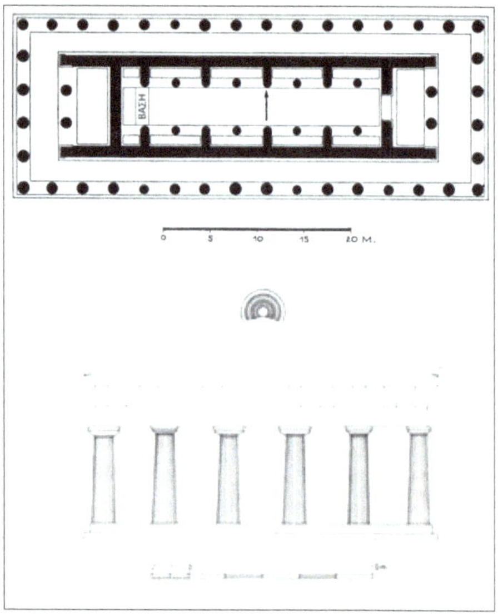

Figure 2. The temple of Hera in Olympia (plan and elevation), circa 600 B.C. Source: Sakoulas 2013.

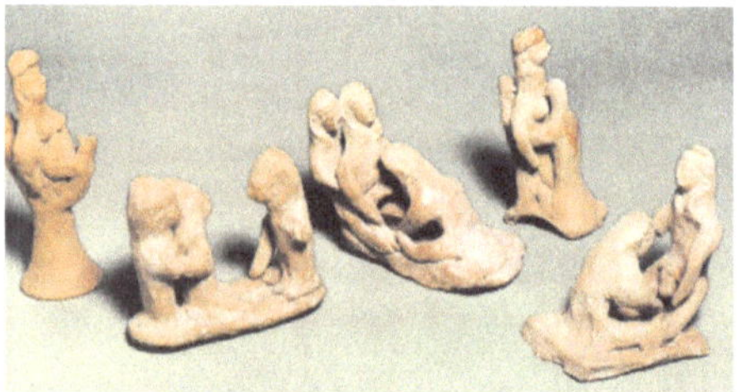

Figure 3. Clay figurines depicting various stages of the childbirth, 6th c B.C. Lapithos Cyprus. Source: Oikonomopoulou 2007.

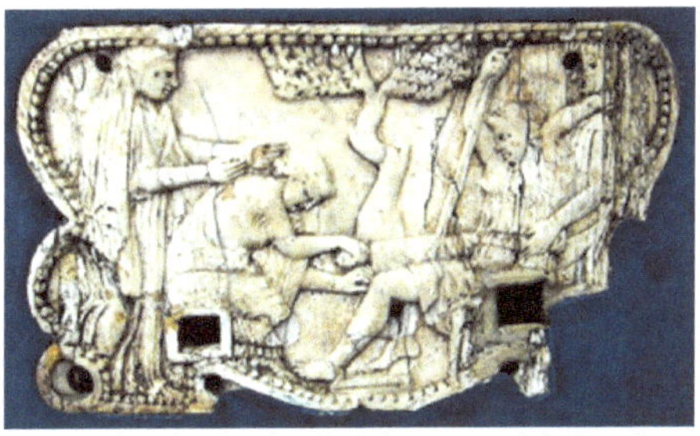

Figure 4. The birth of Meleager or Achilles, Ivory plate, Pompeii, 1st c A.D.

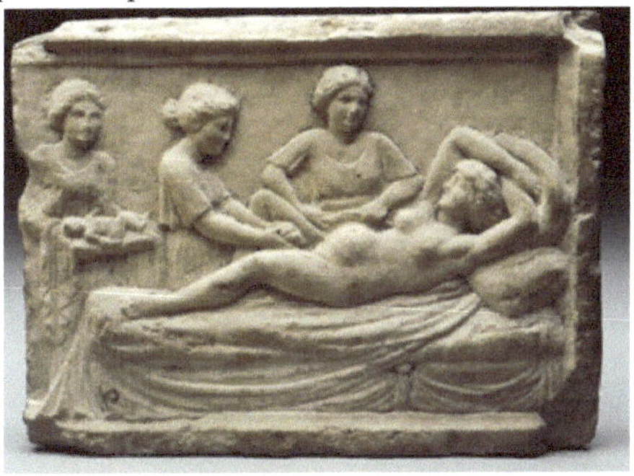

Figure 5. Marble plate, Ostia, 2nd c A.D. Source: Lifo 2012.

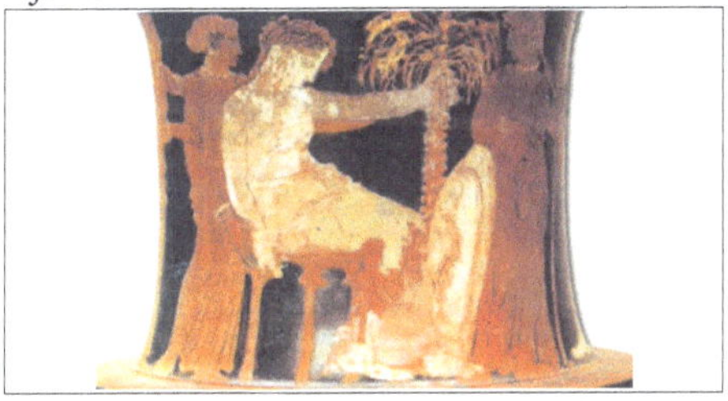

Figure 6. Leto's childbirth in Delos, red compass, 370 B.C. Source: Oikonomopoulou 2007.

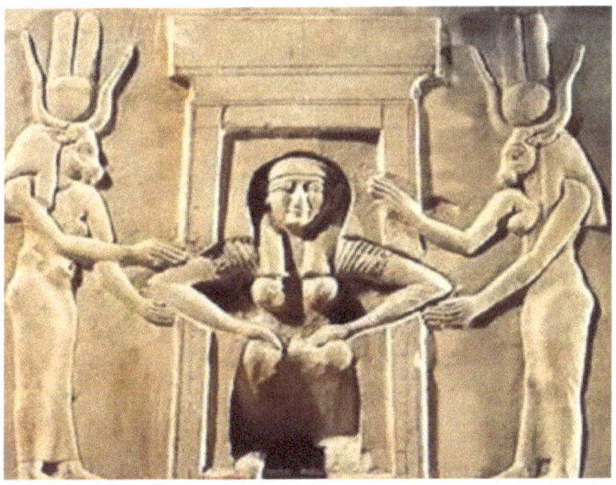

Figure 7. The goddess helps a woman to give birth, Egypt, 330 B.C.

take place in a familiar or an intimate space, as the temple, where evil or demonic forces could not enter. Thus, Hera converted the backspace of the Hereon in a maternity ward, where women, with the help of Eileithyia, gave birth without throes (Oikonomopoulos 2005). It could therefore be claimed, that the concept of maternity wards appears already in mythology. Evidence of this is the design of the Hereons (Figure 2). The Hereon is surrounded by 40 columns, symbolizing the 40 weeks of pregnancy, 40 days of confinement, 40 weeks of required breastfeeding and 40 days of abstention from marital duties. During the Mycenaean period, unmarried women did not give birth in temples or in their house, but under bridges, near cemeteries, in caves, at crossroads or in the fields, as it was considered that such a birth would bring disaster on the fertility of the Earth (Oikonomopoulos, 2005).

Ancient Birth Practices

Many ancient reliefs and figurines depict moments of births, according to the artist's perception of giving birth. Usually three figures (Figure 3), mainly female, are involved in the process: the pregnant woman in the centre and the midwife with her assistant on each side. The space is not determined and the only spatial elements that are distinguished are a bed or the obstetric stool on which the pregnant woman sits (Figure 4).
A red compass from 370 B.C found in Athens, depicts the birth of Leto in Delos and gives an extra element to the space of childbirth. A phoenix supports Leto's hand, from which we can assume that the delivery took place in an outdoor space (Figure 6).

Seeking the spatial aspect of labor in the ancient culture of Egypt, differences were found (Figure 7-8). There are documents that refer to birth at home. Other documents note that delivery used to take place in special buildings that we could call birth-arbors. These structures consisted of a mat roof, supported by wooden columns carved so as to look like papyrus stems. These structures were placed in isolated corners of the estates or in roofs of small houses. According to evidence, a mattress, a pillow and a stool were placed in the spot of childbirth (Thompson, 2010). In fact, hot water was put under the stool, as this facilitated the process of childbirth (Parsons, 2011).

During the Minoan and Mycenaean period, men also began to enter into the field of gynecology. In the same period, Asclepius approached gynecology and obstetrics too. It is noted that he was the first to introduce, in case of dystocia, the delivery in water, which is a new spatial element in the birth process, although it had already been used in Greek mythology (Oikonomopoulou, 2007, p. 51).

First Medical Attempts in Childbirth

From the 6th century B.C. until the appearance of Hippocrates (440 BC) the specialty of Obstetrics was the work of women, when at the same time other medical activities were forbidden to them (Oikonomopoulou, 2007).
Thanks to Hippocrates, during the Classical period, a scientific revolution occurred in medicine. He argued that the duty of the physician was to save both, the pregnant and the foetus. That's why the Hippocratic doctors were involved

Figure 8. Relief from the Temple of Kom Ombo, Egypt, 2nd c B.C. Source: Lifo 2012.

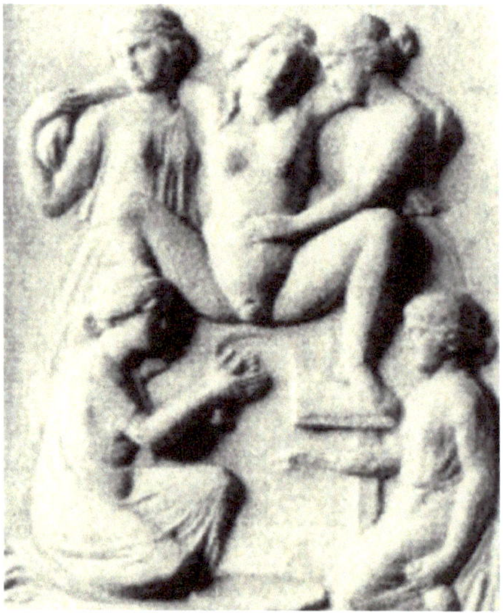

Figure 9. Childbirth in ancient Greece 5th c B.C.

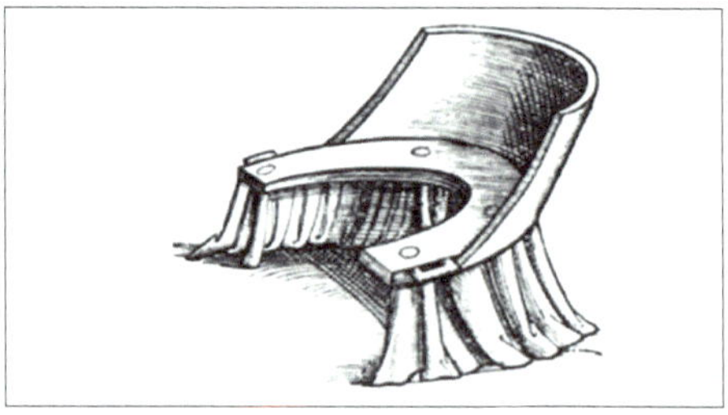

Figure 10. Obstetric chair of Ambroise Pare, 1554. Source: Mantalenakis.

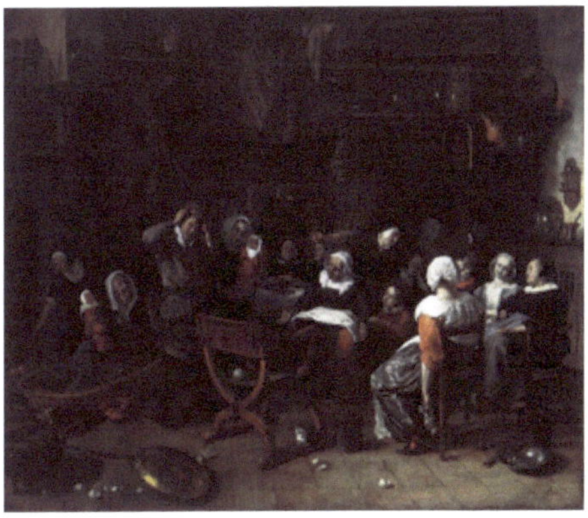

Figure 11. Twin birth celebration, 1668 Jan Steen, Oil on canvas, 89x109 cm Kunsthalle, Hamburg.

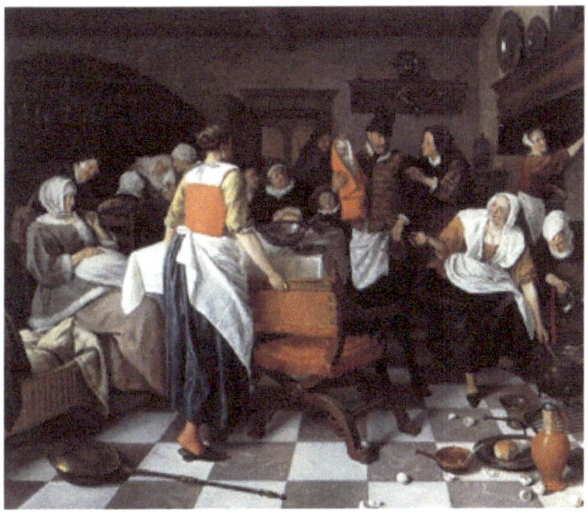

Figure 12. Celebrating the birth, 1664 Jan Steen, Oil on canvas, 89x109 cm, Wallace Collection, London.

only in cases of dystocia, informal or neglected childbirths. The greatest revolution in Obstetrics came from Soranus of Ephesus, during the Roman period. He was characterized as the famous gynecologist of antiquity, who also wrote many books on the subject (trans. Temkin 1996). Regarding required preparations for a normal childbirth, Soranus recommends the following: olive oil, hot water, hot compresses, sponges, pieces of wool, bandages, a pillow, scents for the recovery of mother's strength, a birthing stool, two beds, a suitable room (Lefkowitz & Fant). It is characteristic that Soranus suggests that the birthing process be conducted in an upright posture and while the woman is sitting on the obstetric stool, a round stool, from which a crescent-shaped cavity had been cut off (trans. Temkin 1996).

During a long period, which lasts for most countries until the 1920s, the main place of birth is the home of the pregnant woman. In some cases, for example in Greece, the majority of women gave birth at home until the 1960s, under the supervision of midwives and later of doctors.

Childbirth, during this period, always took place in spaces familiar to the mother, who was surrounded by people of confidence, basically related and of the same sex. A warm protected space - the room of the pregnant woman, a living room, the kitchen, a cellar, a warehouse or a residence of someone familiar and relative - was the space for the pregnant in labor. Regarding the characteristics of space, they cannot be determined, because each house had its own construction and size of rooms (comfortable, rich or poor, simple, etc), according to the social status of the pregnant.

The pregnant woman was usually assisted by the objects available in the space (home etc.) - chairs, tables, beds or its bars and anything else – in order to cope with the delivery. Having discussed with very old women in Greece, we know that on many occasions, in rural areas for instance, women gave birth in the fields, under the trees.

THE HOSPITAL PERIOD

Gradually, the place of birth is changing and moving from the house to a properly, in medical terms, maternity ward. This change is related to the progress of medicine and to the introduction of anesthetic drugs in a controlled medical environment.

Giving birth in well organized hospital units (obstetrics – maternity wards) is, until today, the common birth process. The first evidence of an organized Obstetric Clinic appeared in Britain around 1740 (Furuto, 2013). Since then, the development of hospital based maternity units was rapid. These units were well planned and designed with the continuous advancing knowledge of medical and environmental design factors.

The entire process, the necessary spaces, the equipment, etc. were developed in detail through the years. Design regulations and standards were published from many authorities globally e.g. NHS UK Hospital Building Notes, Canada, Scandinavia, Australian regulations etc. (Vavili 2003, p. 24-31).

A RETURN: GIVING BIRTH AT HOME

Although the majority of women give birth in maternity hospitals or units, women in several regions of the world (e.g. Africa, Latin America and Asia) continue, by necessity or tradition, to give birth in outdoor health care facilities. At the same time, in the so called Western world, a return to giving birth at home is noticed, under a new approach, in order that pregnant women regain control of the delivery, in a friendly, homely environment, usually the mother's house.

The main issue, however, is the suitability of the house, in order to host the delivery process with safety. There are residential centres that are organized, planned and designed, exclusively for childbirth, where the parents with their newborn are hosted for a few days (Gatermann, Vavili 2009 p. 76), Figure 13-14.

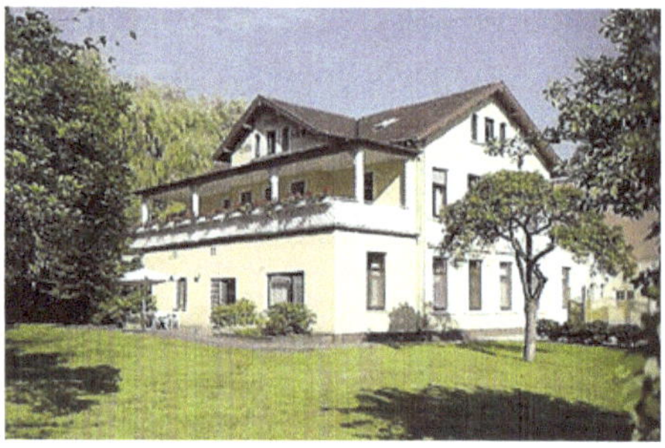

Figure 13. A maternity house, German.

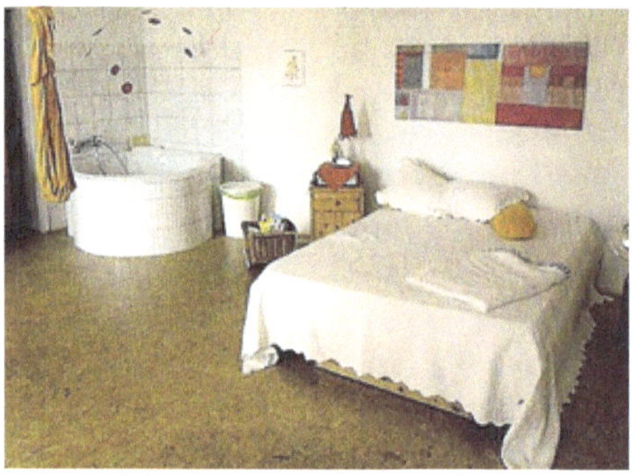

Figure 14. Room in a maternity house. Source: Gatermann 2009.

CHILDBIRTH IN WATER

The new space element, which entered dynamically in the childbirth process over the past decades, is water. Birth in water is not an innovative process, as many may think. Also, as mentioned above, Asclepius was the first who introduced the so-called 'eftokio' bath, which corresponds to the current practices of birth in water.

Undoubtedly, from a scientific point of view, birth in water has recently been recognized in the western world. In fact, the first water birth in Europe, which is known to us, took place in France in 1803. In the 70's, in Russia and France, some midwives and physicians started to examine the ways of delivery of the baby in the water, a beneficial childbirth environment (Furuto, 2013).

Specially designed pools with water at a temperature of 37° C host the whole process of delivery, Figure 15. In terms of architectural design, the water birth room is a carefully designed space, according to specific regulations and standards, size, equipment, temperature, humidity, materials.

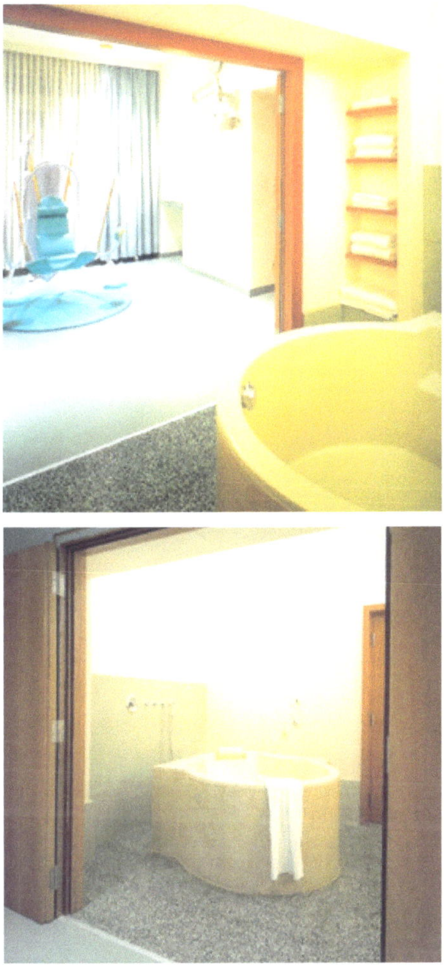

Figure 15. Room for giving birth in water, Golden Cross Hospital, Vienna. Source: Weller.

CURRENT ARCHITECTURAL CONCEPTS

Some people suggest that giving birth at home is an ideal place for delivery. Women tend to choose home birth, mainly in order to avoid the unnecessary medical interventions, common in hospital births and because of the comfortable and familiar environment of home. Yet the question arises: who guarantees the entire safety of the birthing process at home when this location is away from hospital? There are so many aspects to discuss. The suitability of the home's spaces (room size, available furnishing, etc.), the distance of the house from the hospital, the availability of relatives or friends to help during the process, are crucial issues. These questions should concern architects about how to manage, in design terms, issues of childbirth.

Architectural solutions already exist. The architecture of these spaces is based on the principle of the home environment and scale, with familiar furnishing - com-

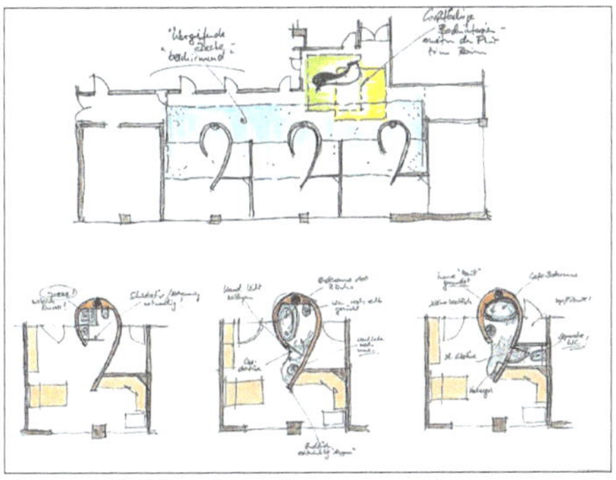

Figure 16. Plan for delivery rooms in a maternity ward. Source: Gatermann 2009.

fortable bed, a place for accommodating the father as well, materials and lighting. Additionally, there is a tub, for childbirth in water, a cot for the fetus, as well as various other items, a style reminding of warmth at home (Figure 17).

A notable example of such a space is the public hospital in Pitivie, in France (Figure 18). There, in the same building, the typical delivery room and the salle sauvage coexist. Simple, minimal lines combined in such a way to accommodate the miracle of human nature. Salle sauvage in Pitivie is designed by women who experienced giving birth there (Odent 1999, p. 29).

Examples of such simple designs are the Maternity House in Zambia (Figure 19), which was built next to a maternity ward and the Woldya Maternity Centre in Ethiopia (Figure 20-21). These centres aim to reduce infant mortality in the above countries. In both cases, the buildings are a one-storey structure that interact directly with the natural environment and are made of materials, which are familiar to local culture and available in each site. The architects created environments familiar to the local population, reminding them of daily living conditions.

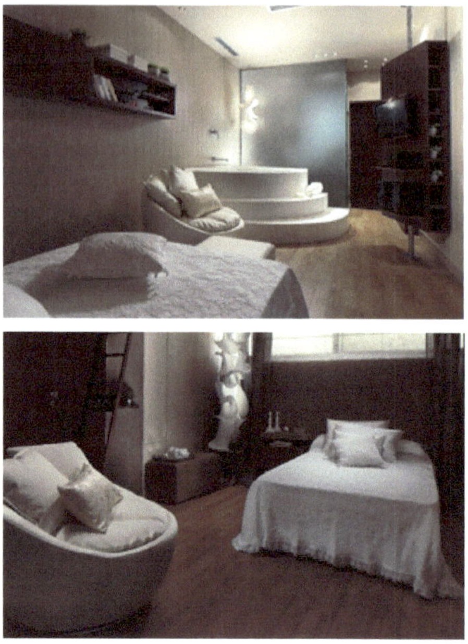

Figure 17. Delivery room 'like at home', Leto Maternity Ward, Athens.

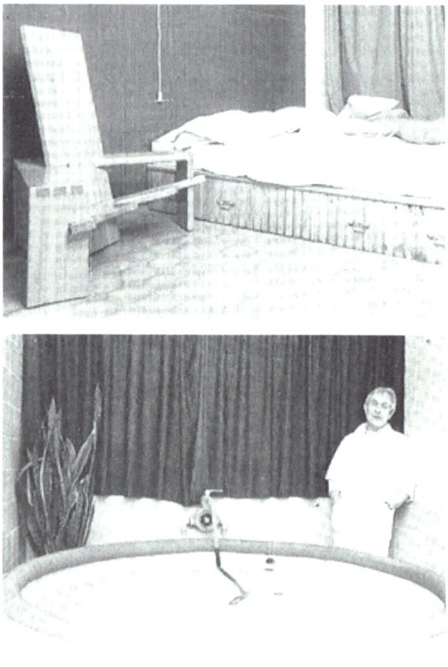

Figure 18. Salle sauvage (above) and the pool in salle sauvage (below) , Pitivie. Source: Odent 1999.

EPILOGUE

This paper is an attempt to trigger some thoughts on delivery spaces and to highlight the significance of the relation between architecture and childbirth. Speaking of the heterotopias of crisis, Michel Foucault said that it is the sacred space or privileged or forbidden place, where people find a shelter when they are in crisis. The pregnant women are in this situation (crisis) during child delivery (Foucault, 1984). The place of birth is 'another' space, as the women prefer

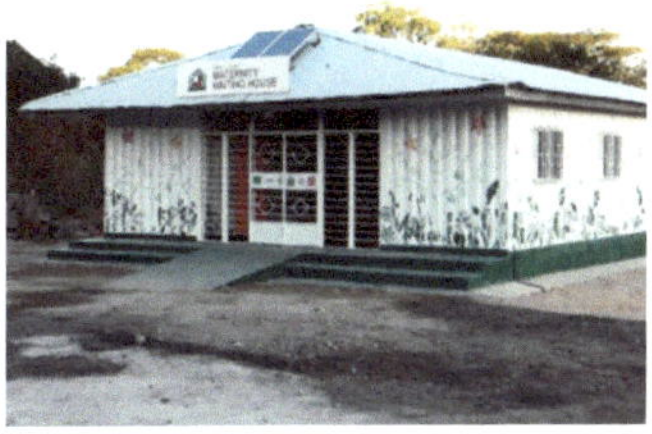

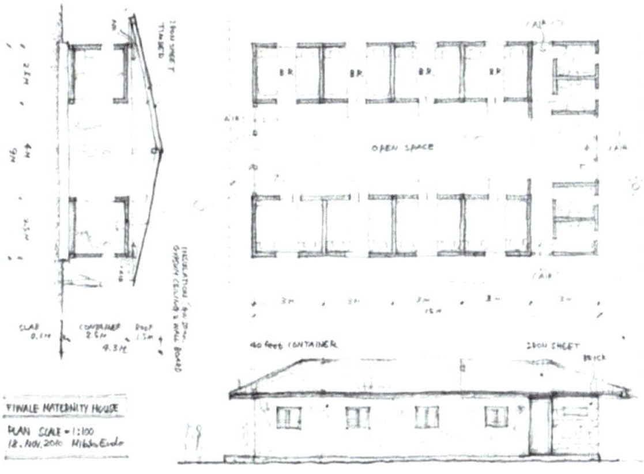

Figure 19. Maternity House in Zambia: photo (above) and plan, section, elevation (right).

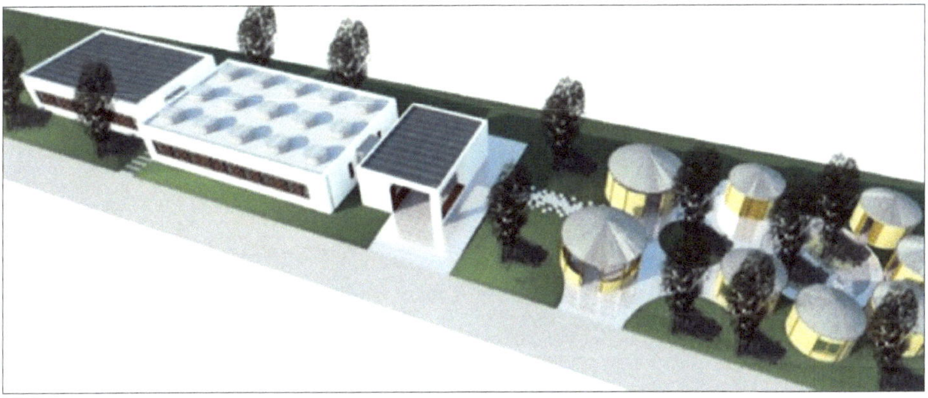

Figure 20. Woldya Maternity Center in Ethiopia.

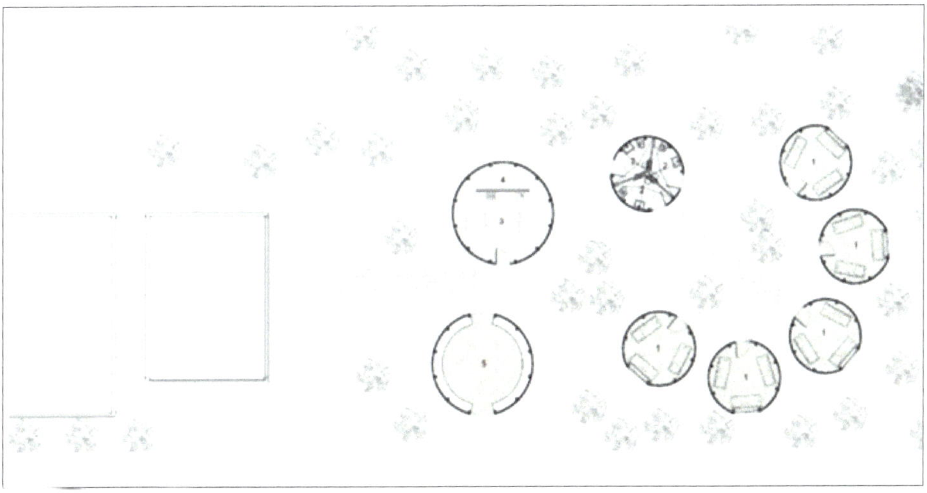

Figure 21. Woldya Maternity Center in Ethiopia (plan).

to be in privacy, isolated - outside of the village or in a special shelter – in order to concentrate and cope with the labor. In this other space, the architect should intervene by designing with respect and care to the pregnant woman and the fetus. The architect has to contribute, sensitively, to the creation of suitable conditions of a unique event. Nowadays, the great challenge is how the architect will find a way to combine the requirements both of the pregnant woamn, for a natural and familiar delivery, and the physicians, for a medically safe process. To achieve that, the architect should start by reviewing the meaning of birth and the current technology in order for architecture to support the entire process.

REFERENCES

Dunn, M. P. 1996, *Soranus of Ephesus (circa AD 98-138) and perinatal care in Roman times*, trans Tamkin, O., John Hopkins Press, Baltimore.

Foucault, M., 1984. 'Of other spaces, Heterotopias', *Architecture, Mouvement, Continuité* 5.

Furuto, A., 2013. Woldya Maternity Centre, *Archdaily*.

Gatermann, C., 2009. 'Designing obstetrics facilities, in F Vavili, *Aspects of Healing Environments*, Ziti Publications, Thessaloniki.

Giannis, A., 2010. *Hesiod-Theogony*.

Lefkowitz, RM & Fant, BM., 2005. 'Childbirth: instructions for the midwife' in RM Lefkowitz and BM Fant, *Women's life on Greece and Rome*.

Lifo, 2012, *The moment of birth. A rare image.*
Mantalenakis, S., *Obstetrics until 19th century in Greek obstetric and gynecolog*, viewed 20 May 2013.

Odent, M., 1999, Childbirth on the way of nature, trans. M Kouladianou, Thymari, Athens.

Oikonomopoulou, Ch. A., 2007. 'Obstetrics and gynecology in ancient Greece', Archeology and Arts, vol. 102.

Oikonomopoulos, Th. Ch & Oikonomopoulou, Ch. A., 2005. The childbirth, the dystokies, the"eftokia and the resuscitation of apneic newborn in vernacular medicine in post byzantine years of the new Hellenism (1453-1953)', *Journal of Issues of Obstetrics and Gynecology*, vol. 3.

Parsons, M., 2011. *Childbirth and children in Ancient Egypt..*

Sakoulas, T., 2013. *Archaic: Architecture in History of Greek and Roman Art.*

Sehosian, J., 2003. *Bio architecture*, Architectural Press, London.

Thompson, CJ., 2010. Pregnancy and childbirth, in Women in ancient Egypt in *Women in the ancient world.*

Vavili, F., 2003. *Guidelines & health care buildings, world hospitals & health care services.*

Weller, CN., 2009. *Hospital architecture + design*, Braun Press.

Wikipedia, 2014. H*ome birth trends in Home birth*, viewed 1 March 2013.

Innovative Materials in Children's Hospital Design

Artemis Kyrkou, Fani Vavili

amykyrkou@gmail.com, faniva@arch.auth.gr
[1]Architect - PhD candidate/Aristotle University of Thessaloniki, Greece
[2]Professor/Aristotle University of Thessaloniki, Greece

Since the Modern Movement of architecture, hospital design has evolved and adjusted to changing needs. Nowadays, it is considered to be a function of multiple variables. It is an architect's duty to design an environment that will propose security and positively affect the patient. The hospitalization process is inevitably a source of stress for an individual. The quality of healthcare facilities' environment is rather crucial for adults but it is even more significant when the patients are children. The design of healthcare facilities for children is a field of architecture that deeply affects the young mind and body of a child during its visit or stay. Much attention should be given to the types of materials used, as children use touch more than adults and are keen to explore everything at ground level. Therefore, the materials used and the way that they are applied is one of the key factors at this point. The needs of the young patients that must be fulfilled are numerous (psychological, physical, social, etc.) but there are also certain priorities that determine the final choices of these materials. Sustainable design has provided strategies to maximize natural light, incorporate non-toxic materials and increase energy efficiency to reduce costs, energy saving and create cleaner indoor environments. On the other hand, new computer systems and sophisticated medical equipment must be combined with an aesthetics that is pleasant for patients, visitors and medical staff. The healing qualities of the space depend on the choice of materials and colours which also need to reinforce the functionality of the space and always support the patients' psychology. The purpose of this paper is to specify the new and innovative materials used in up-to-date children's healthcare facilities design and estimate the way that these materials can fulfil the young patients' needs.

Keywords: *technology in children's healthcare, children's hospital, children's hospital design.*

Introduction

Since the Modern Movement of architecture, hospital design has evolved and adjusted to the changing needs. The hospitalization process causes stress for an individual. This is caused due to the absence of a familiar setting, the insecurity of the future, the fear of unknown medical tests or surgery, the pain, the restriction of social and everyday life that automatically affect the patient (Vavili, 2009). A hospital stay is often associated with negative and depressing thoughts, it is widely known that stress inhibits healing. Health is an overall condition that apart from the physical state depends on environmental, psychological, social and emotional factors. Therefore, the environment can have positive effects both on a visitor but more importantly on a recovering patient.

Children are a unique group, that are still developing perception of body, time and future and who find it difficult to perceive recovery after their present discomfort. The quality of healthcare facilities' environment is rather crucial and more significant when the patients are children.

THE IMPORTANCE OF A HEALING ENVIRONMENT IN CHILDREN'S HOSPITALS

Children's healing environment is a significant parameter in their hospitalization process and can positively affect their recovery. Regarding children's healthcare facilities architecture, quality design and thoughtful planning can approach safety, security and thus the elimination of their fears, which are substantial for their health.

A hospital visit for a child can sometimes be a rather upsetting or even frightening experience, depending on the quality of the healthcare facility and the given medical care.
The hospital environment is at some time the main micro-system of the child and represents an extremely interesting context from the point of view of the health promotion for children and adolescents while in hospital. The environment plays such an active role during the healing process, it reduces patients' anxiety and fears, supporting their needs or even giving them back the chance to keep contact with their family and friends; A safe, secure and stress-free hospital environment would offer care, protection and respect of the child's body and mind as well as friendly atmosphere and understandable orientation. Art, technology and ecology combined all together, can create the exceptional circumstances for a child's healing process and promote its well-being. Through the appropriate design and suitable details, a welcome atmosphere can be composed in which all five senses can be stimulated and make the child feel more comfortable. The term environment in this case includes all of its interpretations; natural, built, interior and exterior.

CHILDREN'S NEEDS AND RIGHTS DURING THEIR HOSPITAL STAY

There are many papers and studies that focus on specifying children's needs and psychological condition during their stay in hospital. Children are highly dependent upon adults for comfort, guidance, and support, therefore during their hospitalization they need. In that case, some of the great challenges that arise are to do with the space in the patient's private room, or ways to create positive distractions that can take the mind (both the child's and the parent's) away from the pain or the stress. The private room should be a pain-free space that the child and its family members can feel comfortable and support the child's emotional needs.

Children's needs during their hospitalization process that are related to architectural design can be divided in two

major categories. The first category is about their psychological balance which is related to the need of family's support, social interaction, security, territorial privacy, comfort, independence, access to outdoors, control etc. The second category is about the activities they can perform at a healthcare facility such as play, rest/sleep, eat, study, surgery/treatment, examination, visiting (Malkin, 1992).
Another very important factor that has an impact on children's healthcare design is the special needs, habits and preferences that each one of the seven age groups during childhood and adolescence has. Starting from foetus, neonate, infant, pre-school, secondary school, transition to adulthood, each stage has its own special characteristics, and own scale and ergonometric features; therefore the healthcare environment has to adapt in order to provide safety and security to everyone.

Furthermore, children during their hospitalization process have certain rights since the UN convention (1989) on the Rights of The Child and the foundation of the EACH (European Association for Children in Hospitals) Charter. Some goals of the EACH charter which are related to the layout and the design of the space are: the right of children to have their parents with them in the hospital, the possibility for children to have their own say in the care plan, opportunities for play and education in the ward, contact with peers and a healing environment.

According to environmental psychology and a study that was performed by Evans and McCoy in 1998 identified and discussed four aspects of the build environment (at the scale of a building) that can potentially influence human health and alter stress levels in individuals. Those aspects are stimulation, coherence, affordances and control (Evans & McCoy, 1998). This classification though, does not include the conditions that are fundamentally potential sources of physical stress. Among the conditions and factors that are potential causes of physical stress, two basic categories have been identified: first the microclimatic conditions of a building and second the ergonomic conditions of use of the space (Del Nord, 2006).

There are numerous studies, reports and papers that try to specify the design elements that can eliminate and reduce stress and at the same time fulfil the needs of the patient. An interesting literature study (2013) by Zanariah et al. that aims to translate quality care factors to quality space parameters comes up with 3 space quality components: technicality (health safety and security), functionality (work flow performance) and aesthetic (psychological aesthetic performance) and 10 space quality parameters which are: lighting, thermal comfort and air quality, noise, safety, space planning, accessibility, way finding, furniture, colour, material and finishes.

Innovative Materials in Children's Hospital Design

The field of architecture for health is at a turning point. Hospital architecture was immediately affected by global economy recession that begun in 2008. Hospitals nowadays are among the institutions suffering from the global economic malaise and many are reacting by laying off staff,

limiting certain services and delaying or even cancelling construction projects (Verderber, 2010). The high costs of construction or renovation prevent private investors from financing.
Moreover, the issue of global climate change has a direct effect on hospital building architecture. The goal is carbon neutrality and regenerative strategies on new constructions and as much as adaptive reuse, preservation and increasing social capital through thoughtful environmental design (Verderber, 2010). The changing priorities of our current situation narrate some underlying trends for the future. The hospital needs reconsideration both as an idea and as a building type (Verderber, 2010). Last but not least, the issue of technology is rather crucial at this point. Nanotechnology, robotics, telemedicine, virtual reality and the rising role of nature in healing are matters that will influence the space and its layout. In brief, hospital gets a new meaning "it is not a place for sickness and sick people but a rather a place for health and recreation" (Lensch, 2006).

One of the most recent trends in children's hospital design that is linked with technology is including interactive elements in the design. In this way, the child would get the feeling of altering the hospital environment and maybe feel more secure by controlling the surroundings. Interactive elements are also positive distractions during the hospital visit or stay. The main aim is to encourage curiosity, wonder, and learning so that the negative feelings are not the dominant ones.

Starting from an interactive patient's room, where a child during its stay can change some features in the room. Modern patient's rooms come with amenities such as pull-out beds for parents to be present at all times, details geared toward children, such as ceilings decorated with a starry night, "headwall and footwall" (Verderber 2010), colourful graphics and artificial lighting that can change with a click of a button (Figure 1). The intention is to make them feel as comfortable as possible during the period of illness.

Lighting (both natural and artificial) is an extremely powerful element in design. It is also an effective parameter for the patient as a powerful regulator of the body and its daily functions. The quality of lighting in hospitals can positively affect the emotional and medical state of a patient; it can also support well-being and stimulate recovery. At spaces such as corridors, waiting rooms and lobbies lighting and video projections on the walls and floors are used in a playful way so that hospitalized children can entertain themselves and reduce their stress levels. An interesting example in this case is the work of Jason Bruges called Nature Trail (2013). It is an interactive project designed specifically for the Great Ormond street hospital, as a means for children to brighten their journey to the operating theatre. The concept of the

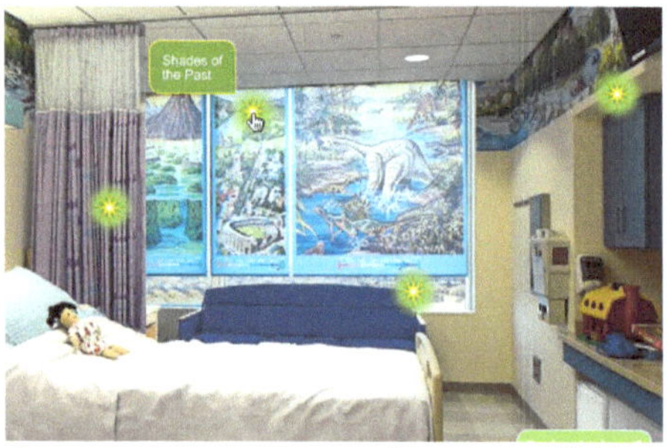

Figure 1. Interactive patient's room at Children's Hospital at Montefiore.

work was informed viewing the hospital walls as a natural canvas- a digital forest, with scenes depicting various forest creatures, including horses, deer, hedgehogs, birds and frogs, to the passerby. It has essentially two main elements; Integrated LED panels and bespoke graphic wallpaper. The LED panels are embedded into the wall surface at various heights in order to be accessible to the eye levels and positions of patients moving along the corridors. Across these surfaces are abstract 'animal movements' which are interactive animated patterns of light that reveal themselves through the trees and foliage of the forest. The artwork consists of 70 LED panels, with a total of 72,000 LEDs (Figure 2).

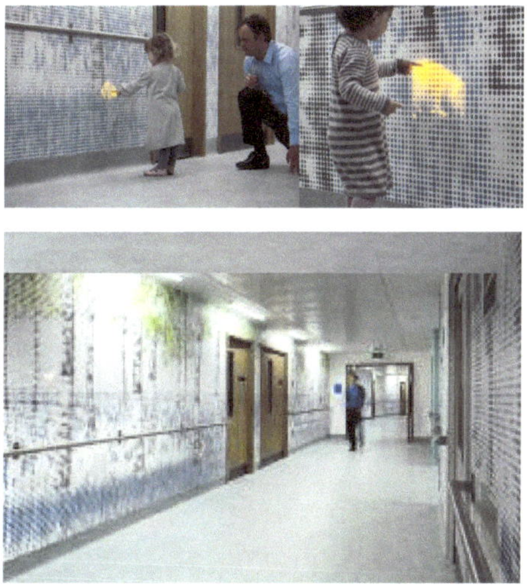

Figure 2. Interactive wall, at Great Ormond Street Hospital, by Jason Bruges studio.

Another example that includes both light and sound (music) is the 'Interactive Musical Wall' by the Moment Factory Studio at the waiting room of Montreal's CHU Sainte-Justine Children's Hospital. This example shows a remarkable way to breathe new life and energy into the very structure of the waiting room. The innovative Interactive Musical Wall gives children the gift of a fun distraction when they need it the most. The permanent installation is a project spearheaded by producer Denise Roberts, who designed the wall to make waiting at the hospital a more pleasant experience for children and families. All a child has to do is place his hands near the wall, and a wall projector connected to motion sensors produces colourful lines and shapes which are accompanied by harmonious musical notes. Those who 'play' the wall can move their hands in same fashion as a conductor, and a different tune is composed every time a child makes his unique motions (Figure 3).

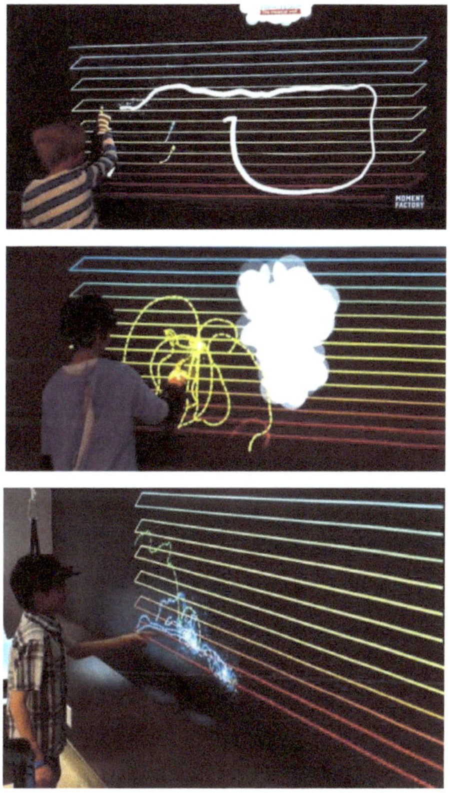

Figure 3. Interactive Musical Wall, at CHU Ste-Justine Children's Hospital in Montreal.

As it is known, art in the hospital environment is very beneficial because it encourages the psychology of patients and positively affects the healing process. Many studies and opinion surveys have proved that visual and performing arts contributed to changes of mood and easing of stress levels. A very unique example of interactive artwork is the hospital sculpture that interacts with human heartbeat by Andrew Small and Steven Almond that was commissioned for the Royal Manchester Children's Hospital in the UK (Figure 4). The sculpture uses digital lighting, medical monitoring equipment and control devices, and it becomes a heart rate monitor when people interact with it. At rest, the artwork 'breathes' in waves of blue light at the average human breath rate. When a person interacts with it by holding the grips, it takes and projects their heart rate in pulses of red light. Infrared sensors around the sculpture create different colour and sequence patterns when their beams are broken, and the sculpture also becomes a clock for five minutes on the hour.

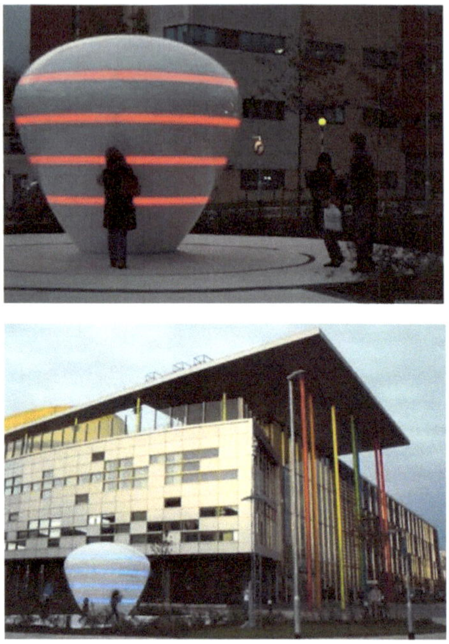

Figure 4. Interactive Artwork, Royal Manchester Children's' Hospital in the UK, by Andrew Small and Steven Almond.

"Several studies show that patients, staff and families are more satisfied with the overall care in pleasant, clean and attractive settings" (National Association of Children's Hospitals and Related Institutions, 2008). Another recent trend is that hospital design (both for adults and children) focuses on creating a pleasant and satisfying ambience experience of the space taking in consideration the overall atmosphere. Stress reduction and stimuli for all the senses through design can be achieved by numerous methods. For example at "The New Martini Hospital" in Groningen (Figure 5). For the layout and furnishing of Martini

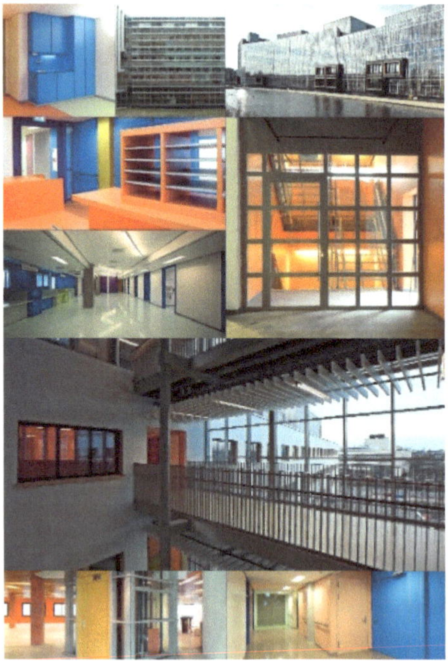

Figure 5. The Martini Hospital in Groningen.

Hospital, Arnold Burger and Bart Vos designed a complete modular-system concept including everything from walls to desks and cupboards. The concept is called IFD, which stands for Industrial, Flexible, and Demountable. Demountable modular walls are used with a small module-size of 30 cm. The technical pipes and cables can be integrated into the walls so that any required combination and layout is possible, even in the arrangement with windows. The walls have different colours, so that it will always be possible to create rooms with different colour schemes, i.e. with a different atmosphere. The modular furniture system is similarly interchangeable. Purpose-made, standardised elements are assembled on site, always in a different way depending on the requirements. As the technical elements integrated into the basic modules are detachable, a change of functions can be realised without having to break anything away. It is possible, to build the desk at a certain stage, and later conveniently add to it, or disassemble the desk so as to use it in a different place or in a different form. The flexible modular furniture system too, has been designed in colour. Apart from the interior the double facades of the building "...allows the windows to open without suffering an increase of noise" (Burger et al., 2006).

On the other hand, when pleasant natural views can't be reached directly (e.g. in examination rooms) design and technology create the proper environment for an ambience experience which will psychologically support the child. For example in order to reduce the need to sedate young patients and improve the patient/family care experience, the radiology department at Children's Hospital of Pittsburgh of UPMC introduced the Adventure Series program, which uses child-friendly, engaging, theme-based room designs; multisensory distractions (e.g., music, videos, aromatherapy); and staff who go out of their way to engage with patients and use age-appropriate techniques to distract and calm them (Figure 6).

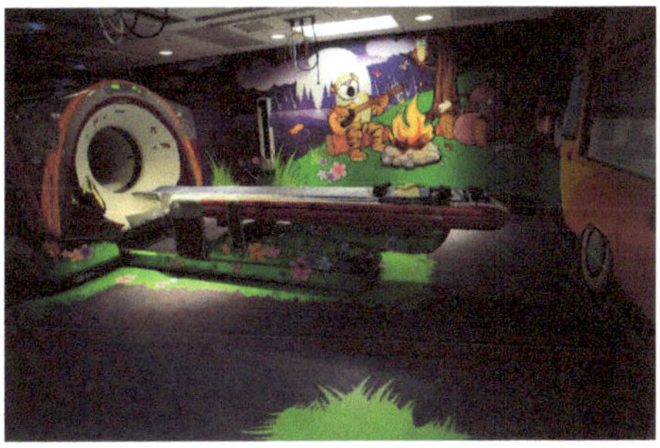

Figure 6. The PET/CT theme room at Children's Hospital of Pittsburgh.

Up to date materials on the floors and the ceilings at patients' rooms but also in other public spaces of the hospital (corridors, waiting areas, lobbies etc.) enable better hygiene and safer movement of the patients. Colourful graphics and playful images on the floors give children the opportunity to feel welcome and at the same time offer positive distractions. At Dell's Children's Medical Centre, Texas "the flooring of natural linoleum and the carpet used is 100% recycled material, its backing is made of plastic bottles" (Verderber, 2010), Figure 7. The floor level is at such height that 'speaks' to a walking child's height or invites them to explore the ground level; In that way design is taking in consideration the scale of the children and offers to them the sense of control of an unknown and strange environment.

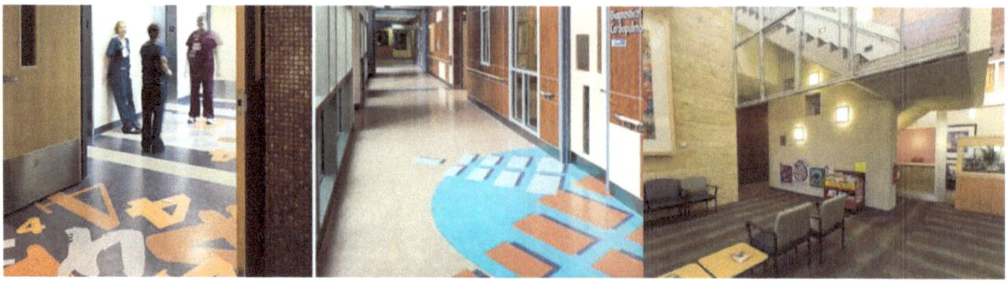

Figure 7. Linoleum and recycled carpet flooring at Dell Children's Medical Center.

The outcomes of contemporary architectural trends in hospital buildings aren't the massive buildings of the past that invaded their surroundings. The exterior of a children's healthcare facility is of great importance. "What children experience at the front door of a hospital, will color the impression of their entire stay". A children's hospital should be "simple and easily understood from the exterior" (Mead, 2005). A very welcome and pleasant building is the example of the Balloch Children's Hospice, in Scotland (Figure 8). "The wave-like formal vocabulary boldly represents the relationship between the ground level and the roof plane. Hospitals will express new formal languages that extend far beyond the rigid orthogonality of the modern machine megahospital" (Verderber, 2006). The wood and the way in which it is applied creates a cosy and warm feeling to the child approaching.

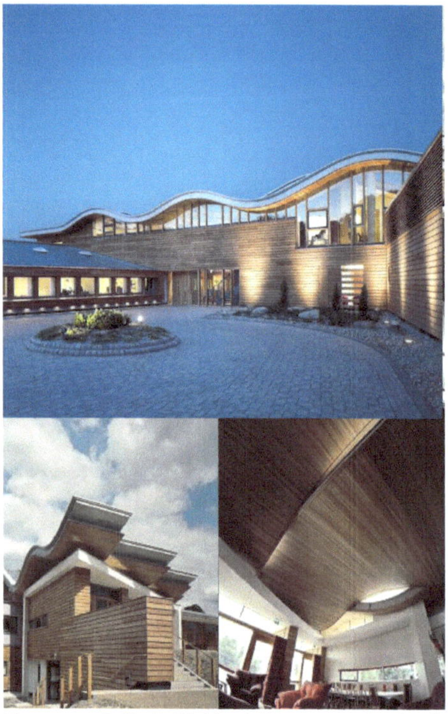

Figure 8. Balloch Children's Hospice, in Scotland.

Another example where the facades of the hospital building create a unique impression is a private clinic in London (Richard Desmond's) (Figure 9). In this case, "...this is unlike any hospital scheme seen before. The façade appears to be animated by the filigree of louvres, apparently in free-fall and designed to evoke the feeling of a wheeling flock of birds. The intervals between the louvre

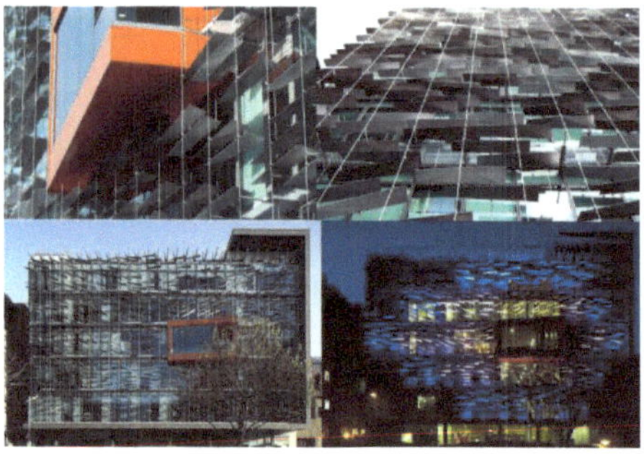

Figure 9. Private Clinic in London.

blades was precisely angled and designed to avoid light spill into the flats opposite and also backwards into the windows of the children's areas." The colour change fittings are controlled inside the building with a Light Projects' designed programme which creates both gradual and fast effects with random colour and intensity spikes. This creates shifting light schemes to fit all aspects of celebration and to create a living, breathing experience. The lighting on the building constantly changes, producing different textures, pastel colours and intensities offering a notable sight to the patients and the passengers.

Conclusions

Promoting better healthcare design requires cooperation between the world of medicine and architecture. It is impossible to foretell what the needs of the future will be but with the help of technology, the creation of pleasant atmospheres, healing environments and thus gradually better quality in children's healthcare facilities is a fact. Never ending innovations in medical science and technology make the design of hospitals even a greater challenge than it already is for architects. Innovative materials, new design aspects and fresh ideas will hopefully help children as much as possible so that the feelings of pain fear and isolation during hospitalization process won't be the dominant ones.

References

Burger A, Afink, G, Kriek, R & Thiadens, G., 2006. *The New Martini hospital: the need for flexibility in the architecture of hospitals,* NAi Publishers, Rotterdam.

Coull, A., 2009. Children's hospital's explorers (CHEX) 10 issues and innovations for children's hospital planning and design – thoughts on designing a children's hospital, *Proceedings of 28th International Public Health Seminar*, Alinea editrice, Firenze.

Coyne, I., 2006. Children's experiences of hospitalization, Journal of Child Health Care, Vol. 10, No. 4, pp. 326-336.

Del Nord, R., 2006. *Environmental stress prevention in children's hospital design*, Motta Architettura, Milano.

Evans, G & McCoy, J., 1998. When buildings don't work: The role of architecture in human health, *Journal of Environmental Psychology*, Vol. 18, ps 980089, pp. 85-94.

Filippazzi, G., 2009. Also walls speak…, Culture for the future of healthcare architecture, *Proceedings of 28th International Public Health Seminar*, edited by Prof. Romano Del Nord, Alinea editrice, Firenze.

Jaspers, F., 2006. *The architecture of hospitals*, NAi Publishers, Rotterdam.

Lawson, B., 2001. *The language of space*, Architectural Press, Great Britain.

Lensch, H., 2006. *The architecture of hospitals*, NAi Publishers, Rotterdam.

Malkin, J., 1992. *Hospital interior architecture, creating healing environments for special patient populations*, Van Nostrand Reinhold, New York.

Mead, W., 2005. *Designing the world's best hospitals*, Images publishing, Australia.

Molenaar, C., 2013. *The colours at martini hospital in Groningen*, Hospital Built and Infastructure, Netherlands.

National Association of Children's Hospitals and Related Institutions, 2008. *Evidence for Innovation*, USA.

Nelson, C., 2006. *Managing quality in architecture: A handbook for creators of the built environment*, Architectural Press, Oxford, UK.

Newman, C., 2009. Children's hospital's explorers (CHEX) 10 issues and innovations for children's hospital planning and design - designing a hospital for children, *Proceedings of 28th International Public Health Seminar*, Alinea editrice, Firenze.

Nicastro, E & Whetsell, M., 1999. Children's fears, *Journal of Pediatric Nursing*, Vol. 14, no. 6.

Paraskeva, P., 2009. Creative spaces for children, *Proceedings of 1st Pan-Hellenic Conference of Art and Environmental Art Education, Foundation of Secondary Degree for Education and Evgenidio Institution*, Athens.

Plappert, J, Gabel, L & Clements, D., 2005. D*esigning the world's best hospitals*, Images publishing, Australia.

Rutter, M., 1981. The city and the child, *American Journal of Orthopsychiatry*, Vol. 51, pp. 610-625.

Simonelli, F, Majer, K & Pinilla, M., 2007. *Health promotion for children and adolescents in and by hospitals, Meyer University Children's Hospital*, Florence, Italy In collaboration with HPH-CA Task Force on Health Promotion for Children and Adolescents in & by Hospitals; Florence, Italy.

Vavili, F., 2000. Children in hospital: A design question, *World Hospital and Health Services*, vol. 36, no. 2, pp. 31-39.

Vavili, F., 2009. *Arts and health facilities*, ZITI Publications, Thessaloniki.

Vavili, F & Stravela, S., 2009. *Aspects of healing environments*, ZITI Publications, Thessaloniki.

Verderber, S., 2010. *Innovations in hospital architecture*, Routledge, New York.

Healthcare Otherwhere – In Singapore

Ruby Lai[1], Chern Siang Jye[2]

ruby.lai@cpgcorp.com.sg
[1] Senior Consultant (Architecture), CPG Consultants Private Limited
[2]Chief Corporate Officer, Agency for Integrated Care, Singapore

Singapore has, up to now, been successful in keeping its expenditure on healthcare to within 4% of its GDP, while providing a high quality of care to its citizens. However, with the increasing ageing of its population, healthcare needs are changing.
Traditionally, healthcare is provided in the acute hospital, but this can be very expensive and is not ideally designed for the varying needs of the population. The Singapore government is embarking on a new wave of healthcare development, and is experimenting with different typologies and infrastructure to gradually evolve its existing towns into aged-friendly habitats, in line with its policy to avoid a "ghetto-risation" of seniors. It is exploring different forms of facilities designed to cater to the different needs of different people: polyclinics, day centres, aged care centres, hospices, community hospitals integrated with acute hospitals, as well as various options for ageing at home. Experiments in public housing attempt to create a "city for all ages", designed to help seniors age-in-place, by providing new infrastructure and services that encourage community bonding and living. This paper explores the various options being developed in Singapore for the aged, chronic sick, terminally ill and people needing rehabilitation care. While the Government is providing substantial aid in terms of infrastructure and training, it requires the cooperation and conscientious aid from both the private and public sectors to carry out the various schemes.

Keywords: *Singapore, healthcare, aged care, integrated development.*

Introduction

Singapore is a nation of about 5.4 million residents. Although it spends only 4% of its Gross Domestic Product on Healthcare, the World Health Organisation (WHO) has ranked Singapore's Healthcare system as the sixth best in the world. However, the challenge to continue providing good healthcare to the citizens is rapidly getting tougher as the population ages.

Singapore has one of the fastest ageing societies in Asia. Currently, about 9% of its population is defined as elderly (65 years and above). By 2030, however, this is expected to grow to about 20%. In fact, in the 2007 Ministerial Committee on Ageing Report, it was projected that by 2050, Singapore would be the fourth oldest country in the world (based on UN Population Division's "World Population Prospects: The 2006 Revision"). Already the nation is feeling a bed crunch as the demand for acute hospital beds is greater than the number of available beds in public hospitals. The government decided to take a coordinated and proactive approach to deal with this problem, and has developed a multi-pronged strategy to cater to the increasing needs of the population.

Current Healthcare System in Singapore

Singapore offers universal healthcare coverage to its citizens, with a financing system based on the twin philosophies of individual responsibility and affordable healthcare for all. The government uses a mixed financing system and multiple tiers of protection to provide healthcare services.

The first tier of protection is provided by the government in the form of subsidies (of up to 80%) of the total bill in acute public hospital wards.

Working Singaporeans and their employers make monthly contributions to the Central Provident Fund (CPF), part of which goes into the Medisave Account where the savings can be used for hospitalisation expenses and approved medical insurance.

Currently, the government uses the "3M + E" framework to help citizens to pay for their healthcare services. These comprise Medisave, Medishield and Medifund, and Eldershield (Figure 1).

Strategies

In March 2007, the government established a Ministerial Committee on Ageing (MCA) with the vision of achieving 'Successful Ageing for Singapore'.

The basic thrust in the government's policies is that individual Singaporeans and their families should be empowered to take responsibility for their social, health and financial needs. The aim is to provide older Singaporeans with information and opportunities to lead healthy lifestyles and remain socially engaged within the community.

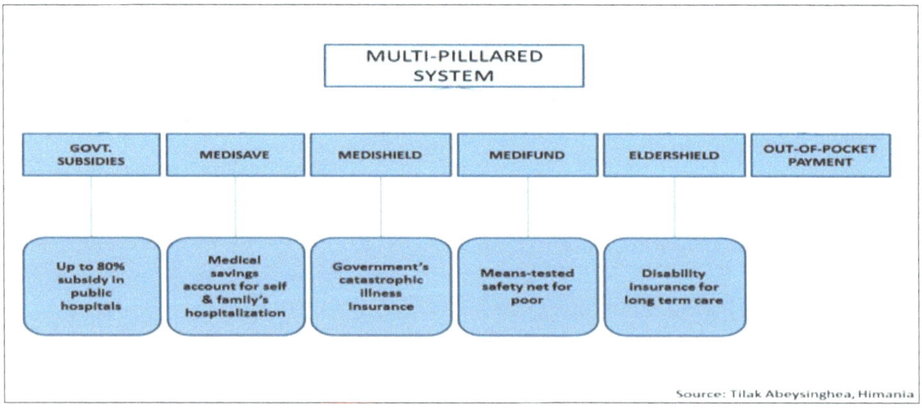

Figure 1. 3m + E framework.

PROVIDING HOLISTIC AND AFFORDABLE HEALTHCARE AND ELDERCARE

The challenge is to provide the most appropriate form of care at an affordable price, and the best way is to ensure a close collaboration between different care givers and institutions so that the patient has varied options while getting continued services. A carefully planned and integrated healthcare system is necessary to ensure this.

An ageing population with higher life expectancy means having to care for more people with chronic and other medical conditions. This would be a drain on the savings of the elderly as most of them would no longer be working and receiving regular income. Many of them would need to rely on their children and other care givers – creating a strain on their finances as well. Being less mobile, the elderly usually have little social interaction with others, and may suffer from loneliness or depression. It is thus necessary to take a holistic approach - to address not only their medical needs, but also their emotional and mental needs. Support for their caregivers is also necessary to help them take care of their elderly dependents.

INCREASING THE NUMBER OF BEDS IN ACUTE HOSPITALS

Singapore's healthcare scene was revitalised in the 1990's when most of the hospitals were rebuilt, and new hospitals added. In the 2000's, citizens enjoyed good healthcare facilities in new hospitals of excellent standards. However, in the last few years, the population has increased dramatically due to an influx of expatriate workers and new permanent residents. In addition, there has been a marked increase in demand by the ageing population. As such, the demand for hospital beds has out-stripped the supply. The government has thus embanked on a spate of constructing new hospitals.

INCREASING THE NUMBER OF BEDS IN OTHER FACILITIES

Adding new acute beds, however, cannot be the only long term solution as acute beds are costly to build and operate, and have a high demand on skilled healthcare staff which is limited in number. In addition, many of the ageing patients do not require acute care and can be better managed in other types of facilities designed for intermediate and long term care. The Ministry of Health has thus turned its attention to the development of other forms of healthcare facilities such as Community Hospitals, Nursing Homes, Hospices and other aged care facilities.

AIC

The Agency for Integrated Care (AIC) was set up in 2009 to centrally coordinate and facilitate the transition of patients from acute care settings to care facilities in the community. One of AIC's new strategies is to engage and support the growth of sub-acute and community care providers to increase the capacity, capability and quality in the non-acute care sectors, and promote better integration of care for the elderly.

Regional health systems

To improve the integration of health services, the Ministry of Health has also restructured the public sector healthcare

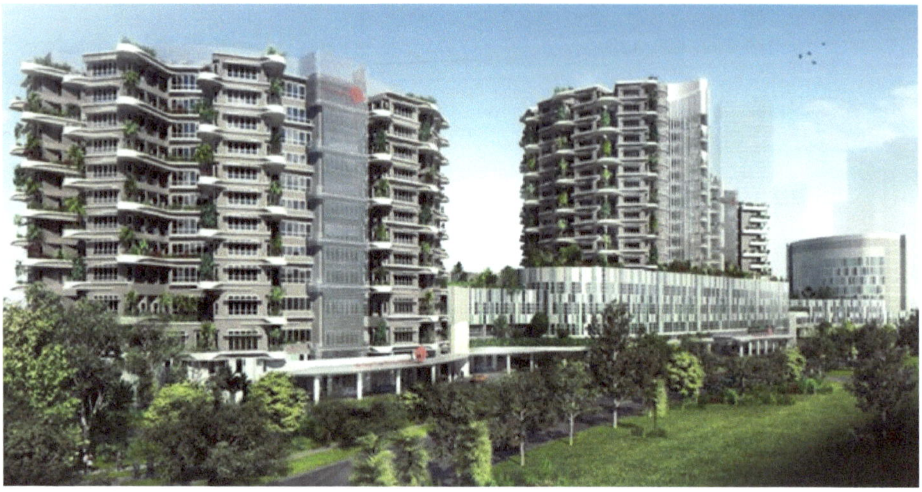

Figure 2. The Jurong Community Hospital (on the left) built within the same development as the acute hospital Ng Teng Fong General Hospital (on the right).

institutions into clusters, comprising an acute care hospital together with a community hospital, working with nursing homes, community care providers, private primary care, polyclinics and other support facilities within each region. A centralised National Electronic Health Record System has been set up to facilitate patient information flow to improve care delivery.

Community hospitals

The term "Community Hospital" in Singapore refers to a step-down care facility where the patient receives rehabilitation and intermediate care. Currently there are five community hospitals operated by Voluntary Welfare organisations (VWOs).

The government has decided that future Community Hospitals should be adjoined to a public sector acute hospital to promote greater integration of care, and to reap economics of scale for operations and scarce medical and healthcare manpower.

The first such integrated development is the 400-bed Jurong Community Hospital (Figure 2) which is built together with the Ng Teng Fong General Hospital. Four other community hospitals are in the pipeline – the Yishun Community Hospital will be beside the Khoo Teck Puat Hospital, the new Seng Kang General Hospital will have a Community Hospital attached to it, the Outram Community Hospital will be built within the campus of the Singapore General Hospital, and the site for the future Woodlands General Hospital (expected to complete in 2021) will also contain a Community Hospital and a Nursing Home.

Community Hospitals will not be the only type of healthcare infrastructure to be integrated with the acute hospital.

The new acute hospitals (and their sister community hospitals) which are planned and under construction, are located within dense residential areas.

Nursing homes

The government will spend $500 million to build 10 new nursing homes, 39 senior care centres and 56 senior activity centres by 2016. Many of these will be located within or near public housing areas, to ensure easy accessibility.

Much care is being taken in the design of the new nursing homes to create interesting spaces. In land scare Singapore, the new nursing homes are high-rise and must cater to the vertical movement of patients. Communal spaces and gardens are thus introduced within each floor to make such spaces easily accessible to the residents, and encourage them to be more mobile and sociable. As most of the residents are not very mobile, attempts are being made to have social and rehabilitation spaces designed within each floor so that patients do not need to be transferred via lifts to centralised facilities below. The wards are designed so that patients can move from one facility to another within the floor, and the openness of the design will encourage the patients to leave their bed and mix with the other residents on that floor. In this way, the residents are encouraged to be more active, and hopefully will improve enough to return home.
The new nursing homes will also be designed to include wards for seniors with dementia.

The new nursing homes will not only be built to cater to the long term patients staying in the nursing home. The plan is to transform nursing homes from a purely residential care facility for those needing care, into a development that is integrated into the social and day care needs of other residents living in the neighbourhood.

Other providers

Currently about 85% of hospital beds are in the 15 public hospitals and specialty centres, while the rest are in the 10 private hospitals. The government's role as the dominant health care provider allows it to influence the supply of hospital beds, the introduction of high tech / high-cost medicine, and the rate of cost increases in the public sector, which sets the bench mark in terms of pricing for the private sector.

ENABLING AGEING-IN-PLACE

In order to encourage more elderly to stay at home instead of moving into nursing homes and other long-term healthcare institutions, the government has looked into various programmes such as streamlining of daycare centres and day rehabilitation centres, befrienders and home help services, etc. to better enable ageing-in-place. The plan is to at least double the outreach of home-based healthcare services, expand the number of day social and rehabilitative care places, and increase manpower and resources to Seniors Activity Centres by 2020.

Polyclinics

Subsidised primary care is mainly provided in government-run polyclinics. To increase the coverage, new polyclinics are being planned. These, together with the wide network of GPs under the Community Health Assist Scheme CHAS will provide the public with good access to primary healthcare services.

Specialist Centres

There are certain types of illnesses associated more with the elderly. Specialist centres for Geriatrics, Dementia and Parkinson's Disease are being set up. Despite the best efforts at primary prevention, a proportion of the population will develop dementia. It is therefore important to provide services for these patients to ensure early detection and provide necessary treatment and support. Day Care Centres with dedicated Dementia Care Centres provide nursing care and therapy for persons with dementia as well as respite for their caregivers, and new Senior Care Centres will have the capability to provide dementia day care services.

Parkinson's Disease is currently one of the most common neurodegenerative conditions seen in Singapore, and is common in the elderly. The new Parkinson Centre is the first centre to be built which will provide therapeutic, physiotherapy, occupational and voice therapy programmes and activities for people living with Parkinson's and related illnesses. It will also serve as a training centre to support and train caregivers and healthcare professionals to better care for such patients in the community (Figure 3).

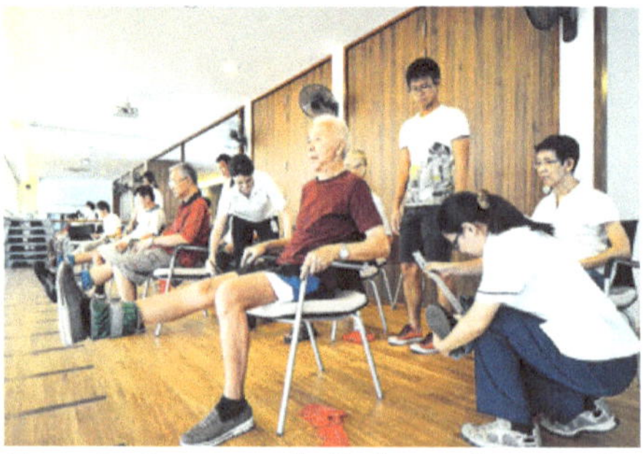

Figure 3. Patients at the Parkinson Centre in Bishan.

Integrated Approach

To enable the elderly to be more mobile, various ministries were tasked to improve their services and infrastructure. The public transport system reviewed their facilities and added elevators and accessible vehicles. The Building and Construction Authority developed a Barrier-Free Accessibility (BFA) Masterplan in 2006, and further redeveloped and enhanced the BFA Code to become the Code on Accessibility in the Built Environment, promoting Universal Design (UD) principles to the industry, encouraging developers and consultants to adopt the principles in their designs. UD features are now incorporated into all public parks and facilities. As part of their actions to help the elderly receive more effective care and support, the government revamped two key services: Senior Care Centres and Home-based Care.

Senior Care Centres

Many of the healthcare facilities currently work in silos – day care centres, rehabilitation centres, polyclinics, etc. However, the elderly often need services across the various facilities – thus they have to be shuttled from one facility to another. Senior Care Centres are a new typology that first integrated the health (active rehabilitation) and social care (maintenance rehabilitation, social day care) services. They are being designed to provide basic day care for the frail elderly, including those who are wheelchair-bound, and those with moderate to severe dementia. In addition, these centres will provide specialised services and programmes such as rehabilitation and dementia programmes for those with higher care needs. Information, referral and care coordination services will also be made available to both the elderly and their families. These centres will be designed to improve the delivery of community care to the elderly, and their progress will be tracked, services coordinated and specialised services brought to them in the same place.

One such centre has been set up at Braddell Heights (Figure 4-6). It offers integrated care for the frail elderly as well as dementia therapy. The services are also provided for those who are not day-care clients, but wish to participate in maintenance exercises to retain their physical and mental functionality. It is located together with a child care centre and other community services so that it is a community hub where the whole family can get together to use its facilities. Over the next few years, S$100 million will be invested in these centres, and by 2016, there will be 40 Senior Care Centres which can serve more than 2,500 elderly persons requiring day care.

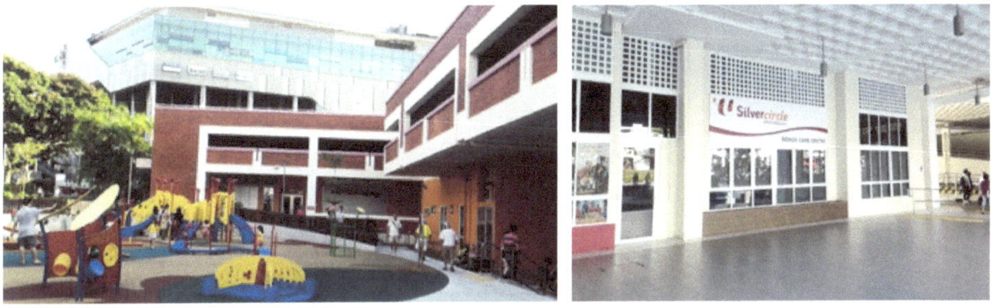

Figure 4. Braddell Heights Community Hub, Child care centre located together with Elderly Day Care Centre.

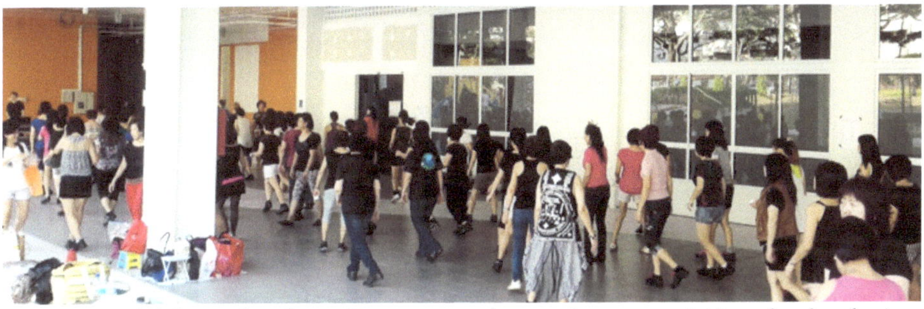

Figure 5. BHCH, Senior Care Centre. Large communal spaces allow group activities such as line dancing.

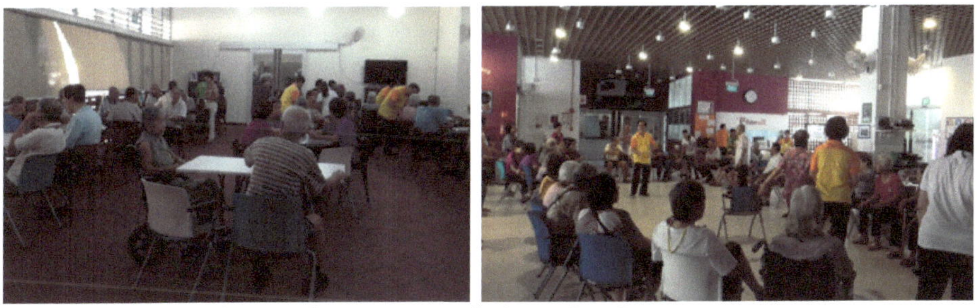

Figure 6. BHCH, meal time and activity time at the Senior Care Centre.

Integrated Development at Admiralty

A new development being constructed at Admiralty is another variation in the integration of healthcare facilities within the community. This new development will have a shopping centre, a food centre, a supermarket, senior and child care centres, medical centre and 2 blocks of studio apartments specially designed for seniors, with senior activity centres (Figure 7).

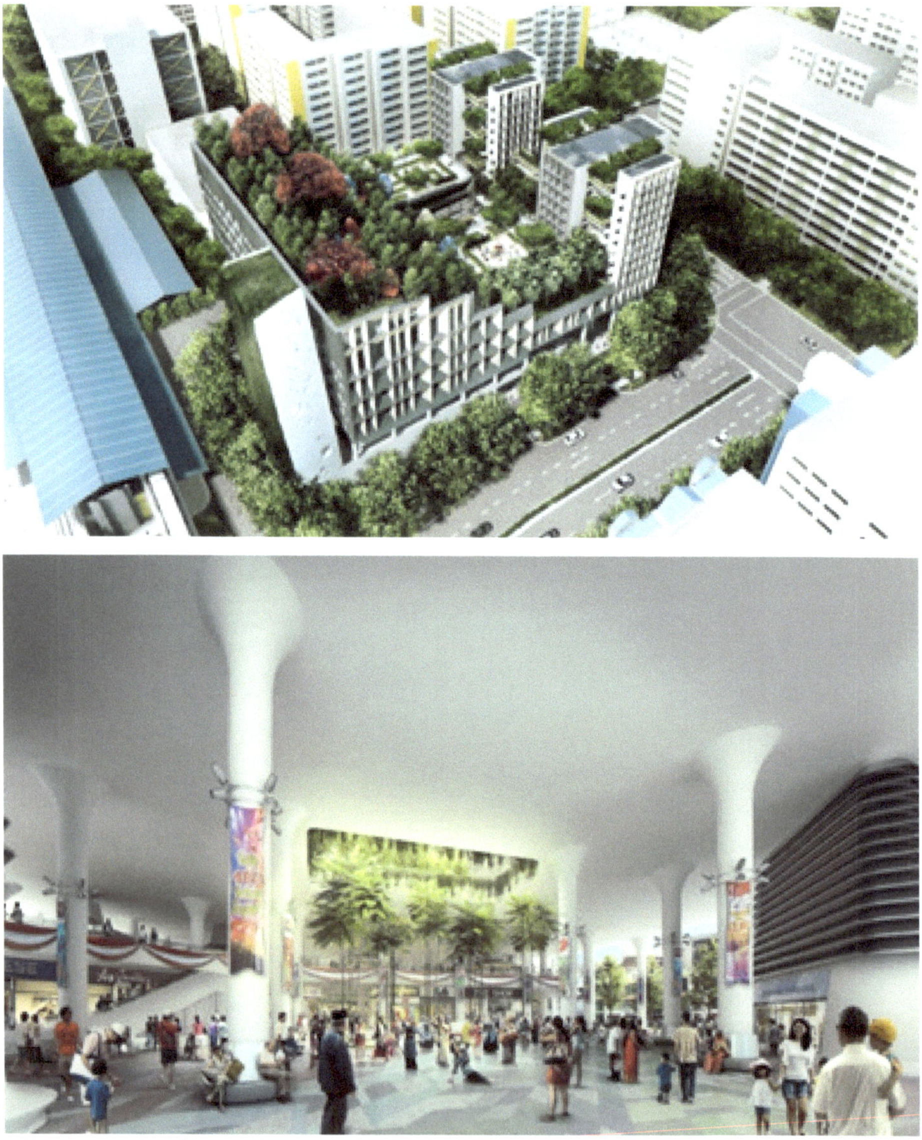

Figure 7. Integrated development. Source: Ministry of National Development. Aerial perspective of the new integrated development in Woodlands (top). Perspective of the People's Plaza for the community (below).

Improvements to Public Housing

The Housing Development Board (HDB), the sole provider of public housing (housing 85% of the population) is one of the government agencies that has been taking the lead in enhancing facilities for the elderly. Major redevelopment programmes have been undertaken in the existing housing developments to improve access such as reducing levels within the homes, increasing widths of corridors and doorways, and providing at least one wheelchair accessible bathroom within the housing unit. A Lift Upgrading Programme was introduced to ensure all public housing are well served by elevators.

City for All Ages (CFAA) Project

In 2011, residents above 60 years old in Marine Parade constituency were polled on what they needed in their homes and neighbourhoods to make life easier and safer for them. This led to the birth of the "City for All Ages" initiative which has spread to other townships. Audits of the flats and town environment were carried out, from the viewpoint of what would be appropriate for an active elderly person, by officials, occupational therapists and residents to identify areas for improvement. Certain precincts were selected to test out the ideas proposed, and then implemented in other areas. It is a ground-up, people-centric approach where individuals identified what was required, and proposed solutions (Figure 8).
The aim is to create a people-initiative across the island to make the city a senior friendly one, and the best place for the seniors to grow old in.

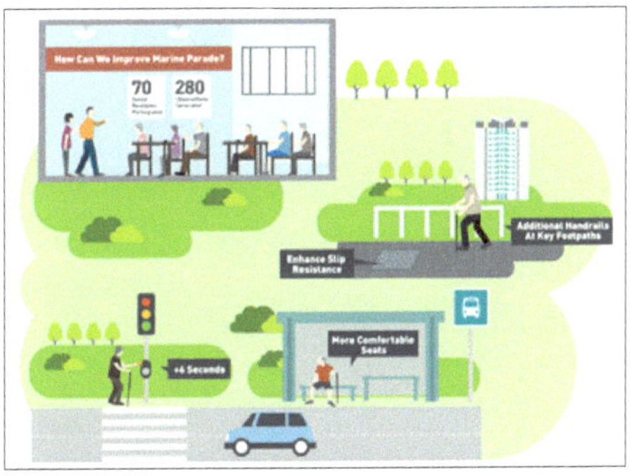

Figure 8. City for All Ages (CFAA) scheme.

Studio Flats for the Elderly

The Housing Development Board is developing studio apartments incorporating elder-friendly features such as emergency pull cords and grab rails. These 35 to 45 sqm sized apartments are with shorter leases of 30 years to make them more affordable, and will allow retirees to free up money for living expenses by selling their existing homes and moving into the relatively cheap and easy to maintain apartments. These apartments are placed within the same block as other types of flats to promote interaction between younger and older residents.

Enhancement for Active Seniors (EASE)

Introduced by the Housing Development Board under the Home Improvement Programme to improve the safety and comfort of seniors living in their public housing apartments. Residents pay a very heavily subsidised rate for improvements such as slip-resistant treatment to their bathroom or toilet floor tiles, grab bars within the apartment, ramps to negotiate level differences, etc. (Figure 9).

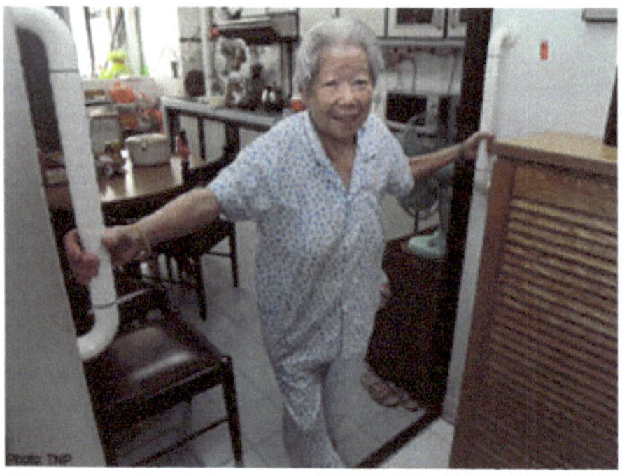

Figure 9. Grab bars installed in the homes help the elderly move around.

PROMOTE ACTIVE AGEING

Research has shown that an individual's well-being is improved if they lead healthy and happy lives, and this may even reduce the risk of the onset of chronic diseases.

Singapore Programme for Integrated Care for the Elderly (SPICE)

SPICE was introduced by AIC to provide comprehensive integrated centre- and home-based services to support caring for the frail elderly. It enables those who have high care needs and are eligible for admissions into nursing homes to recover and age within the community. A multi-disciplinary team comprising medical, nursing, allied health and ancillary professionals provides the various healthcare needs for the patient including primary and preventive care, rehabilitation services, personal care and social and leisure activities. These services are delivered both at the centres and at the patients' home, depending on their needs.

AIC partners voluntary welfare organisations to operate SPICE centres. The centres will collaborate with the acute hospital and general practitioners nearby to form a seamless model of care.

Communal spaces for the elderly

To encourage the elderly to live within the community, several public housing estates have encouraged the residents to create social spaces for the elderly (Figure 10-11).

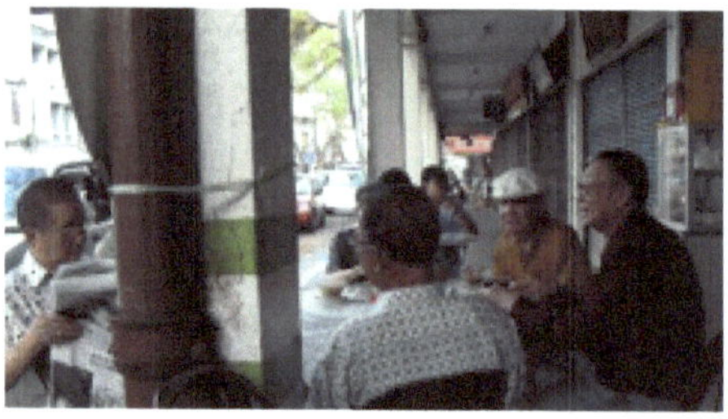

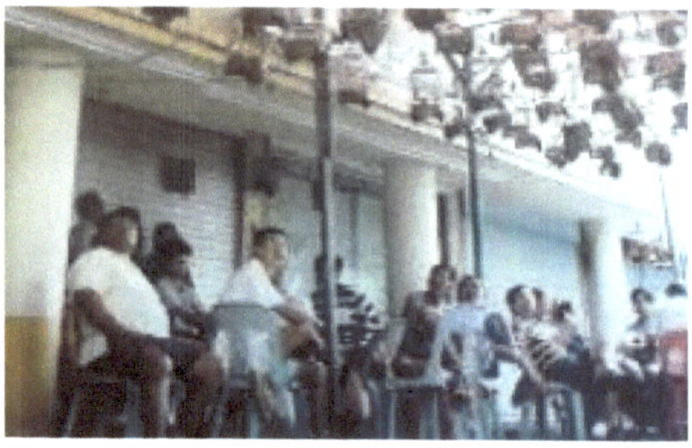

Figure 10. Solutions for the elderly: some elderly residents gathering at the local coffee shop (top); a favourite past time for some of the elderly is relaxing with their birds (below). Source: Ministry of Social and Family Development – Examples of Urban Solutions for Ageing.

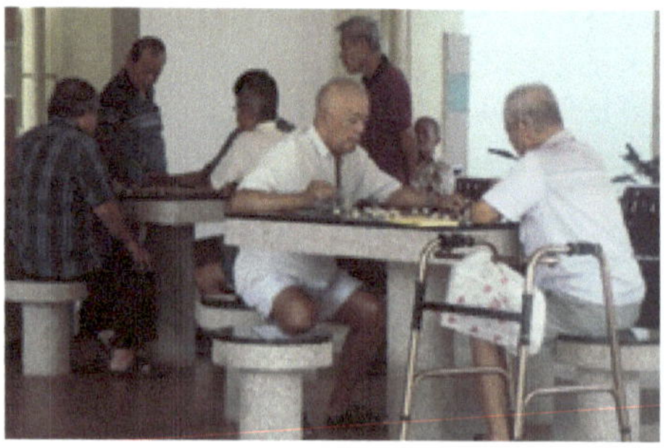

Figure 11. Having a quiet game at the void deck below their apartment. Source: R. Lai.

IMPROVING AFFORDABILITY

While services are being improved for the elderly, it is important to ensure that it remains affordable. Some methods to ensure this are to encourage right-siting of care, introduction of fixed rates for outpatient charges for the lower income group, and enhancing the 3M Framework.

Enhancing the 3M framework and right-siting of care

The use of Medicare was mainly approved for expenses for inpatient care in hospitals. This encouraged the utilisation of acute healthcare services. In 2013, it was decided to allow the use of Medicare over a greater continuum of care, and encourage the right-siting of care so that people will use more outpatient service, instead of occupying more expensive acute hospital beds.

Increasing means-testing levels

Since 2009, the Ministry of Health started Means Testing as a way to determine the level of subsidy for Singaporeans and permanent residents when they use public hospital facilities. This is a way to provide more subsidies for the lower income group.

Increasing subsidies and encouraging more support from Voluntary Welfare Organisations (VWOs)

To ensure that the services are affordable, subsidies for community hospitals, nursing homes, centre-based care, and home care were raised. Subsidies for chronic care were also raised, and efforts have been made to expand home nursing, home medical and ensuite home personal care services.

SUMMARY

By promoting healthy living and encouraging the people to be more self-reliant and responsible for their own health, the government tries to keep the cost of healthcare down. People are encouraged to stay at home and use day care services or home care services as much as possible, instead of moving into nursing home or other institutions.

The right siting of health care is important to prevent excessive expenditure in acute hospitals. People are being educated to realise that healthcare is available not only in the acute hospitals. Many schemes have been introduced to help the Singaporean maintain a healthy life within affordable means by seeking healthcare in the right places.

REFERENCES

Gan, KY., 2013. *Committee of supply speech by Minister for Health – better health for all (Part 1 or 2)*, Singapore.

Gan, KY., 2013. *Speech by Minister for Health at the launch of friends plus and friends special @ St Hilda's Link*, Singapore.

Himania,TA & Lim, J., 2012. *Singapore's healthcare financing: Some challenges*, Singapore.

Ibrahim, MF., 2013. *Healthy together, anytime, anywhere – making the connections*, Singapore.

Khalik, S., 2013. *Nursing homes will be near your homes, The Straits Times*, Singapore.

Khor, A., 2013. *Committee of supplys Speech by Minister of State for Health – better care for our seniors, progress in community mental health and woe's health,* Singapore.

Lam, PM., 2013. *Government Parliamentary Committee (Health) Report on Improving Healthcare Affordability for Singaporeans*, Singapore.

Ministerial Committee on Ageing: Report for 2007, 2008, Singapore.

Ministry of Health, 2013. *New plans for integrated development in Woodlands unveiled to better address community needs*, Singapore.

Yacob, H., 2012. *Speech at committee of supply debates,* Singapore.

Planning and Design Related to a Critical Global Community Need - Mental Health Care: A Much Needed Focus

Philip Patrick Sun

ppsun@aol.com
AIA, ACHA, NCARB, CEO and Executive Director, Asian Community Mental Health Services, USA

38% of those who need mental health care receive it in the USA. Worldwide it is worse. Low to middle income countries have a gap between 76-85% and high income countries only meet 35-50% of the need.
The measure of disability adjusted life years (DALYs) shows neuropsychiatric conditions cause losses which are higher than cardiovascular disease and cancer. Because of complex interactions and co-morbidity between mental health and physical health, the disparities are believed to be even much higher. Additionally, almost one million people die due to suicide each year and this is the third leading cause of death among the young.
The 'front line' and first priority on mental health care reported in WHO's Mental Health Report 2001 is provision of mental health treatment through primary care.
This paper focuses on an example of planning and process for outpatient facilities for this critical need and how this is much different than physical health operations and settings. Interdisciplinary research, analysis, design and evaluation processes included physicians, therapists, case managers, patients (clients/consumer), researchers and health care planners/architects. Data, hypothesis, analysis of operational, physical/environmental conditions, patient interviews and surveys led to modeling and design approaches for healthier environments.
Mental health is most devastating for the poor worldwide. Lessons learned include examples of positive and detrimental environments which are fundamentally different than physical health. This paper also suggests the link between integrated approaches improves outcome and built environments.
Because mental health fundamentally involves psychological and environmental perception the quality of the design or architecture for treatment is arguably more important than the design for other clinical care settings. This paper is about the approach toward planning and design which recognizes resilience, ecology and value also known as Hope, Strength and Resilience.

Keywords: *significance of mental health, mental health care vs. physical health care, integrated planning and development, lean methods, mental health design attributes.*

INTRODUCTION

In the majority of health care (physical health), the problem is observable either by the naked eye or through technology. This is not the case with behavioral health or mental health.
We, as health care architects have for generations concentrated on physical health projects which have dominated the landscape of health care projects. Hospitals, health centers, clinics, long term care facilities have been the majority concentration while life expectancy for the serious mentally ill is reportedly reduced by 10-20 years, worse than that for heavy smoking.
The World Health Organization reported in 2003: "It is becoming evident that when mental health services are available there may be reductions in the costs of physical health care, increases in productivity and reduced demands on other social services and the criminal justice system (e.g. Conti & Burton 1994, Smith et al. 1996, von Korff et al. 1998). Some of these offsets may not be observed for a considerable time. In respect of interventions for children, for example, the payoffs are associated with the avoidance of mental, social and legal problems in adulthood.

Mental health is a complex subject in the USA because it includes substance abuse, inpatient care, residential care, outpatient care, and homelessness. Its effects are broad and affects productivity, families and society, safety and the justice system, co-morbidity with the larger health care system.

In the United States, Chris Weiss researched and wrote that "one of the biggest untreated problems in the United States affecting everything from social relationships to employment is mental health. Many do not receive the care they need, mostly for financial reasons."

He added: "Around 25% of adults experience a mental health issue in a given year, yet less than 1 in 3 adults receives services. According to the CDC, around 50% of Americans will experience some mental health issues over their lifetimes. The rate of mental health issues in the U.S. is abnormally high, and lack of treatment options is only making this worse.

Health Care in itself often lacks the political punch necessary to achieve change. As such Mr. Weiss added "The estimated impact in terms of loss of productivity in the workplace is around $63 billion. Only a small percentage of these diagnoses consist of severe problems such as schizophrenia, but the impact of other more treatable forms of mental disorders is undeniable".

The Substance Abuse and Mental Health Services Administration recently released the results from its 2011 national survey on mental health. One of the most disturbing results in this survey is that only 38% of individuals with mental health issues have received appropriate services.

The volume of expense in total health care and for mental health care can be compared in the following charts. In 2008, the total per capital cost for health care was over $7500, the highest in the world (Figure 1).

In comparison, the per capita expendi-

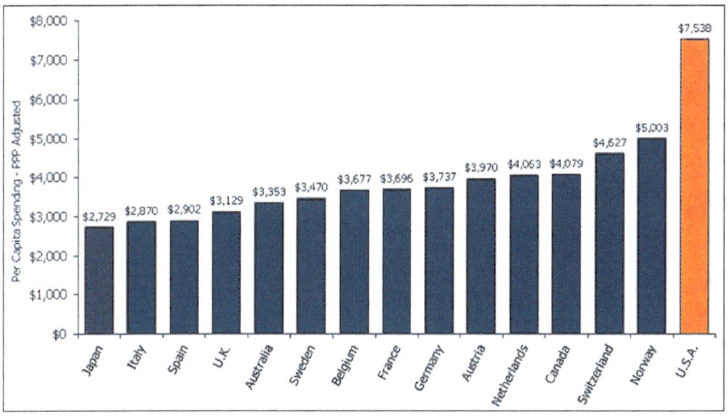

Figure 1. Per Capita health care spending. Source: Kaiser Foundation.

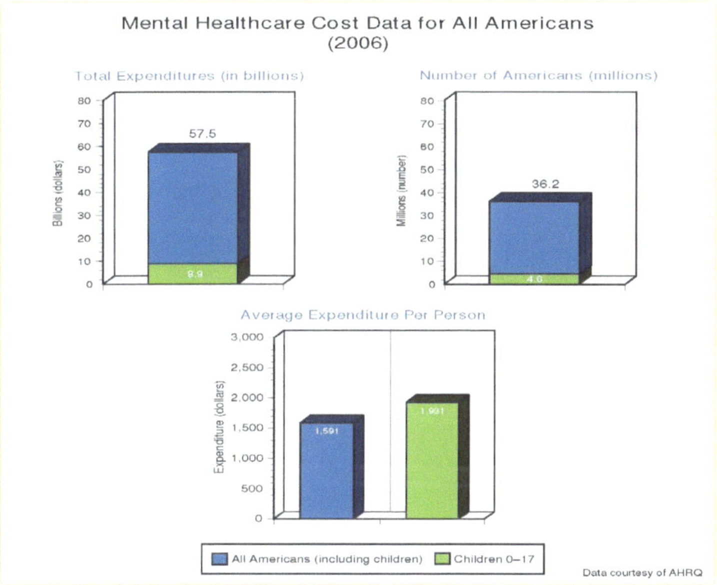

Figure 2. Mental health expenditures. Source: Agency for Healthcare Research and Quality's (AHRQ's) Medical Expenditure Panel Survey (MEPS).

ture in 2006 for mental health was between $1500 and $1900 respectively for adults and children (Figure 2).

The National Institute on Health reports: "The Substance Abuse and Mental Health Services Administration (SAMHSA) examines the mental health treatment each year through the National Survey on Drug Use and Health (NSDUH). In 2008, 13.4 percent of adults in the United States received treatment for a mental health problem. This includes all adults who received care in inpatient or outpatient settings and/or used prescription medication for mental or emotional problems" (Figure 3). And

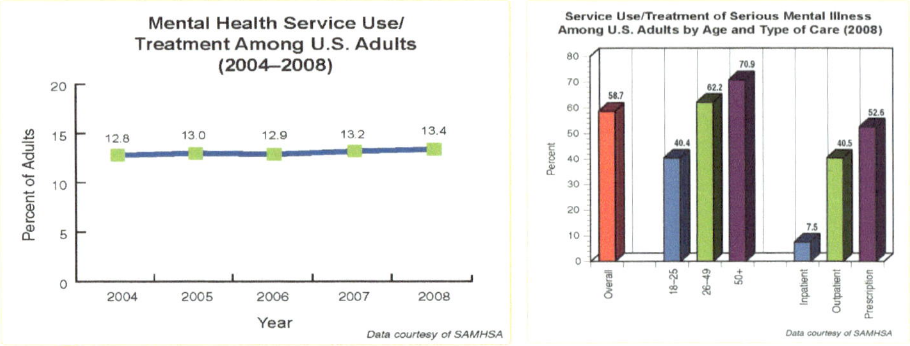

Figure 3. Mental health use and serious mental health among adult. Source: SAMHSA.

"SAMHSA's National Survey on Drug Use and Health (NSDUH) also found in 2008 that just over half (58.7 percent) of adults in the United States with a serious mental illness (SMI) received treatment for a mental health problem. Treatment rates for SMI differed across age groups, and the most common types of treatment were outpatient services and prescription medication."

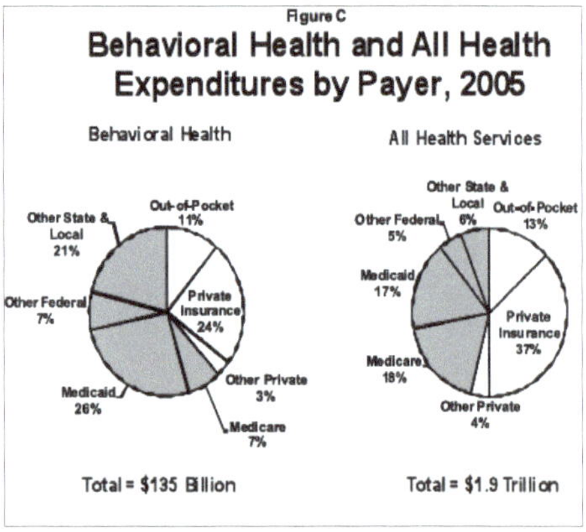

Figure 4. Behavioral health and all health expenditures by Payer 2005. Source: SAMHSA.

Another comparison of the size of mental health expenditures is shown by a study commissioned by the Kaiser Foundation in 2010. It was found that in 2005 mental health expenditures in the USA totaled $135 Billion while total health care expenditures totaled $1.9 Trillion (Figure 4).

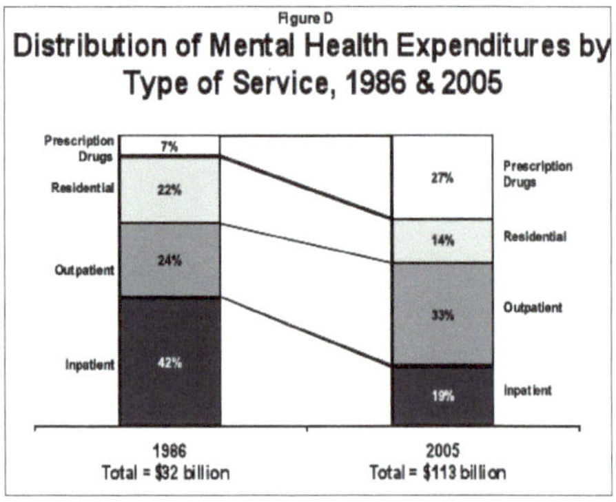

Figure 5. Distribution of mental health expenditures by type of service, 1986 and 2005. Source: SAMHSA.

Clearly, mental health and outpatient is an important part of health care but not the dominant part of the health care industry in the United States.

CONTEXT

Mental health care has migrated from inpatient and residential institutionalization at 64% in 1986 to 33% in 2005 and managing patients through outpatient care and medication (prescription drugs) at 33% in 1986 to 60% in 2005 (Figure 5).

Since this movement was gradual and community and often non-profit based it did not create large design projects or programs. As this began to change, the role of a community based response to mental health did not lend itself to large projects and as such attracted less attention. As such the development of the design guidelines and examples of outpatient mental health facilities are not as well documented. Some of the most complete work is included in the Department of Veterans Affairs Office of Design and Construction Design Guidelines dated 2010. Other major health care organizations and universities have developed design guidelines but we have not found sections dedicated to mental health. As such, this paper will later discuss the methodology used to help guide planning and design through participatory involvement of the providers and patients/clients.

Changes in national legislation have brought greater attention to mental health and the need for outpatient services. As health care issues and access to health care have occupied much of the demand for change in health care policy in the USA, mental health has been a part of the change. By 2010 over 40 million in the USA did not have health care insurance. That figure has been on the increase. In addition, coverage has not covered several items such as preexisting conditions and mental health. That has now changed with the implementation of the Patient Protection and Affordable Care Act (PPACA).

Access is Now Mandated: The new access to mental health care has created a drive to provide new directions and programs for delivery of mental health care services. Early intervention and delivery of mental health care to the general population has always been important and now access to mental health care is mandated. The PPACA has now mandated access and the programs for outpatient mental health care are intended to have greater impact in reducing rates of hospitalization and incarceration and improve community health and security. In addition, the national funding agencies are focusing on the integration of mental health and physical health.

Integrated Care Models: In the USA there are two major agencies which are responsible for Federal programs in primary care and for mental health care. They are respectively the Health Resources Services Administration (HRSA) and Substance Abuse and Mental Health Services Administration (SAMHSA). One of the new programs being tested is called Primary Care Integration (PCI).

The program has involved funding to primary care facilities known as Federally Qualified Health Centers (FQHC) and not for profit mental health agencies. Many of the mental health agencies have provided care for the same patients as FQHCs and the match seemed quite reasonable. Thus what seems intuitively simple also begins to uncover attributes which set these two types of care apart and exposes care models and environments including design criteria.

This focus on integration of physical health or the typical primary care operations and mental health outpatient care has brought focus to the differences in operational models and facilities.

"Health is a state of complete physical, mental and social well-being, and not merely the absence of disease or infirmity."
World Health Organization 1948

"A sad soul can kill you quicker than a germ."
John Steinbeck

DIFFERENCES BETWEEN PHYSICAL HEALTH CARE AND MENTAL HEALTH CARE IN THE OUTPATIENT SETTING

On one hand, the patient is the same person but the way care is delivered in the physical health operation is quite different than in the mental health environment.

1. In mental health the patient is often referred to as the client or the consumer. This distinction may seem minor at first but it carries deeper into the relationship between the patient and the doctor or the client and the provider or the consumer and the clinician.

2. In physical health the symptoms are usually "physically" apparent either through direct observation or tools which allow for imagery to confirm there is a physical aliment. This is not the case with mental health conditions. The assessment process is most important and prior to this there should be no assumption.

3. *Primary Care*: in physical health the treatment and cure are to eliminate the physical abnormality and allow the body to heal or go back to a recognized state of normality. This may take a single or a few treatments but the cure is the objective.

4. *Mental Health*: in mental health the objective is considerably different. The treatment is not an occasion but a plan. The objective is stabilization and maintenance which is more likely than not long term.

5. *Frequency*: in primary care (physical health) a continuum of care may result in the patient seeing the doctor four times a year. That is considered a pattern which provides adequately for health maintenance. In mental health the client may see the doctor or clinician/therapist, and often does, three to four times a month. The frequency of visits is entirely different. This difference suggests how the space is perceived and patterns in operations and orientation affect the client/patient (Figure 6-7).

6. *Design focus*: the focus on functional planning of the rooms and equipment for physical health is usually in developing the space to efficiently address the functions for the physician and nurse. In mental health the concentration is more centered on the patient and patient behavior (such as using neutral colors and limited or small patterns to reduce any distractions), including safety and security (items should be bolted down or not included in the room) when dealing with the severely mentally ill (SMI). Natural light is greatly desired in both mental health and physical health settings and in both settings it is considered a healing attribute.

7. *Furnishings and focus*: the standard treatment room in physical health and its parameters are also different. In

the case of a mental health treatment room, the serenity of the space should dominate and the treatment is primarily through discussion. Seating therefore takes precedence to the exam table. That said there are the attributes of focus and safety for both the patient and the clinician as mentioned above.

8. *Electronic medical records*: the advent of the computer and electronic health records has resulted in a desire to complete the record and notes as soon as possible so that billing can take place as soon as possible. It is not uncommon to have the provider focused on the computer while asking questions to the patient and glance between the patient and the computer. In mental health the focus is the patient and while there may be a computer in the room, the focus is entirely on the patient, as it should be. It is now encouraged that the physical health provider complete and close notes while the patient is in the exam room or as soon as possible. Notes are completed after the session in most cases in mental health often with time to contemplate the session.

9. *Visit/session time*: the mental health 'session' is typically 50 minutes. The primary care visit/encounter/session has been driven by a business model which requires the provider to see approximately 20 patients per day to financially break even. That results in an approximate 20 minute visit time per patient, and the physician time is anywhere from 7 ½ to 10 minutes under this model. The remainder of the time in physical health contact or encounter is by the nurse and support staff (Figure 8-11).

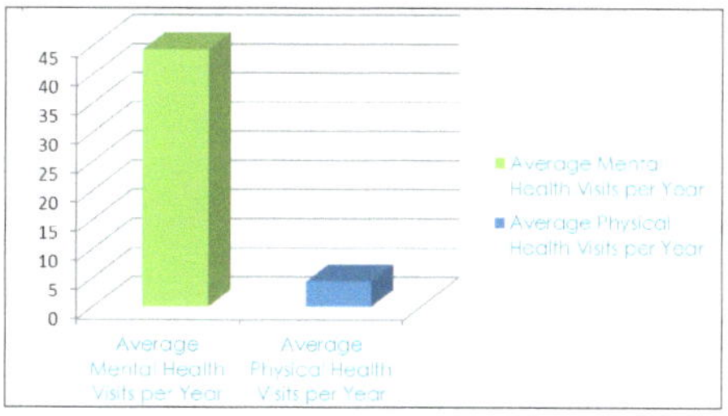

Figure 6. Average mental health visits per year and physical health visits per year for primary care integration patient. Source: ACMHS and AHS.

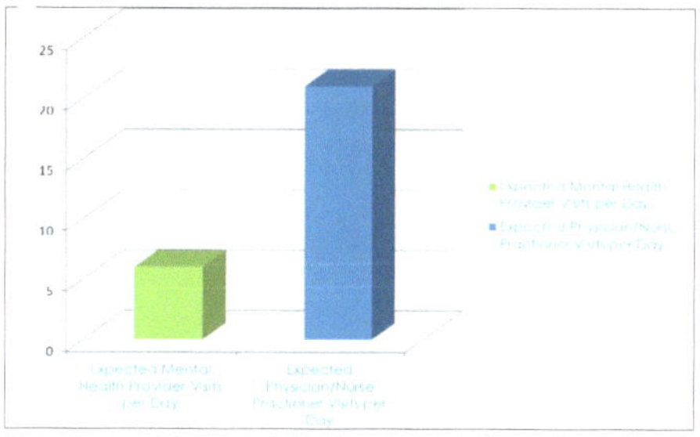

Figure 7. Expected daily activity load for providers in mental health vs. expected daily activity load for physician or nurse providers in physical health. Source: ACMHS and AHS.

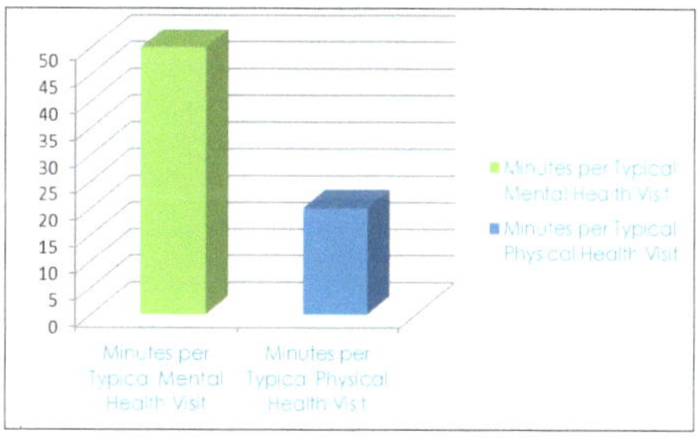

Figure 8. Minutes for typical mental health vs. physical health visits. Source: ACMHS and AHS.

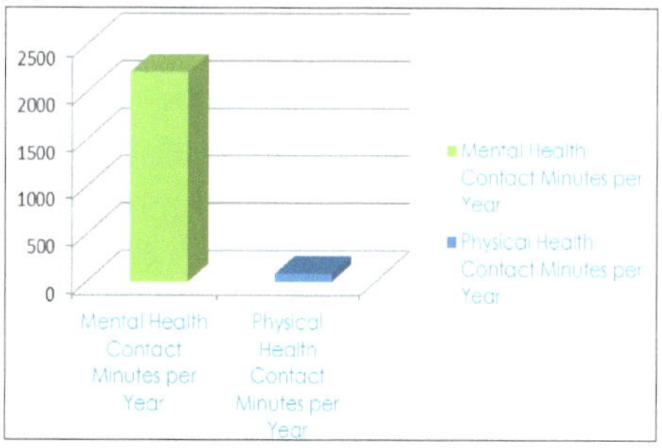

Figure 9. Client contact minutes per year for mental health and patient contact minutes per year for physical health. Source: ACMHS and AHS."111

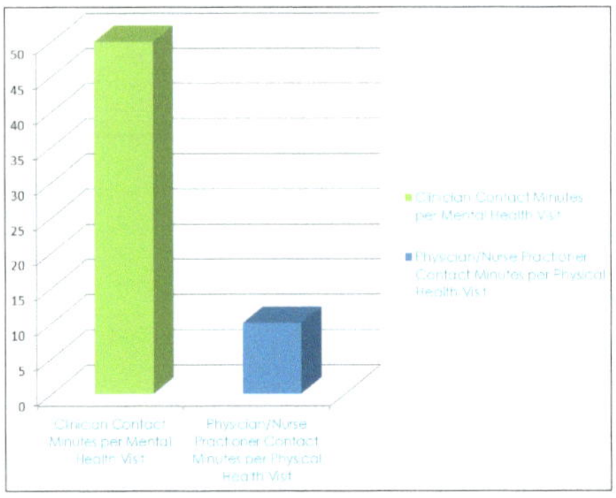

Figure 10. Clinician contact per visit with client in mental health vs. physician or nurse practitioner contact per physical health visit. Source: ACMHS and AHS.

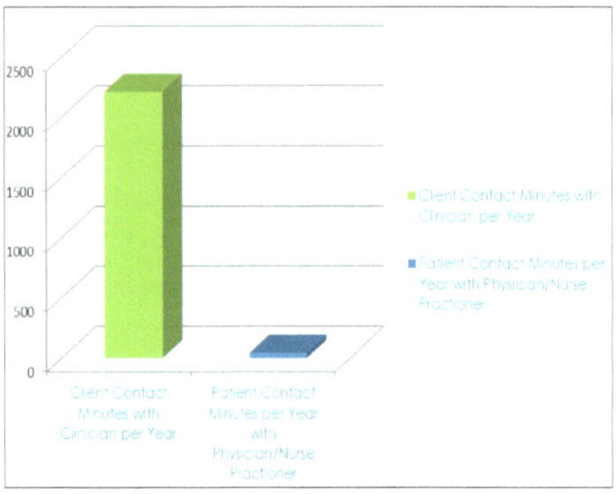

Figure 11. Client contact with clinician per year in mental health vs. patient contact with physician or nurse practitioner in physical health. Source: ACMHS and AHS.

THE CASE STUDY

The case study involves a non-profit which provides mental health and disability services. The Asian Community Mental Health Service (ACMHS) is a nonprofit organization established over 40 years ago in 1974. Organizations such as these are often referred to as agencies. The patients or clients in this agency are predominately Asian and have severe to moderate mental health care needs. ACMHS has a staff of approximately ninety composed of psychiatrists, psychologists, case managers, therapists, and a few support staff. Three major activities dominate the agency: mental health assessment and counseling, developmental disability case management, and outreach to the community to assist in better use of community resources.

The clients or patients are both adult and children and there are approximately 672 mental health clients and 1231 developmental disability clients at any one time. The developmental disability clients are almost entirely seen off site during home visits and planned encounters. The outreach events are also handled off site in almost all cases (Figure 12).

Recently, the agency has developed an integrated form of care delivery with a local primary care agency, Asian Health Services (AHS), thus offering physical health services to the severely mentally ill. Of the approximate 270 severely mentally ill, approximately 130 elected to join the group which provides physical health services.

A unique attribute of this agency is the diversity of the Asian population served. The staff composition also reflects the community in language and cultural competence (Figure 13).

The facilities of the agency total approximately 17,000 square feet on three floors of an older and historically registered building in Oakland, California (Figure 14). The agency has been in this facility for over thirty years, moving from suite to suite over the years. The agency currently occupies space on all three floors of the building. The physical health setting is in the same building but is in retail space leased by the primary care provider.

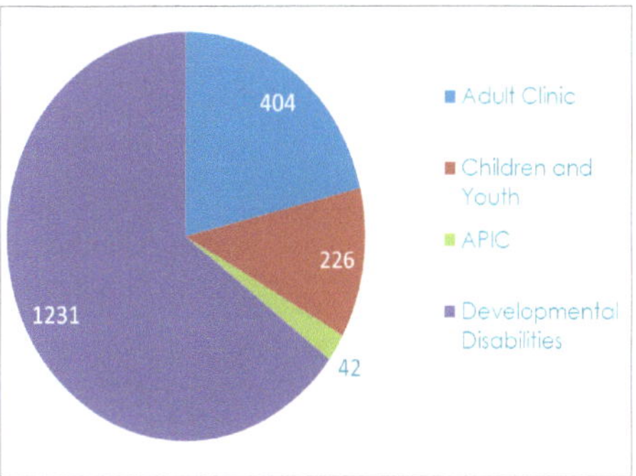

Figure 12. Distribution of ACMHS clients by program. Source: ACMHS.

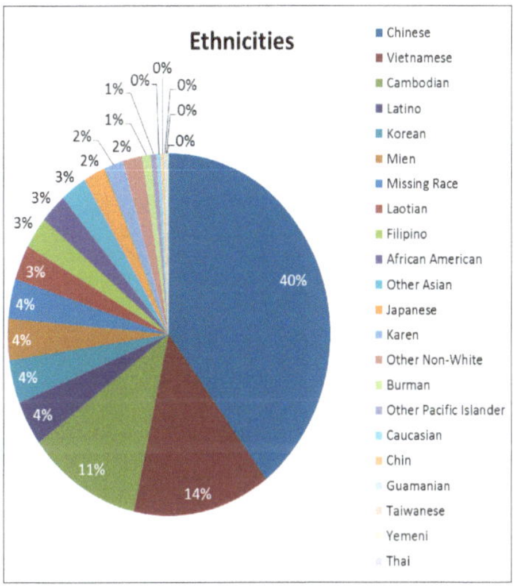

Figure 13. Distribution of ACMHS clients by ethnicity. Source: ACMH.

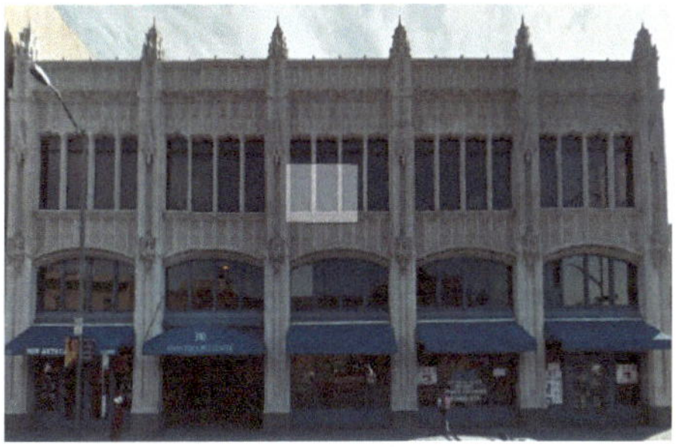

Figure 14. ACMHS at 310 8th Street, Oakland CA. Source: ACMHS.

The design component of this paper involves the comprehensive planning process to survey, analyze, program and plan their physical environment for a better experience by patients and improved care for patients.
The planning and design process proceeded along Lean and Integrated Project Development methodologies. A six step process shown below is based on decision points of Figure 15.

Decision Point 1: the formality of the decision management system allowed the project to stay focused. The underlying methodology for planning came from three sources, Bioteaming Manifesto by Ken Thompson and Robin Good for organizing communications; Problem Seeking by William Pena for planning methodology; and Toyota Way by Jeffery Liker for management principles.

Organizing for planning is critical to a successful effort.

Borrowing from Bioteaming Manifesto, communications were of a 'blast' mode rather than selecting specific individuals and directing information or questions to them. As much as possible all staff were included in all notices, correspondence and issues through being copied in email. Data and information was stored in a shred drive on the computer server, but staff was not directed to go to the server, they were sent the information. The server stored information for retrieval.
Managing the undertaking requires clarity as to who will have data input privileges, strategic input, subjective input and finally decision making power. In this case, all staff were invited to all

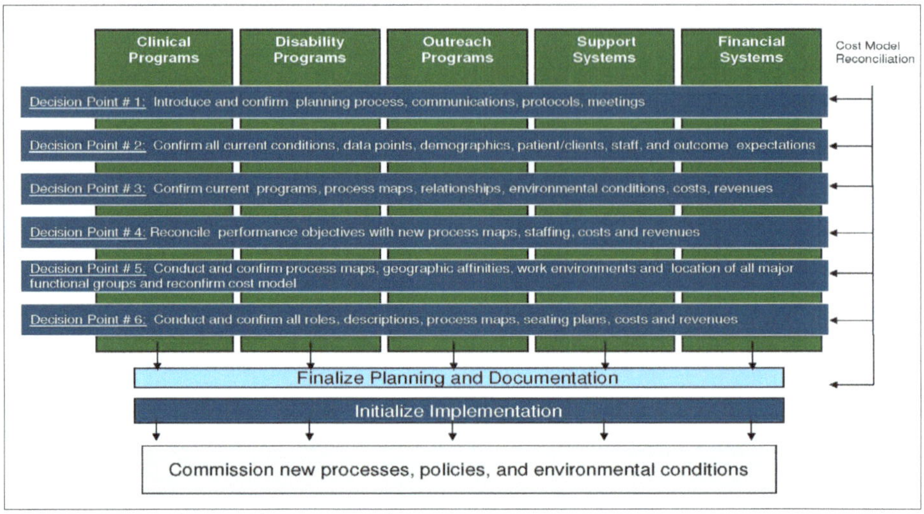

Figure 15. Integrated six step decision point planning process.

meetings for input, review and comment, and the supervisors and managers were expected to be in attendance. The Executive Director made all final decisions and participated in all meetings which greatly accelerated the process.
In addition the data and thoughts were all captured or posted 'on the wall' and created a transparency in the planning process such that for all staff who could not make it to the meetings would be able to understand the direction and detail of the planning and its' progress. In addition there was a separate section of wall relegated to issues and all staff were invited to pin up thoughts and issues which were discussed for resolution so that planning would be based on a solid and well resolved foundation.

Decision Points 2 through 4: the organization of data so this process could achieve success was based on the five areas contained in Problem Seeking, mentioned earlier. These five categories are shown in Figure 16.

1. Establish **Goals**
2. Collect & Analyze **Facts**
3. Uncover & Test **Concepts**
4. Determine **Needs**
5. State the **Problem**

Figure 16. Problem seeking data organizational structure. Source: Problem Seeking by William Pena.

Data containing demographics, disorders, patients, staff, expenses, comparative analysis regarding other agencies, projections, were all captured and tested in the planning sessions. A critical step in the planning process is to have a shared memory of data based on facts not assumptions. Without this, the decisions made are subject to change because of a different basis of understanding the facts regarding the matter.
While there was considerable computer based data analysis it has been found that a system of "low tech – high touch"

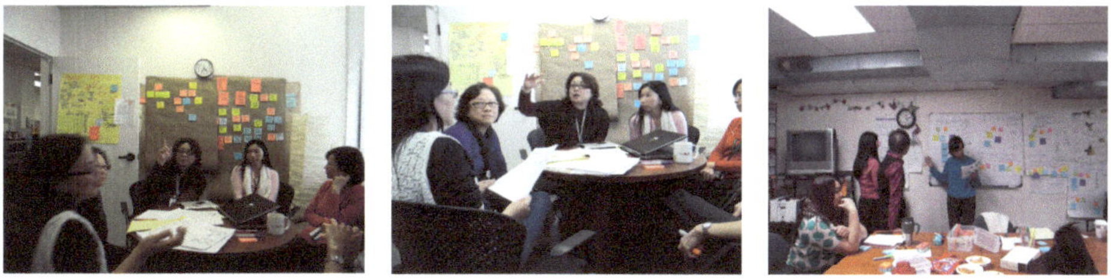

Figure 17. ACMHS programming, planning, process mapping sessions. Source: ACMHS.

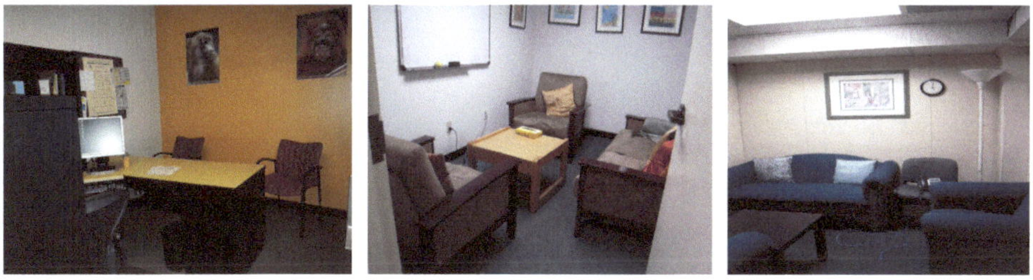

Figure 18. Alternative counseling spaces – PATH office vs. ACMHS rooms.

graphics and communications was more effective in opening up conversation with staff, providers and consumers. As such, the analysis cards are limited to one thought each, with the ability to focus on one issue or fact and the group can agree or disagree. Thus keep or dismiss the information as relevant to the planning.

Post-it notes were used to help analyze current activities, processes and flows. Groups large and small met to validate and confirm information and to develop concepts for process maps and planning criteria (Figure 17).

Part of the analysis and confirmation stage involved the space, environmental conditions, and operational models for space use. There are two basic forms of facility organization for mental health counseling/treatment facilities. In simple terms, there are shared treatment or counseling rooms where the clinician or provider meets with the patient/client and the clinician's office is elsewhere; such as at ACMHS. In other settings, the clinician has an office where the patient is seen; such as the PATH program in Oakland, California. In other settings there are shared spaces or counseling/treatment rooms (Figure 18).

At ACMHS there are a series of rooms, all different. As a part of an effort to review the effectiveness of the operations, processes, and to be able to establish guidelines for planning an evaluation of the treatment spaces was conducted. Using an integrated and lean process, the survey of spaces was developed which included clinicians and clients/patients as participants. Two processes were used. Both an interview process and a voting process were used to establish preferences and opinions.

The entire clinical staff was asked to participate along with the Consumer Advisory Board composed of client/patients. For the graphic voting technique each participant was given five dots of five colors. Each color represented a range from excellent to poor. They reviewed

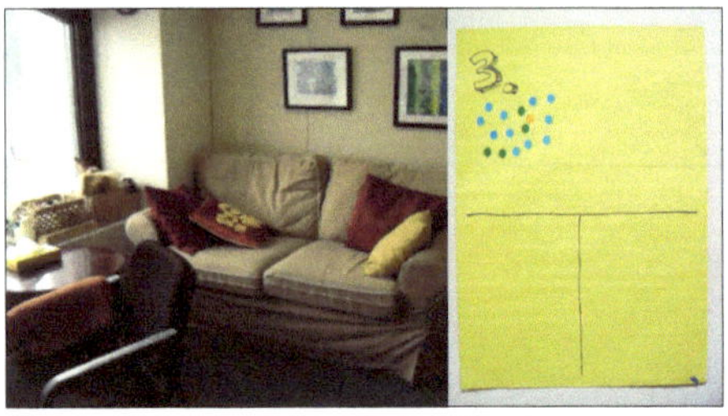

Figure 19. Evaluation of the favorite counseling space, Room 3. Source: ACMHS.

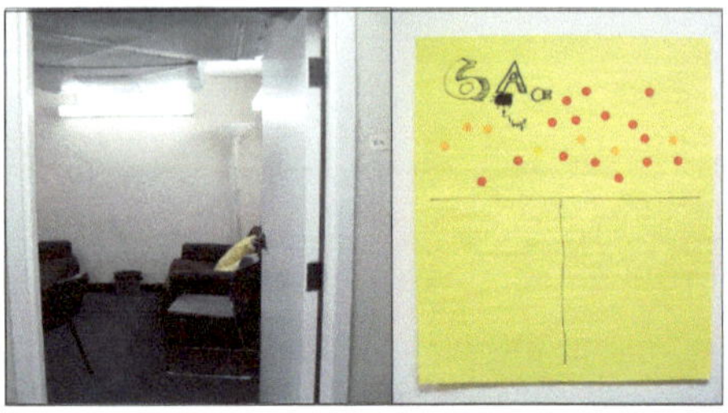

Figure 20. Evaluation of the most disliked counseling space, Room 6A. Source: ACMHS.

and scored eleven rooms by placing the dots on a scoring sheet in front of the room. The fact that they were given five dots and not eleven was planned. The participants were to evaluate the ones they liked and most disliked.

In addition to the dots, a large pouch was also placed in front of the room. Comment cards and writing instruments were available next to the pouch. Comments were encouraged. Room 3 received the highest number of excellent blue dots while room 6A had the poorest marks - red dots (Figure 19-20).

The comments were primarily in five major categories on both the comment cards and in the interviews and were as follows: Lighting, Room Size, Furnishings, Equipment, Color. Aside from general comments, nothing became a particular driver for planning and design. Natural lighting (windows to the exterior) was a major desire. The room sizes, while all different were not an issue. Furnishings continued to favor lounge chair seating as opposed to an office like seating. While the room with natural lighting, Room 3, was favored the second most desired room was one with bright colors, Room 10 (Figure 21).

The process led to a plan for a future

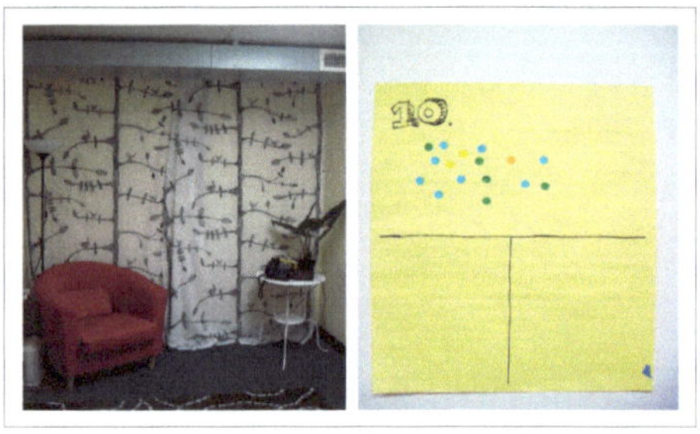

Figure 21. Evaluation of the second most liked counseling space, Room 10. Source: ACMHS.

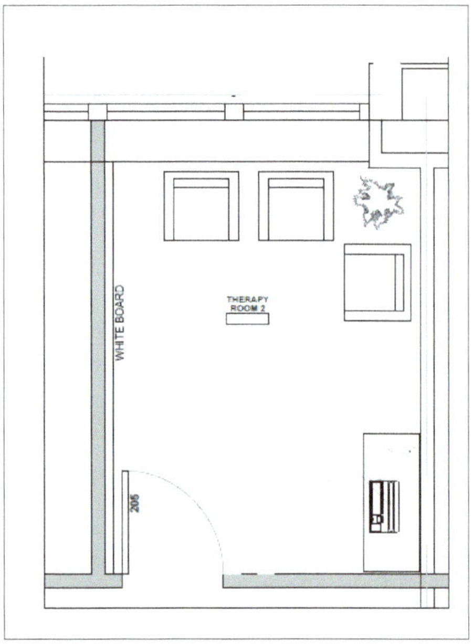

Figure 22. New planned ACMHS counseling space with a yellow arrow showing the ability for the clinician to leave the room quickly if the client became violent. Source: ACMHS.

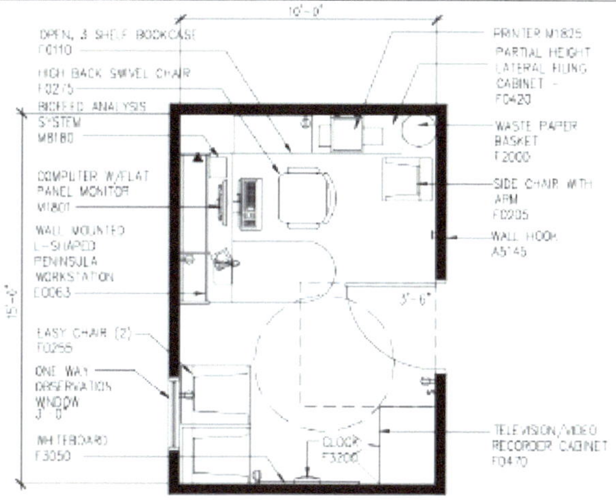

Figure 23. Example of a VA design guideline space showing the difficulty for the clinician to leave quickly if the client shown as the red arrow blocks the clinician shown as the yellow arrow. Source: Veterans Administration, Office of Design and Construction, Design Guidelines.

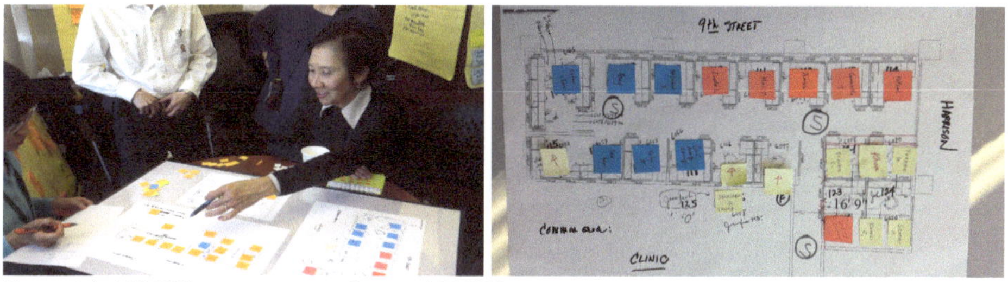

Figure 24. ACMHS gaming session. Source: ACMHS.

treatment or counseling room. The conclusion is a simple yet elegant room shown in Figure 22. The location of the clinician near the door is a critical element for safety and need for the clinician to be able to exit in an emergency. Other plans were analyzed from published guidelines were unacceptable because of these same issues where the clinician can be blocked from exiting (Figure 23).

Decision Point 5: following the development of the typical counseling room the process used 'gaming' to establish locational and affinity plans for the operational groups and then the spaces within those groups (Figure 24). Gaming led to the formation of conceptual responses including the development of additional naturally lit treatment/counseling rooms (shown in purple) and a larger and more inviting waiting/reception room (shown in beige), as shown in Figure 25.

Decision Point 6: the final process is a review of the conceptual plans and reaffirmation of all the previous decisions including restatement of goals, confirmation of facts which drive patient loads, tests of concepts including the process maps for each function, review of needs including staffing and resources, and finally the confirmation of the statements of the problem which then lead into final reviews and design documentation (Figure 26).

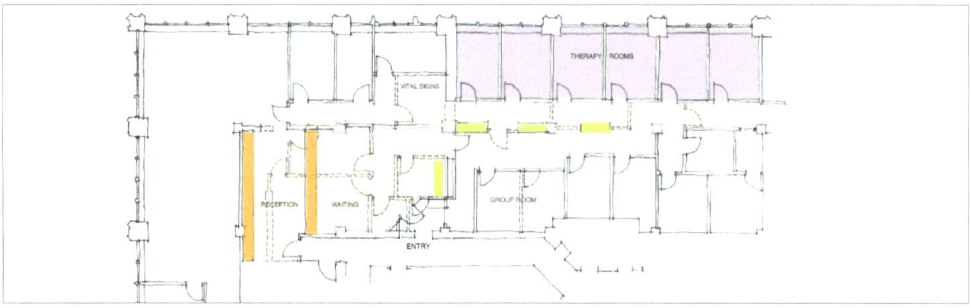

Figure 25. Conceptual plan for new treatment/counseling rooms and a new waiting/reception room. Source: ACMHS.

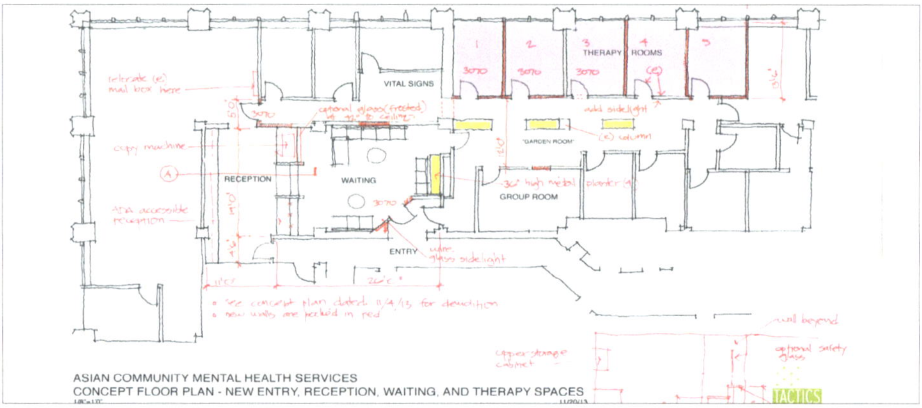

Figure 26. Review and Confirmation of Conceptual Plans. Source: ACMHS.

SUMMARY

While this paper has not provided comprehensive guidelines for mental health facilities, it has highlighted the following:

1. Mental health is an important part of communities and health care. And now mental health care is an equal to primary health care as defined by the new Patient Protection and Affordable Care Act.

2. Mental health care operations and facilities are different than physical health or primary care and as such require different responses.

3. Counseling and treatment space in mental health care facilities must be developed with a concentration on the behavioral health client and the security of the clinician.

4. Lean and integrated processes such as Problem Seeking and Bioteaming methodologies are well suited to the evaluation, analysis, and decision management which leads to effective planning and design of mental health facilities.

5. Interactive participation and transparency of all information by posting on the walls so that all parties can participate is important to durable decisions.

Diseases of the soul are more dangerous and more numerous than those of the body ~ Cicero

Case Study - Revitalization of Army Facility Complex for the Purpose of Mental Care Hospital – Idrija, Slovenia

Gabrijel Arko, Andrej Bohinc

andrej.bohinc@gmail.com, info@a-arhitekt.com
Atelje-arhitekt d.o.o., Slovenia

City of Idrija, one of the UNESCO heritage sites (mercury mine), is the location of the case study. The site was built in 1933 for the purpose of military defence complex and later in 1953 changed its purpose into health care facility. In 1994 the complete reconstruction of the complex began. The site located on the top of the hill above the city consists of five buildings. The nursing wards in buildings L and S were reconstructed from 1994 to 1997. The remaining building A (which will be presented in more detail) was reconstructed in 2009-2010. The purpose of the reconstruction was to create a suitable space for in- and out- patient therapy and daily activities covering the total of 3,251 m² gross area including the outside terrace. The building was carefully refurbished and special colouring scheme was made in accordance with the program and available budget. Designing projects like this is a challenge for every architect searching for sustainable way of creating a new environment out of the existing building. Reconstructions are usually a more difficult way of creating a project, especially if you have to deal with health care with its emphasis on functionality and long-term cost. The intention of the project team was to create buildings and environment, in general, for people with mental health problems where they can feel appreciated and part of the community through delivering programs for revitalization, working areas, recreational facilities, open hospital wards and space for out-patients during day care, all with one goal to try to deinstitutionalize the existing system of mental health following the guidelines of Psychiatric hospital of Idrija Spes, Amor and Libertas in translation hope, love and freedom in the end.

Keywords: *healthcare, mental healthcare, reconstruction, Slovenia.*

Introduction

The paper starts with general data regarding country and its health care system and continues with the case study of revitalization of army facility complex for the purpose of mental care hospital in the town of Idrija, Slovenia with the basic data, program in general, statistics, historical background, description of the site, a more detailed description of reconstruction of the last central building A of the complex and description of works in progress with conclusion. Designing projects like this is a challenge for every architect searching for sustainable way of creating a new environment out of the existing building. Reconstructions are usually a more difficult way of creating a project, especially if you have to deal with health care with its emphasis on functionality and long-term cost. In this project we were also dealing with a certain stigma that surrounds mental health in general, not only the patients and working staff but also us as architects. In order to break the silence on this matter we decided to meet the challenge and create a beautiful setting for the patients as well as for the staff and visitors.

FACTS ON SLOVENIA

Slovenia is a small country (20,273 km^2) located in Central Europe between Austria and Hungary in the north, Italy in the west, Croatia in the east and the Adriatic Sea in the south.
In 1991 Slovenia, formerly a constituent part of Yugoslavia, declared independence.
In 2004 Slovenia entered the EU – European community and the NATO.
In 2007 Slovenia entered EURO zone and introduced EURO as its official currency.
In 2010 Slovenia entered the OECD.
The population estimate for 2010 is 2,005,136 (7/2010 est.).
The main demographic characteristics in Slovenia are low birth rate, a low fertility rate and a low rate of population growth. The birth rate decreased from 13.1 per 1,000 inhabitants in 1985 to 8.97 per 1,000 inhabitants in 2010.
Life expectancy at birth in Slovenia for total population is 76.92 years (2010 est). (73.25 years for males and 80.84 years for females. (2010 est)).
Proportion of health care budget to GDP is 8.3% .
Total health spending per capita is 2,329 USD in 2008.

SLOVENIA HEALTH CARE SYSTEM

Main system of financing and coverage

The base is a compulsory health insurance system. Slovenia maintains a Bismarck-type health care system which was introduced for workers as an extension of compulsory accident insurance system in 1888. The health insurance of Slovenia (HIIS) was created as a public and not-for-profit entity strictly supervised by the state and bound by statute to provide compulsory health insurance to the population.

Voluntary health insurance

Voluntary health insurance was introduced in 1993. It was designed to diversify funding sources. There is no substitute or voluntary full-coverage schemes since opting out of the compulsory system is not permitted. Voluntary insurance in Slovenia can provide supplementary insurance and covers co-payments within the compulsory system levied on certain services and/or additional (non-standard) health care benefits depending on individual insurance policies.

Health care delivery system

Health care capacity is structured at three levels: primary, secondary and tertiary.

At the primary level, health care centres provide health care to the population of one or several communities. Specialist care at the secondary level is organized in regional general hospitals, hospitals covering specific specialities and specialist out-patient practice organized within hospitals or health care centres or as independent practices (private specialist practices – see above). The tertiary care level includes university hospitals and institutes performing highly specialized services, education, research, transfer of knowledge and development. Tertiary care services are generally organized on national level.

Social care

Community nursing services are organized in all local communities and are based in health care centres. Homes for elderly and disabled people provide long-term health care. The level of care for chronically ill and incapacitated patients is relatively high in these institutions. Nearly all these homes are public. Most of post-war architecture was based or organised within existing buildings, not primarily engineered for hospital purposes, which were reconstructed several times during decades. Most of modern health care buildings were built in the 1960s, starting with the construction of University Clinical Centre in the capital of Ljubljana. Today very few hospitals are being built. Most of them are reconstructed.

Psychiatric care

Mental health is part of primary health care system. Actual treatment of severe mental disorders is available at the primary level. There are community care facilities for patients with metal disorder.

Non-governmental organizations and associations are provideing out-patient community care for their patients. Together with the psychiatric profession they are involved in the preventive, mainly anti stigma programs with housing facilities with support, day centres, vocational rehabilitation development, sheltered employments and educational facilities for patients and carers. There are all together six regional psychiatric hospitals and one psychiatric clinic. All have wards for general psychiatry, psycho-geriatrics and the treatment of alcohol addiction. (Source: Mental Health Atlas 2005, WHO Geneva).

Case study: Psychiatric Hospital Idrija. Reconstruction of the Existing Building Complex

Program in general

Hospital provides mental health treatment and care for people with acute or non-acute mental disorders. Hospital is also responsible for professional and organizational development of psychiatric science in general and represents a training base for staff working in or out of the hospital. As part of its operations hospital provides general psychiatric care, elderly psychiatric care, treatment of alcoholism and other substances addiction, adolescent psychiatric care and forensic care.
Out-patient activities include special psychiatric treatment to patients in hospital and outside hospital, in dispensaries, in the community, day hospital and at home.

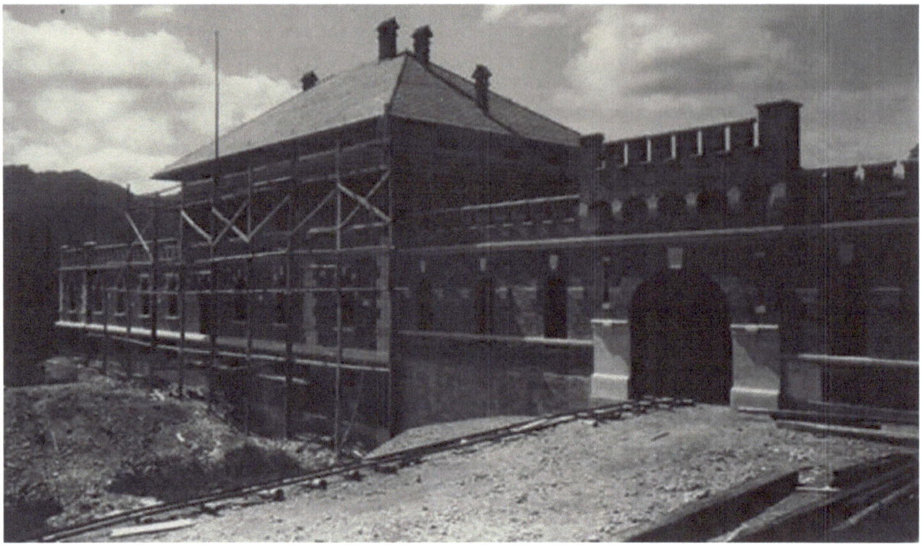

Figure 1. View of the original building – military defence complex.

Statistics

Number of beds: 175 in 2009.
One, two or four patient bedroom depending on the program.
Average duration of stay: 39.11 days in 2009.

Historical background

In between years 1928 and 1932 Kingdom of Italy built a powerful military defence complex "Caserma di fanteria Costantino Brighenti". The complex of military buildings was opened on 5th April, 1933 and was considered to be the greatest Italian army complex, built on the Italian eastern border with Yugoslavia, originally designed to house 4,000 Italian soldiers (Figure 1).

After the Second World War in July 1953 the government decided to rebuild the complex for the needs of mental health services. Hospital had 450 in-patient beds available. In one room there were six, seven or ten patient beds. Average length of stay was 365 days. PH Idrija is now the second largest psychiatric hospital in Slovenia. In the period from 1994 to 2010 hospital renovated all nursing facilities with 220 beds, activation therapy facilities, hospital pharmacy, laboratory, dispensary, hospital kitchen, etc.

Description of the site

The site located on the top of the hill above the city of Idrija consists of five buildings. Three of them belong entirely to the psychiatric hospital, the entrance building is partly owned by private residents, ground floor by Psychiatric Hospital. The remaining building is used as a service area. The nursing wards in buildings L and S were reconstructed from 1994 to 1997. The remaining building A was reconstructed from 2009 to 2010. In this time Psychiatric Hospital Idrija has renovated cca. 9,124 m^2 or 90% of all areas that are exclusively intended for in-patient care (Figure 2-4).

Reconstruction of the last pavilion A in 2010

The purpose of reconstruction was to create a suitable space for in- and out-patient therapy and daily activities covering the total of 3,251 m^2 gross area including the outside terrace. Due to its nature the building was carefully refurbished and special colouring scheme was made in accordance with the program and the available budget. Program of the building was determined by the user and followed the following order:

- the basement consists of service areas, wardrobes for the staff, working therapy for the patients (carpenters);
- the ground floor consists of kitchen and dining area for patients and staff;
- the first floor consists of activation therapy, library, computer room and outside terrace.

The attic consists of day hospital with individual therapy, examination room, multipurpose hall and office space for the administration in the attic. The construction itself included complete reconstruction of the attic including floors, walls, ceilings, appropriate thermo insulation and renovation of the roof. Levels below kept the bearing walls. Everything else was made anew according to the program, including new staircase, elevator, toilets and appropriate fire prevention sectors. Windows and the facade were renovated according to the National Heritage Preservation Institute (Figure 5-8).

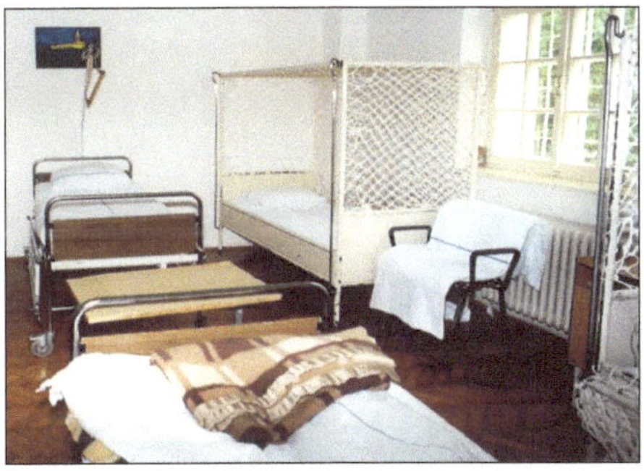

Figure 2. View of the typical patient room before the renovation began.

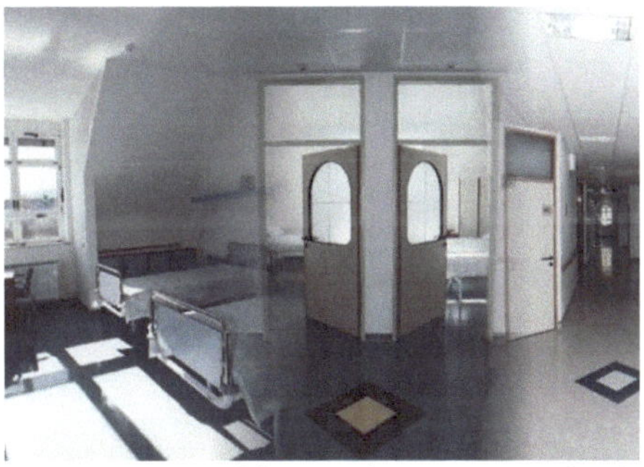

Figure 3. View of the typical patient room after the renovation of the S building in 1997.

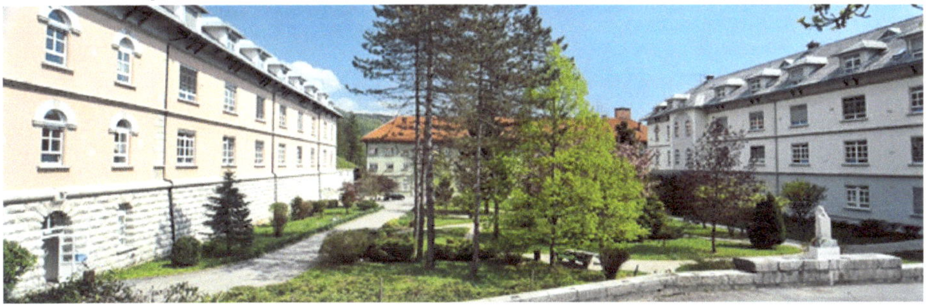

Figure 4. View from the A building of the renovated courtyard and adjacent buildings L and S with nursing wards.

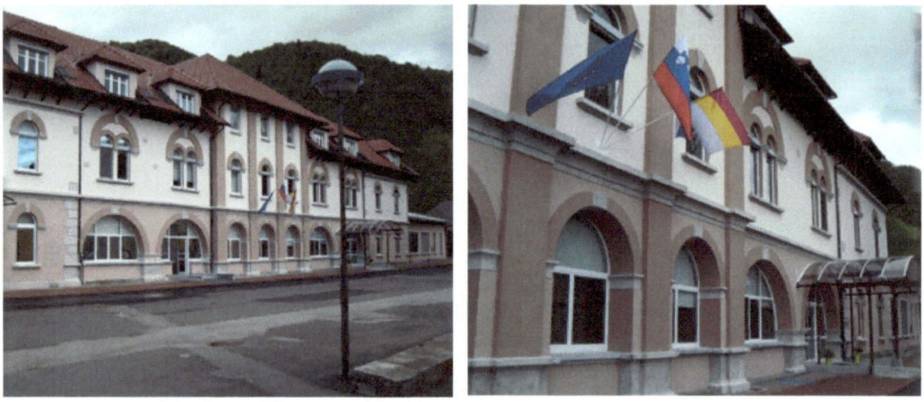

Figure 5. View of the front of the renewed building A.

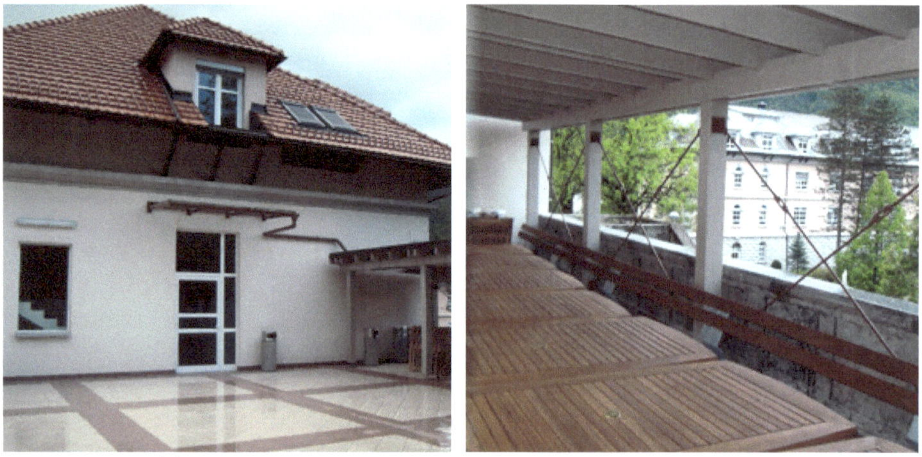

Figure 6. View of the terrace.

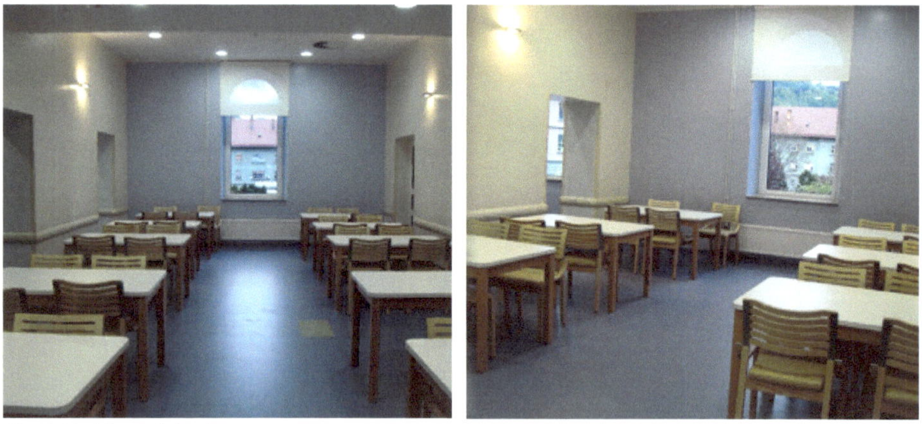

Figure 7. View of the dining room.

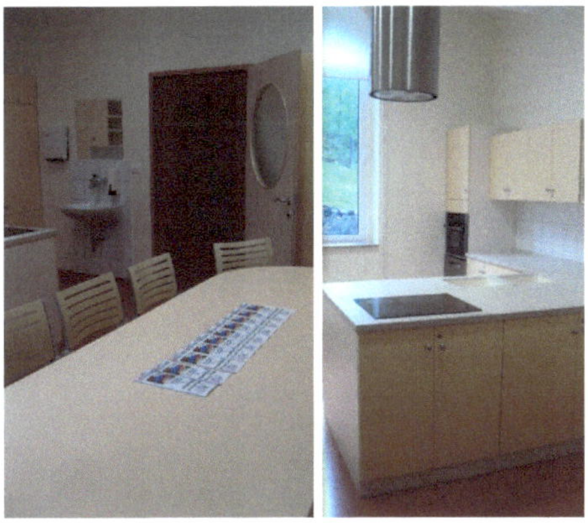

Figure 8. View of the working therapy room.

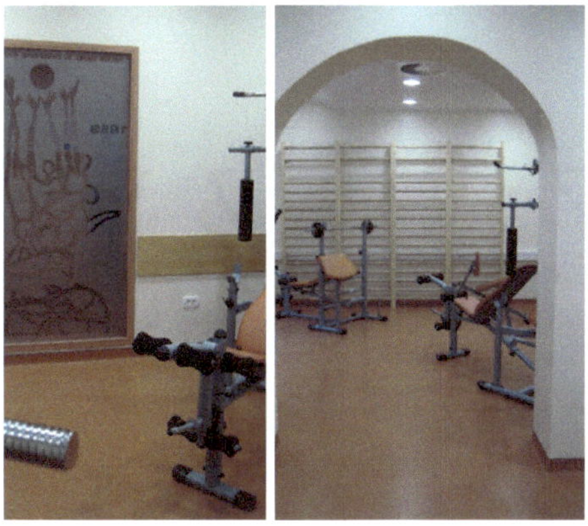

Figure 9. View of the working therapy room– fitness.

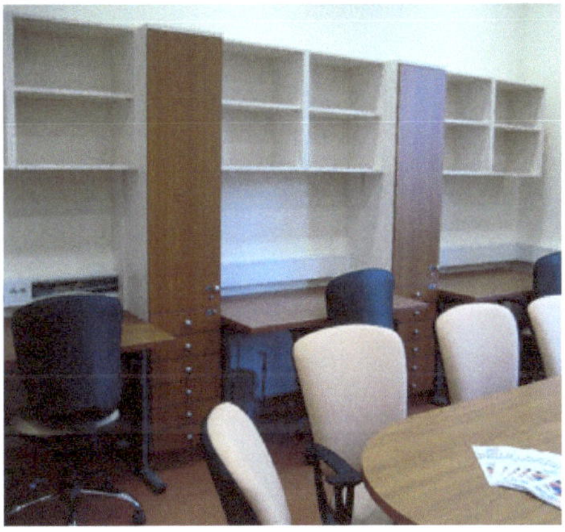

Figure 10. View of the working therapy room.

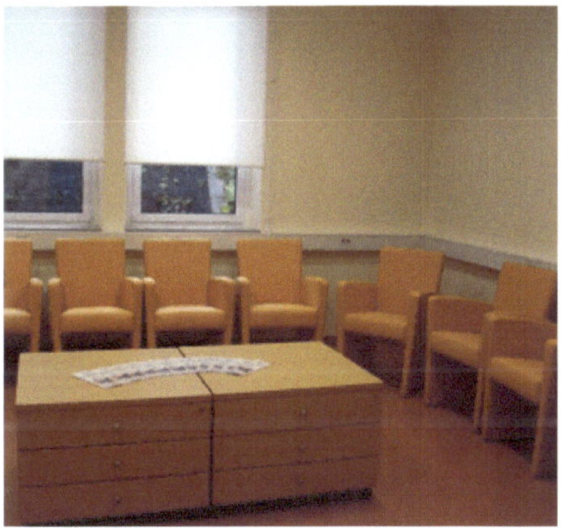

In between years 2010 and 2014 renovation of biochemical laboratory in hospital was finished.

The general dispensary unit from Idrija was relocated to the main hospital building. The asbestos roofing on all central hospital buildings was replaced.
Reconstruction of the auxiliary building, that includes service area, warehouse, visiting relative's area with small shop and a gallery, is currently under reconstruction.

Conclusions

The intention of the project team was to create buildings and environment, in general, for people with mental health problems where they can feel appreciated and part of the community through delivering programs for revitalization, working areas, recreational facilities, open hospital wards and space for outpatients during day care, all with one goal to try to deinstitutionalize the existing system of mental health.

REFERENCES

European observatory on Health Care system, *Health Care systems in Transition*, Vol.4., No.3., 2002.

Photos: personal archive Atelje-arhitekt d.o.o., Arhe d.o.o. Ljubljana, Slovenia. Psihiatrična bolnišnica Idrija, Ustvarjalnost in duševne motnje, 2010.

Trstenjak Anton, Psihologija barv, Ljubljana, Inštitut Antona Trstenjaka, 1996
Tušar Bogdan, Psychiatric hospital Idrija presentation material.

WHO (2005). Geneva, *Mental health Atlas.*

www.cia.gov
www.oecd.org
www.pb-idrija.si

Draft Guidelines for Mental Health Infrastructure

Awaatief Railoun

RailoA@health.gov.za
Hons BA (Cur) Registered Nurse, National Department of Health, Facilities and Planning, Infrastructure Unit, South Africa

The Mental Healthcare Act no 17 of 2002 was promulgated in 2002 and with this Act there was very little guidance for its implementation. Since then, the Mental Health Policy Framework and the National Strategic Plan 2013-2020 was developed and approved by the National Health Council in July 2013 and the development of Draft Guidelines Norms and Standards for Infrastructure in 2014.

For the past eleven years, provinces implemented the Mental Health Act as best as they were able to without the guidance from the National Department of Health. Hence, this resulted in mental health being delivered in not fit for purpose mental health units in health facilities in South Africa.

South African health care facilities are situated in various districts, in all the provinces. Mental health is a special area of a wide range of clinical areas that is offered by these health facilities. When the Mental Health Act no 17 of 2002 was promulgated, the mental health service was implemented but there were no technical guidelines as to how the facilities that render these services should look or how they should be designed. Thus, most health facilities that render mental health are in a very bad condition. This is reflected in a health facilities audit that was done in 1996 by CSIR and those reports indicated that all the mental health facilities and some general health facilities needed to be replaced.

Keywords: *mental health, healthcare facilities, South Africa.*

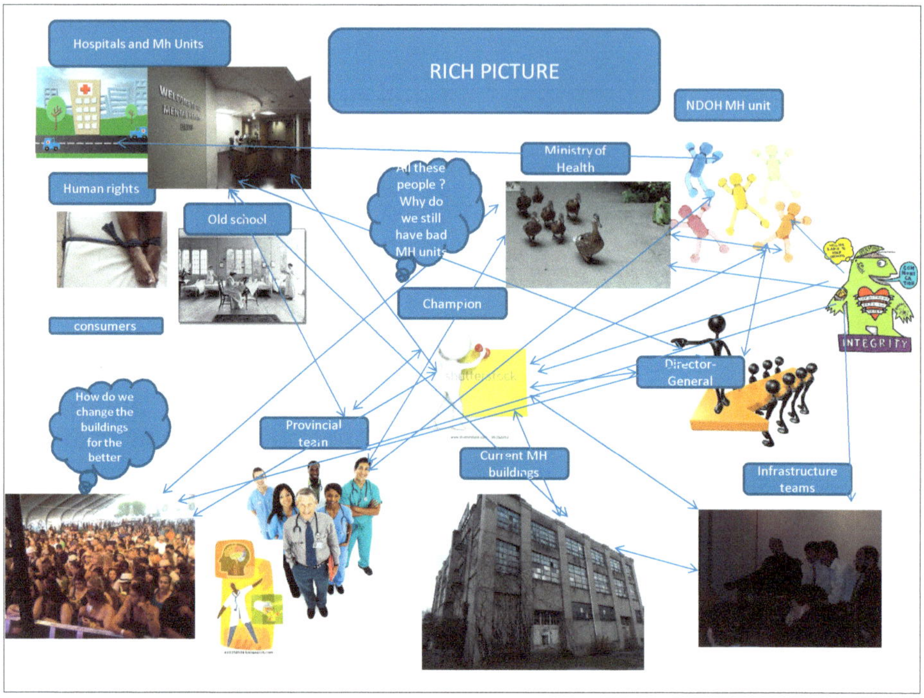

Mental Health Strategic Framework 2013-2020.

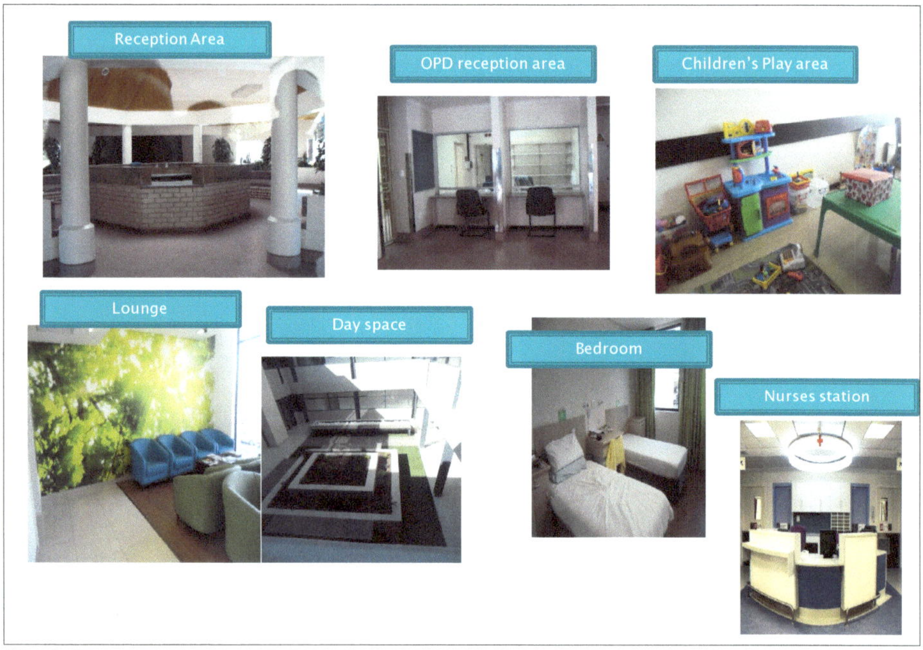

New look.

Planning and Design Healthcare in Developing and Newly Industrialized Countries

Session introduction

Designing facilities for care and health promotion in developing and newly industrialized countries is a great challenge for designers and researchers specialized in the healthcare sector. The task requires having a vision that stretches from the general framework of health policies to construction detail, in an area where all the design choices have a variety of implications that affect the different project scales.

This session highlighted how in emerging countries it is necessary to identify the most suitable types of buildings for healthcare linked to the political and economic healthcare plan. The types of existing buildings in developing countries should be compared to project models already adopted in other parts of the world. Classifying the existing facilities is the first step in providing a knowledge base for the development of plans to improve and implement care buildings. It is therefore necessary to apply the analysis methods, both qualitative and quantitative, developed in academic research.

Spontaneous building types developed over time are models that can give designers valuable suggestions for maximizing the use of resources in the area. The spontaneous architectural buildings take into account the climatic characteristics of the area and make the most of the orientation of the rooms to ensure proper lighting and natural ventilation. In this context the use of local materials is a choice that helps to give the facility a familiar look, respects the identity of the places and uses the resources available near the building construction sites. Furthermore, the use of local labour in the construction of the works is an important factor that helps to increase the ability to recognize and have confidence in healthcare environments.

Strengthening primary healthcare and activities related to the promotion of health is an important step towards achieving the desired equity of care. In this scenario the designer has the dual task of interpreting the needs of the local population and playing an active role in the development programs implemented by the political authorities, identifying the types of intervention possible on existing assets or developing new configurations to meet the changes imposed by the evolution of care.

Urban Primary Health Care for Poor and Disadvantaged Population in Bangladesh
Addressing Planning and Design Issues

Jasmin Ara Begum

jasmin.arch@aust.edu
Professor, Department of Architecture, Ahsanullah University of Science and Technology (AUST), Dhaka, Bangladesh

The rapid urbanisation caused mainly by rural-urban migration with a population growth rate of 5% is posing a threat to the living environment and health in the urban areas of Bangladesh. Around 60% population of Bangladesh will reside in urban areas by the year 2050. The national health policy, 2011 stressed the need for providing urban primary health care, especially for poor, disadvantaged and unemployed persons. The demography and epidemiology, behavioural pattern, living norms and so on of urban poor are quite different in Bangladesh. So, special attention needs to be given while planning and designing urban health care facilities for poor and disadvantaged populations. However, there are no clear guidelines for planning and design of health care facilities in general and urban health care in particular in Bangladesh. The paper will focus on urban primary health care facility planning and design issues and guidelines. The paper begins by looking at the existing health care planning and design of public health facilities in Bangladesh, identifying problems and important issues specific to urban areas. It will also try to gather knowledge from other developing countries. A sample case study will be carried out to identify the problem areas which could be developed further for future study. The final section explores ways of developing guidelines taking account of problems identified through case study and literature search with recommendation on planning and design of urban primary health care, especially for poor and disadvantaged populations.

Keywords: *Urban Primary Health Care, urban poor, planning, design, guidelines.*

Introduction

In 2011, with a population of 152.51 million and 939 persons per square kilometre, Bangladesh was the eighth largest nation and one of the poorest countries in the world. The population doubling time is 25 years which shows a rapid increase in population. The rapid urbanisation caused mainly by rural-urban migration with a population growth rate of 5% is posing a threat to the living environment and health in the urban areas of Bangladesh. Around 60% of the population of Bangladesh will reside in urban areas by the year 2050. The national health policy of 2011 stressed the need for providing urban primary health care, especially for poor, disadvantaged and unemployed persons. The demography and epidemiology, behavioural pattern, living norms and so on of urban poor are quite different in Bangladesh. So, special attention needs to be given while planning and designing urban health care facilities for poor and disadvantaged populations.

There is a lack of organized data, adequate research, planning guidelines and standards in relation to health facilities. There is also a lack of communication between user, client, and planning and design team. Improving this situation is essential for the proper development of health facilities in Bangladesh. Proper interaction, communication and programs between private, volunteer and public health services are also needed to avoid duplication of facilities.

Despite the great effort of the Government and non government organizations, the existing primary health care facilities could not achieve their desired goal due to lack of resources, faith on the part of the users, proper planning and design guidelines. The existing problems and priorities of health care and the need for planning and design guidelines are the underlying reasons for choosing the subject as an area for study.

The aim and objectives of the research were the following:

1. To conduct a physical and functional evaluation of sample urban public primary health centres to get feedback information for planning and design of future health centres and to improve the existing facilities.
2. To identify planning and design problems, issues and guidelines of urban PHC facilities in Bangladesh.
3. Based on a literature survey and sample survey of existing urban PHC facilities, identify planning and design issues and develop recommendation.

The overall aim of this paper is to present the important findings of the evaluation in the area of planning and design of urban PHC facilities for the poor and disadvantaged population in Bangladesh. The proposed planning and design guidelines would be useful for future planners, designers and users of PHC facilities in Bangladesh as well as other developing countries.

HEALTH SITUATION IN BANGLADESH

The demographic profile of Bangladesh indicates a high percentage of young and dependent people (Figure 1). The crude birth rate and infant mortality rate are very high compared to other countries.

The Table 1 shows the basic health statistics of Bangladesh.

The main causes of health problems in Bangladesh are a low level of nutrition and social economy which are further deteriorating due to rapid population growth and high illiteracy. Malnutrition and infectious diseases occupy a

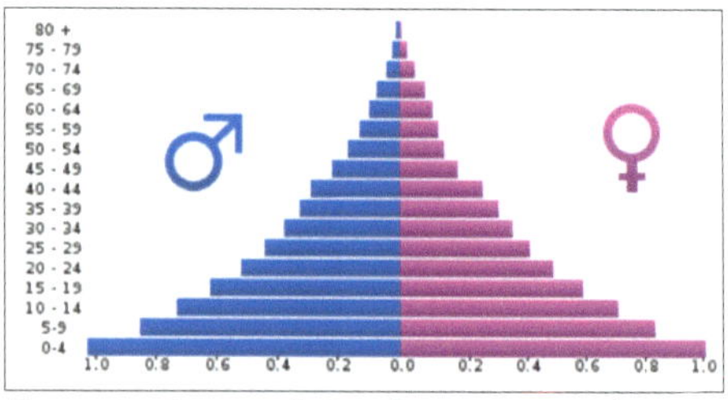

Figure 1. Image of Population Pyramid 2005, Bangladesh.

Health Parameters	Statistics	Health Parameters	Statistics
The % of the population under the age of 15 and above 65	36.2 and 6.5	Total expenditure as a % of GDP	0.63 in 1981-82 3.1 in 2006
The sex ratio of the population In 2007	105 male to 100 female	No of doctors No of nurses	1 per 4719 1 per 8226
Life expectancy at birth	45yrs (1965), 65.4yrs (2007)	No of beds	0.3
Life expectancy of Male and Female:	64.4 years and 66.0 years	No of gov. hospitals No of private hospitals	671 1005
The birth rate, death rate, annual growth rate in 2007	2.06%, 0.56%,1.41%	No of teaching hospitals No of post graduate instit.	14 5
The under-5 mortality rate and maternal mortality rate	54 per 1000 30 per 1000	Upazilla Health Complex UHFWC	402 1362
Total fertility rate	2.47	Specialized hospital	31

Table 1. Source: BBS, 2008.

high rate etiologically. Malnutrition is widespread among children and expectant and lactating mothers. Over half of the population is considered to be below the poverty level in terms of minimum caloric requirements (2122 kcal per person per day). The average daily calorie intake per person in Bangladesh reduced from 1964 kcal in 1965 to 1894 kcal in 2006 (Food Security Atlas 2006). Heavy rainfall during monsoon and inadequate drainage system accelerates the spread of communicable diseases. About one-fifth of the total admissions suffered from the group of conditions comprising injuries, accidents, burns and fractures.There is a great scarcity of health resources in Bangladesh. The per capita expenditure on health is probably one of the lowest in the world.

EXISTING HEALTH CARE PLANNING AND DESIGN

Since the independence of Bangladesh, there has been significant progress in health outcomes with an emphasis on Primary Health Care (PHC) and an improvement in health indicators.

At present, health services are delivered in three distinct patterns:

i. The centralized public system based upon the concept of Regionalized Health Care with a system of referral from the small sub-centre all the way to the urban based hospital.

ii. Scattered private services ranging from community co-operative health insurance plans to individual private physician care, non government organizations (NGO), private clinics and nursing homes.

iii. Traditional services based upon folk beliefs and herbal treatment.

The public health care system in Bangladesh consists of four levels of care, i.e. primary, secondary, tertiary and specialized health care built on a regionalized model. Each of the regions with the teaching hospital at the apex of the organization has similar facilities and is expected to be self sufficient as far as primary, secondary and tertiary care are concerned.

i. Primary level health care is delivered through Health and Family Welfare Centres (HFWC) with one in each union domiciliary level, Upazilla/ Thana Health Complex (UHC/THC) with one in each Upazilla. These are the first referral level and integrated health and family planning services with field workers for every 3000-4000 population and 31 bed capacities in hospitals.

ii. Secondary level health care is provided through 100 bed capacities in a District Hospital. Facilities provide specialist services in internal medicine, general surgery, gynaecology, paediatrics and obstetrics, eye, clinical, pathology, blood transfusion and public health laboratories.

iii. Tertiary Level health care is available at the medical college hospital, public health and medical institutes and other specialist hospitals at the national level where a mass wide range of specialized as well as better laboratory facilities are available.

The government of Bangladesh pays for one third of the national health system from taxes and international subsidies. In order to develop a national insurance program, a number of NGO's have started to offer micro-credit medical programs.

URBAN PHC FOR A POOR AND DISADVANTAGED POPULATION

Bangladesh is facing rapid urbanization mainly due to rural-urban migration driven by better job opportunities, rural poverty, climate change and so on. The urban population rose from 19.8% in 1990 to 36.7% in 2008 with roughly 34.6 million (2006) people now living in urban areas. Urban areas with poor infrastructure can barely cope with this continuous urban population growth. Poor rural migrants mostly settle in slums, squats, or pavements with poor and unhealthy living conditions. There were more than 9000 slums in Bangladesh in 2005, mostly in Dhaka city, as recorded by a slum mapping project. The number of poor, disadvantaged and slum dwellers in urban areas is continuously growing.

SURVEY METHODOLOGY

The survey method and questionnaire was designed by the author based on the method used for her PhD research on Primary Health Care facilities (PHC) in Bangladesh (Begum 1994). Both the structured and unstructured questionnaire was carried out to get a comprehensive idea on functional facility and user opinion. The survey was conducted in January and February 2014.

SURVEY FINDINGS AND ANALYSIS

The patients and visitors get to the health centre by walking, rickshaw, auto rickshaw, car and bus. The services provided from the five UPHC centres are summarized as follows:

- MCH (including delivery of normal and caesarian cases, pre and post delivery care, MR, DNC and post care, Immunization, Care for new-born)
- General medical (male and female)
- Emergency
- Family Planning (F.P.)

- Treatment of viral and infectious diseases
- Pathology
- Counselling
- Field level services (preventive and promotive).

Out-patient Areas

Out-patient areas are the first point of contact between the people and the health facility. The out-patient areas of the centre have general medical care for male and female patients, MCH including under-five clinics, F.P. clinics, infectious disease and counselling services. Around 30 to 120 patients visit out-patient department per day in 5 different centres. The visiting hour for OPD is 9 am to 4 pm. Patients can walk in directly or visit on an appointment basis. They are registered at the front desk of the OPD. Services in the OPD are provided by MBBS doctors, paramedics and assisted by nurses (Figures 2-3). The counselling services covers violence against women, caring pregnancy, Family planning and Child care. All the health centres have dispensary facilities.

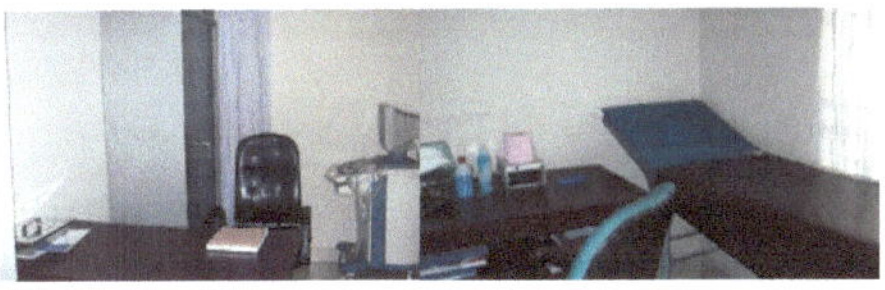

Figure 2. Out-patient consultation and examination.

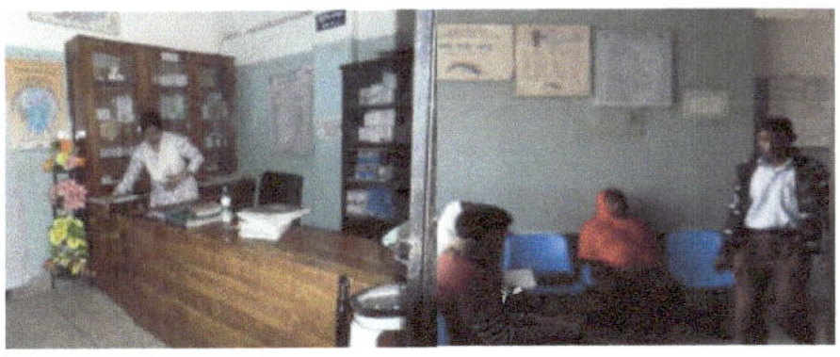

Figure 3. Out-patient reception and waiting.

In-patient accommodation

Patient accommodation consists of usually 6 to 12 beds, one for male patients and one for female and children. In addition there are 1 to 2 beds in a cabin for general inpatient, post operative recovery or for ante-natal and post natal care. During the survey, it was observed that the beds in 2 clinics are underutilized. One of the UPHC has no in-patient facilities (Figure 4).

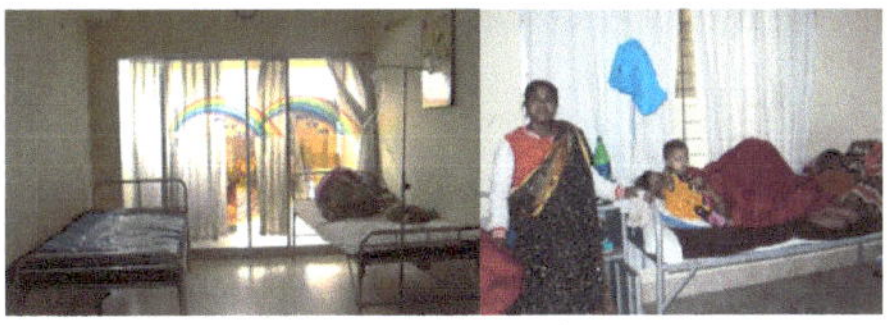

Figure 4. In-patient accommodation.

Patients are supervised regularly by 3 to 6 doctors and 6 to 15 nurses. The nurses work in 3 shifts: 9-15, 15-21 and 21-9. The ward areas have nurse-base/work station, usually close to bed areas. There are provisions for new born babies with a baby cot and one attendant; mostly the mother stays with the baby.

Laboratory

Routine laboratory tests of blood and urine are carried out in the laboratory space. Samples are collected in the laboratory. There is usually a toilet close to the laboratory (Figure 5).

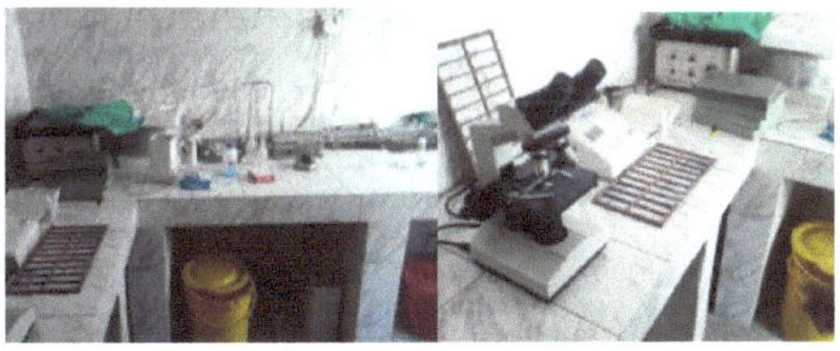

Figure 5. Pathology room.

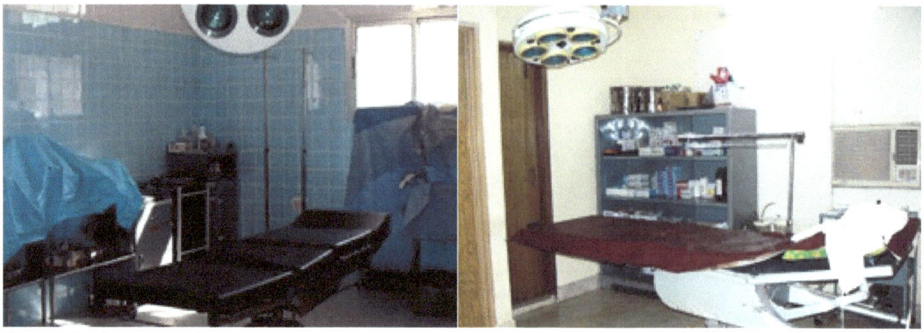

Figure 6. Operation theatre.

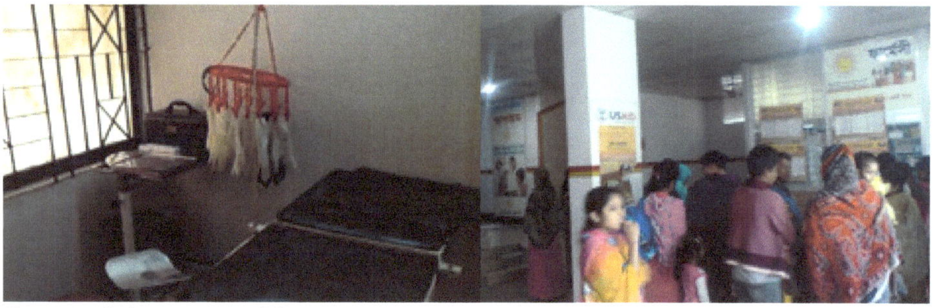

Figure 7. Delivery room and dispensary.

There were no Radiology or X-Ray facilities in any of the five health centres.

Operation and Delivery

Operation theatre functions mostly between 9 am to 9 pm. Types of cases dealt with are mostly general surgery, obstetrics and caesarean cases. There are 1 to 2 beds for recovery. The O.T.s have unit type air conditioners with adequate light and ventilation (Figure 6). The maintenance of O.T. and delivery rooms are generally poor and unhygienic (Figure 7). The maternity unit is attended by staff nurses. All the facilities like labour room, sluice, supply, disposal, ante natal and post natal beds are there with baby cots. The cleaning system is not at a satisfactory level.

Emergency

The daily average number of emergency patient is 2 to 10. The types of cases constitute mostly accidental cases, respiratory and abdominal cases (Figure 8). The health centres have their own ambulance service.

Support Services

There is a kitchen in all the health centres. Laundry of hospital linens is done out of house. Supply of drugs, vaccines, dressing, instruments, medical supplies and stationeries is bought as per requirement, usually after every 3 months. Hospital waste is collected and disposed in separate bins (Figure 9). Sterilization of theatre linen, O.T. instruments, gowns, masks and other items are done regularly.

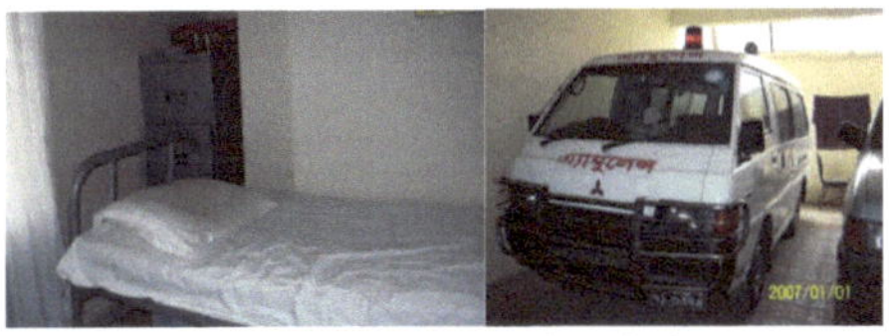

Figure 8. Emergency room and ambulance.

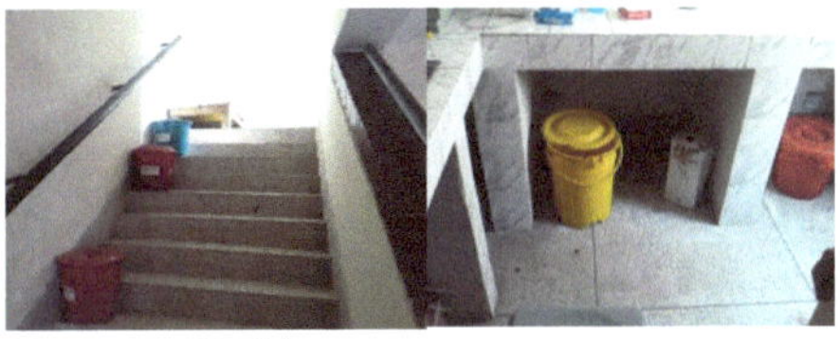

Figure 9. Health centre waste.

They have their own autoclave machine. Some disposable items are also used like gloves and syringes. The staff of the centre identified lack of adequate storage which forced them to store in different places, often causing congestion within activity spaces and circulation problems. All the UPHC centres, being in the capital city, have proper gas, electricity and piped water supply. The electricity is supplied by the Power Development Board.

The majority of clinics have no clear link with the upper levels of care that would be beneficial for patients to get referral to higher level of services. One study shows the patients attendance over the year and peak times. As a primary health care centre, the clinics provide services in the area of preventive, promotive and curative care.

The UPHC centres are mostly operating in rented premises. Thus, discussion on design intentions and design was not possible. Certain changes in the use of spaces were obviously made to satisfy the centres functional needs.

Segregation of sexes was worked out in the in-patient areas by separating male and female wards and also toilets for male and female patients are separate. The waiting area in the out-patient department is combined for both sexes which remains over-crowded most of the time.

Health centre waste is generally separated in different coloured buckets to separate sharp and infected items from non-infected items. The city corporation collects the non-infected waste on a daily basis and Prisom Bangladesh collects the infected and harmful items on a weekly basis. All the activity areas are cleaned by sweeping and mopping using disinfectants. The buildings are maintained by annual servicing and painting and quality of maintenance varies among the centres. There was not a single toilet which wheel chair users could use. A number of centres also do not have any lift or ramp for the use of differently able patients.

CONCLUSIONS AND RECOMMENDATIONS

The physical and functional evaluation was carried out on a full working day using a questionnaire, direct observation, photography, data entry and informal discussion with the users. A separate survey was conducted in a slum area by the author, to have a brief idea on user's background information.

The methods mentioned above helped to get a comprehensive picture about the UPHC centre in Bangladesh. The consequent analysis of the survey and other related information revealed the following conclusion and recommendations.

In order to decide the location of UPHC centres, it is necessary to map areas where poor and disadvantaged people reside in different urban areas. The catchment population for different UPHC centres may vary and the size and services may also vary according to demographic and epidemiological characteristics of the target population.

The surveyed UPHC centres are all functioning in rented premises and are not purpose built designed buildings. The Government of Bangladesh along with different NGOs had to address the immediate need for UPHC centres. But for long term planning and design, with the growth of population, changes in function, services and medical technology, the providers of UPHC centres will have to think about purpose built urban health facilities which can serve its catchment population for the life-time of the building.

Creating demand of UHC centres is another issue that needs to be addressed for proper utilization of services. The survey showed that the health centres could not attract a large number of the target population due to lack of knowledge about the services on the part of the users, health awareness, service provision, cost of health services and so on. Health Education is a mandatory part of UPHC centres. It is also necessary to identify users by their respective UPHC centres, that means bringing all users under the health care network.

Improving the living environment and healthy life style of the users is also important for better health care of the target group. Generally poor living environments, unsanitary built environments, water and sewerage system and climatic impact have an adverse effect on the health of poor people. So improving the living conditions of poor people needs to be addressed in time.

The rented premises lack a lot of desired qualities, an UPHC centre should have. In addition to the above broad issues, the following design issues are identified for the future planning and design of UPHC centres.

- The use of an outdoor planted yard or courtyard provides natural light, ventilation and excellent natural views to all the functional spaces. It helps to maintain a calm and peaceful environment which is physically and psychologically necessary for the recovery of patients.

- Ease of movement for the users (e.g. patients, staff and services) is an essential prerequisite for health facility design. The location of individual department and inter-departmental relationships is important for the planning and design of any health care facility. These relationships also need to be maintained even after future growth and change takes place.

- Use of appropriate disabled accessibility standards.

- Privacy of female patients should be acknowledged.

- Maintenance cost should be kept as low as possible.

- Low noise level, calm and quiet environment, especially for in-patient areas.

- The lack of adequate storage spaces in different functional areas caused storage in the corridor and within activity areas. It is also noticed that a health centre needs enough storage space to keep activity areas clean, tidy and usable.

- Multi-purpose spaces, in-door and outdoor, which are used for health education, training, recreation, meeting and a number of related functions are also essential for PHC facilities. None of the surveyed health centres had such meeting areas.

- Psychological healing of mother, children and other age groups by a healthy building environment is not taken care of in any of the surveyed UPHC centres. A number of them do not have natural light, ventilation and a view to nature outside. A good out-door and in-door relationship is essential for a healthy environment and natural healing process.

- Abundance of natural light and ventilation in each and every functional space require less use of artificial light and ventilation, thus reducing the operating costs of the centre.

- Use of Green Building concepts and technologies would reduce construction and maintenance costs. Waste management, rain-water collection, use of solar energy and other technologies could also reduce lifetime overhead and maintenance costs.

- Possibility for growth and change.

- Consideration of socio-cultural aspects of the users. The belief of the users in traditional medicine can be respected to bring users to the health centres.

The survey, physical and literature, with subsequent analysis undertaken, is believed to be useful for the future planning and design of PHC centres in Bangladesh and other developing countries . The successes and shortcomings of the functional UPHC would help to develop guidelines for use of PHC facility planners, designers and organizers and ultimately lead to more efficient built environment and users' satisfaction.

REFERENCES

Afsana K. and Wahid SS., 2013. Health care for poor people in the urban slums of Bangladesh, *The Lancet*, Vol. 382, Issue 9910, pp. 2049 – 2051.

Bangladesh Bureau of Statistics, 2005. *2005 Statistical Yearbook of Bangladesh*, 25th edition.

Bangladesh Bureau of Statistics, 2008. *2008 Statistical Yearbook of Bangladesh*, 28th edition.

Begum, JA Dr., 1994. *Primary Health Care facilities in Bangladesh – A method of planning and design taking account of limited resources, local technology, future growth and change*, unpublished PhD thesis submitted for the degree at the University of North London, UK.

CIA., *The World Fact Book*, viewed 20 October 2010.

Postill, J., 1983. Physical and functional evaluation of existing facilities, in WHO, *Approaches to planning and design of Health Care facilities in developing areas*, Vol. 4, WHO, Geneva.

Thwin, Aye Aye et al., 1996. *Health and demographic profile of the urban population of Bangladesh: An analysis of selected indicators*, International Centre for Diarrhoeal Disease Research, Bangladesh, ICDDRB, special publication no. 47.

Uddin MSG, & Kabir M., 2011. Factors associated with child health in urban areas of Bangladesh, *Journal of Scientific Research*, Vol. 24, no. 2, pp. 145-154.

UNICEF., 2010. 2009 Multiple Indicator Cluster Survey, Bangladesh, Volume 1, *Technical report*, UNICEF.

World Health Organization (WHO) - Bangladesh., 2008. *World Health Statistics 2008*.

Emerging Trends in Public Health Facilities Planning and Design: Nigerian Case Studies

Adekunle Olusola Adeyemo

arcade2000ng@gmail.com
University of Ilorin Teaching Hospital, Nigeria

Public Health Facilities in Nigeria are classified as Primary, Secondary or Tertiary controlled by Local, State and Federal Government respectively. Primary Health Care provides general health services of preventive, curative, promotive and rehabilitative nature to the population and the National Primary Health Care Development Agency developed the Ward Minimum Health Care Package to be provided for the population. The typologies in use include: clinics, dispensaries, health posts, maternities and model primary health care centres. For secondary healthcare which is to provide specialized services to patients referred from the primary health care level through out-patient and in-patient services of hospitals for general medical, surgical, paediatrics, obstetrics and gynaecology patients and community health services, there are comprehensive health centres and general hospitals. There are teaching hospitals, Federal medical centres and other specialized healthcare facilities for tertiary healthcare which are to provide highly specialized services to care for specific disease conditions or specific groups of patients. Earlier studies have shown that there is lack of adequate health facilities in various parts of the country as in other parts of the developing world. There is the need to study the design typologies developed over time for the various facilities as well as the emerging trends. The aim of this paper is to examine the various design typologies that have been developed over the years for public healthcare facilities with focus on how they meet their objectives according to the National Health Policy. The methodology is the visit and documentation of the facilities as well as interaction with stakeholders. The results, apart from providing a documentation of public healthcare facilities in Nigeria, provides examples from which other developing countries can learn in the quest to provide qualitative healthcare for their citizenry.

Keywords: *Public health facilities, design typologies.*

Nigeria: Geography, Demography and Political Administration

Nigeria is a country on the West Coast of Africa. Nigeria has a land mass of 923,768 Km^2 and a July 2013 projected population estimate of 174,507,539 (Wikipedia 2014), and an annual growth rate of 3.2%, making it the most populous black country in the world. Nigeria operates a Federal System of Government with three levels; the Federal, the

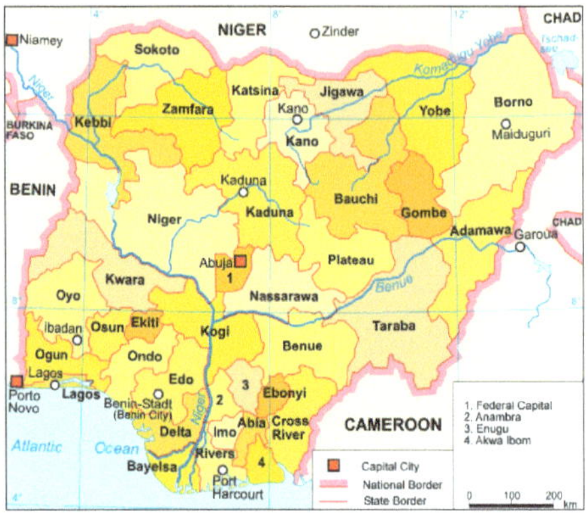

Figure 1. Political map of Nigeria. Wikimedia, 2014.

State and the Local Government Areas/Councils (LGAs). There are 774 LGAs within the 36 states and Federal Capital Territory (FCT) Abuja. The 774 LGAs are further sub-divided into 9,565 wards. The states and FCT are grouped into six geo-political zones. The ward is the smallest political structure, consisting of a geographical area with a population range of 10,000 to 30,000 people. There are on average, ten (10) wards per LGA.

THE NIGERIAN HEALTH CARE SYSTEM

According to the National Health Policy, the National Health Care system is 'a comprehensive health care system, based on primary health care to every citizen of the country within the available resources so that individuals and communities are assured of productivity, social well-being and enjoyment of living' (FMOH 2010 p. 9). It is a three-tier system of health care involving the Federal, State and Local Governments. While local governments are responsible for primary health care, state governments are responsible for secondary care and the federal government is generally responsible for tertiary Care.

Primary Health Care

In the National Health Policy, primary health care provides general health services of preventive, curative, promotive and rehabilitative nature to the population as the entry point of the health care system. The provision of care at this level is largely the responsibility of local governments with the support of State Ministries of Health and within the overall national health policy (FMOH 2010). The National Primary Health Care Development Agency in 2007 developed the Ward Minimum Health Care Package strategy by which Primary Health Care (PHC) facilities are to provide intervention in at least seven key areas: control of communicable diseases (Malaria, STI/HIV/AIDS, TB), child survival, maternal and new-born care, health education and community mobilization, nutrition, non-communicable disease prevention and provision of essential drugs.
Some of the primary health care centre building typologies in use include: clinics, dispensaries, health posts, maternities and model primary health care centres. The nomenclature for the PHCs seems to be evolving as a greater understanding is gained on the facilities and some of the facilities are being upgraded.

Secondary Health Care

The secondary health care level provides specialized services to patients referred from the primary health care level through out-patient and in-patient services of hospitals for general medical, surgical, paediatrics, obstetrics and gynaecology patients and community health services. It also serves as administrative headquarters supervising health care activities of the peripheral units. Secondary health care is available at the district, division and zonal levels as defined by the authorities of the State. Adequate specialized support services such as laboratory, diagnostic, blood-bank, rehabilitation, and physiotherapy are provided, albeit not in all instances. Common secondary health care building typologies in use include: comprehensive health centres, cottage hospitals and general hospitals.

Tertiary Health Care

Tertiary health care consists of highly specialized services, designed to provide care for specific disease conditions or specific group of patients. Appropriate supporting services are incorporated into the development of these tertiary facilities to provide effective referral services from the secondary health care facilities.

Building typologies for tertiary health care are: teaching hospitals, federal medical centres and other specialized health care facilities like separate neuro-psychiatric, orthopaedic, eye and ear hospitals. The federal government has 20 teaching hospitals, 22 federal medical centres and 13 speciality hospitals (FMOH website 2014).

NEED AND AIM

Earlier literature including Akande (2004), Adeyemo (2005), and Akpomuvie (2010) have shown that there is a lack of adequate health facilities in various parts of the country as in other parts of the developing world. There is a need to study the design typologies developed over time for the various healthcare facilities at different levels and their adequacy to fulfil their purpose. There is also the need to observe emerging trends in facility planning and design.

The aim of this paper is to examine the various design typologies that have been developed over the years for public health care facilities in Nigeria with a focus on how they meet their objectives according to the National Health Policy. It also surveys the trends aimed at addressing the various needs and challenges arising as these facilities are being put to use.

METHODOLOGY

The Case Study method, which is a form of qualitative descriptive research, is used in the study. The particular type can be described as illustrative case studies (Becker, Bronwyn et al. 2012). It involved the visit of some of the typical health care facilities at the different levels and documentation of the facilities by means of photographs and floor plans. Stakeholders in the facilities were also interacted with using question outlines developed from the objectives they are to fulfil according to the National Health Policy.

SCOPE AND LIMITATION

The scope of the study is the common building typologies for primary, secondary and tertiary health care in Nigeria. It is limited to some of the common typologies presently in use but it is by no means a documentation of all the typologies. Nevertheless, the case studies documented are typical and follow the same principles as the others.

CASE STUDY 1: BASIC HEALTH CENTRE AND MATERNITY

Classification: Primary health care facility.
Facility documented: Oke Ogun basic health centre and maternity, Upper GaaAkanbi.
Location: Akanbi III Ward, Ilorin South Local Government Area.
Date commissioned: 1993.
Architect: Not known.

The Basic Health Centre is by far the most common primary health care facility in the country. It is a building with an outdoor area for waiting, health talks and immunization, a consultation/treatment room, a drug store and a general store. Its sanitary facility is usually a detached pit latrine. The consultation/treatment room is the centre of activity in the facility, serving multiple functions. The general store in the facility documented was used to keep maternal and child health (MCH)/delivery kits for the midwives service scheme (MSS). Usually meant to serve not more than a ward, the typology is one of the earliest developed with the adoption of primary health care in the country (Figure 2-3).

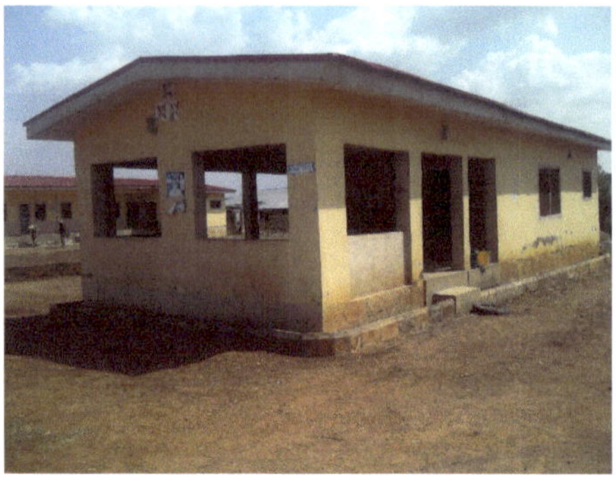

Figure 2. Basic health centre.

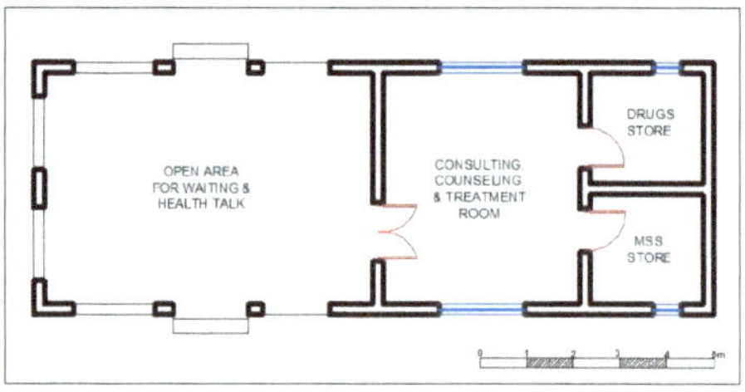

Figure 3. Basic health centre floor plan.

The maternity building is on the same site as the basic health centre in the facility documented but this is not always so. The building has open areas for health talks during ante-natal visits, a laboratory, family planning room, a pre-natal/lying-in ward, a delivery Room and a post-natal ward/recovery room. There is a room which should have been the consulting room but since it is with the basic health centre, is presently used by the health inspectors. There is also a store and sanitary facilities within the building (Figure 4-5).

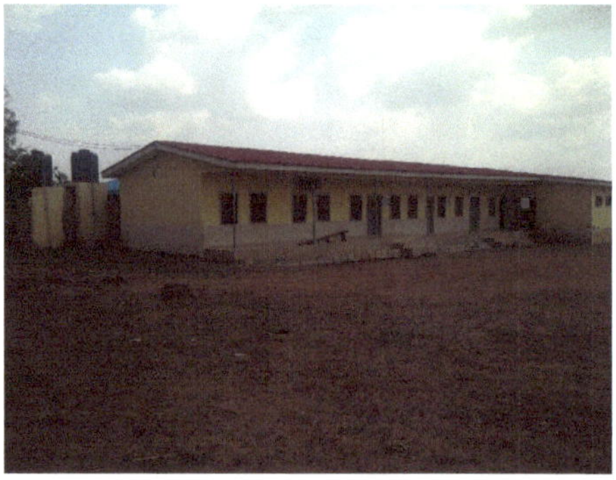

Figure 4. Maternity.

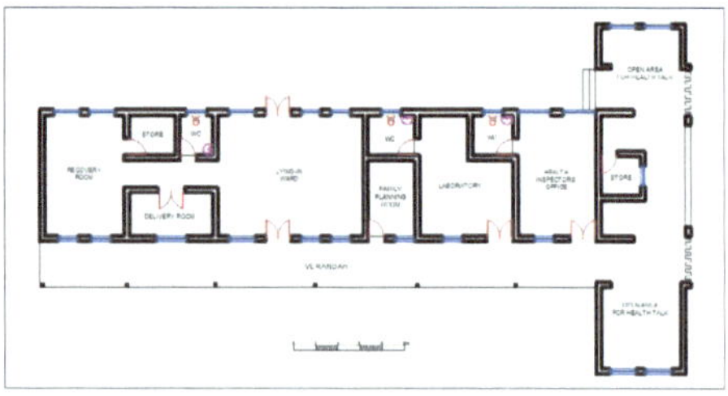

Figure 5. Maternity floor plan.

CASE STUDY 2: DISPENSARY AND MATERNITY

Classification: Primary health care facility.
Facility documented: Dispensary and maternity, Oke Oyi.
Location: Oke Oyi Ward, Ilorin East Local Government Area.
Date commissioned: 1994, Renovated 2013.
Architect: Not known.

The dispensary and maternity facility is a typology meant to serve just those two purposes. It is a building with an outdoor area for waiting, health talks and immunization, a consultation/dispensing room which has windows through which drugs can be dispensed, an antenatal room which opens into a palpation room.

The palpation room opens into a labour ward leading into a delivery room. It has a toilet to serve the labour ward and 3 external toilets opening from the veranda of the building. Usually meant to serve not more than a ward, the typology also has an office for health inspectors and two stores (Figure 6-7).

CASE STUDY 3: PRIMARY HEALTH CARE CLINIC

Classification: Primary health care facility.
Facility documented: Kulende Primary Health Care Clinic, Kulende.
Location: Akanbi V Ward, Ilorin South Local Government Area.
Date commissioned: Upgraded 2013.
Architect: Not known.

The primary health clinic is an upgrade of the basic health centre, dispensary and maternity. It is usually meant to serve a ward especially where there is another basic health clinic in that ward. It encompasses all the functions usually performed by the former and more: a general waiting area which has around it the records room, revenue collection, nurses' station laboratory and pharmacy; palpation and consulting rooms; the waiting area for the consulting room has benches constructed of masonry; an HIV counselling and testing (HCT) room, injection and dressing rooms, immunization room, a direct observation therapy (DOT) room and a family planning room with an insertion room (Figure 8-9).

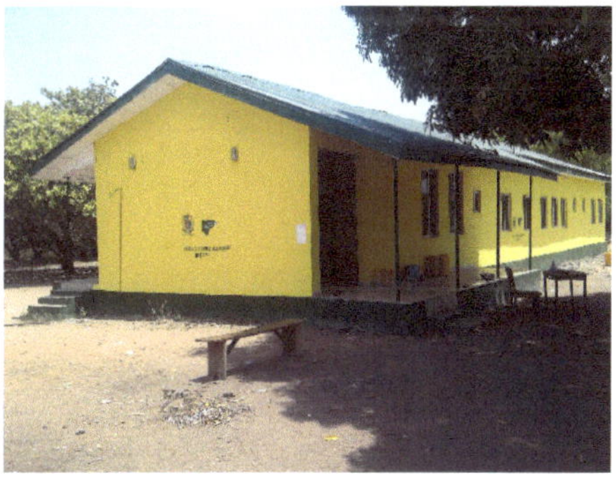

Figure 6. Clinic and dispensary.

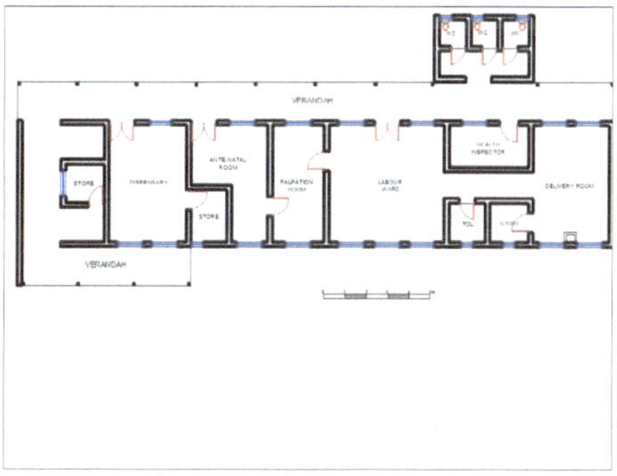

Figure 7. Clinic and dispensary floor plan.

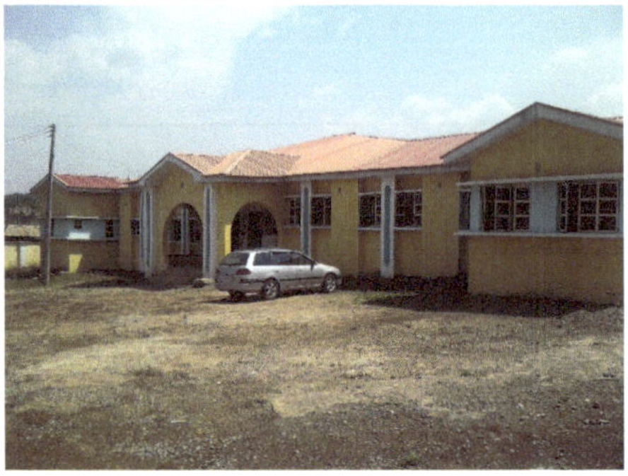

Figure 8. Primary health care clinic.

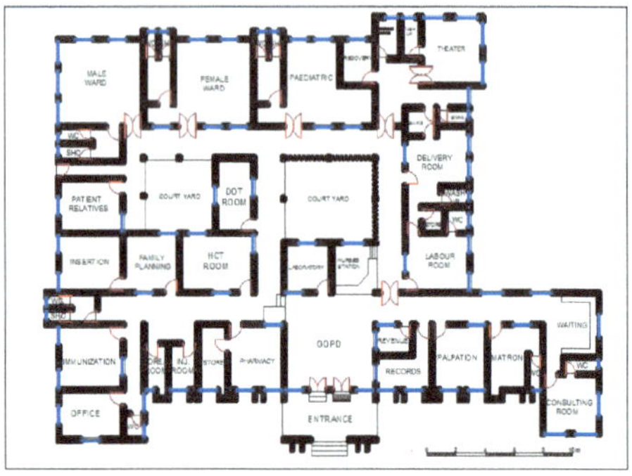

Figure 9. Primary health care clinic floor plan.

CASE STUDY 4: MODEL PRIMARY HEALTH CARE CENTRE

Classification: Primary health care facility.
Facility documented: Model Primary Health Care Centre, Oke Ose.
Location: Oke Ose, Ilorin East Local Government Area.
Date commissioned: 1996.
Architect: Not known.

The Model Primary Health Care Centre serves as a referral centre for the smaller PHC facilities spanning across several wards. The Oke Ose Model PHC documented serves three: Oke Oyi, Oke Ose, and Alalubosa wards. It has an extensive waiting area which is used for health talks especially during ante-natal clinics, within which there is a nurses' station, records and revenue points. There is an emergency room with 3 cubicles which has a door linking the Doctor's office/consulting room.
The facility has a two room out- patient department (OPD) for injection, dressing and observation and a family planning room sharing the same sub-waiting with the OPD. There is an ante-natal ward, a labour/delivery room and a post-natal ward/nursery (Figure 10-11).

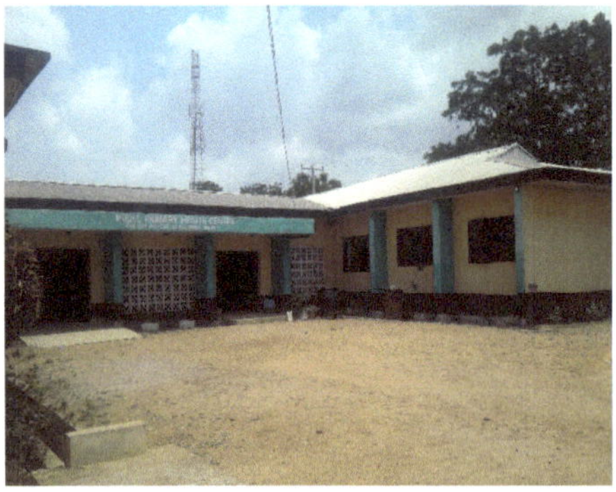

Figure 10. Model Primary Health Care Centre.

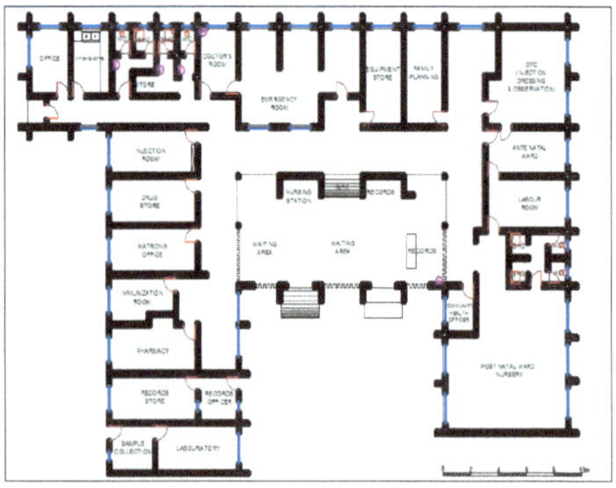

Figure 11. Model Primary Health Care Centre floor plan.

CASE STUDY 5: COMPREHENSIVE HEALTH CENTRE

Classification: Secondary health care facility.
Facility documented: Comprehensive Health Centre, Ijagbo.
Location: Ijagbo, Oyun Local Government Area.
Date commissioned: 1992.
Architect: Kwara State Ministry of Health.

The comprehensive health centre is the first level of secondary health care facilities. They usually serve medium size semi-urban towns and are owned by the state government. The one documented serves Ijagbo, one of the major towns in Oyun Local Government Area. Although it was originally called a basic health centre, further understanding of its function led to its subsequent re-classification. The facility has two major waiting areas, one for the general out-patients department (GOPD) which is used for health talks and the other for the pharmacy which is also closer to the wards. The GOPD waiting area has an emergency room and record office around it. The facility has two consulting rooms unlike primary health care centres which have one, and an administration office which is not usually present in primary health care centres. There is an immunization room and a data room essentially for records. It was learnt that what was now used as a data room should have been used as a theatre. The maternity section has an ante-natal room, a delivery room and a maternity ward. The centre has male and female wards, a pharmacy with its store and a laboratory with waiting area, phlebotomy room and blood bank (Figure 12-13).

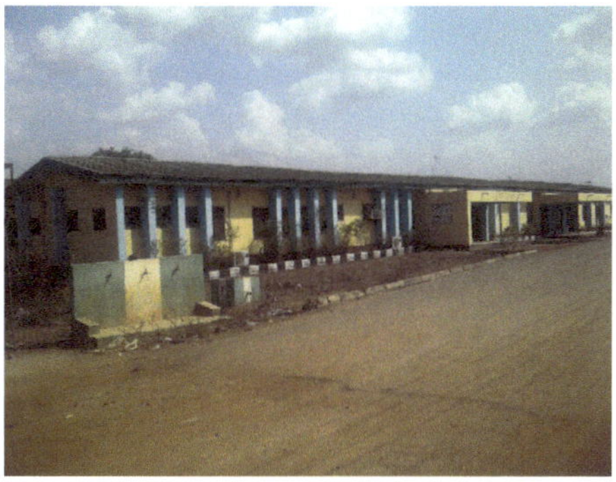

Figure 12. Comprehensive Health Centre.

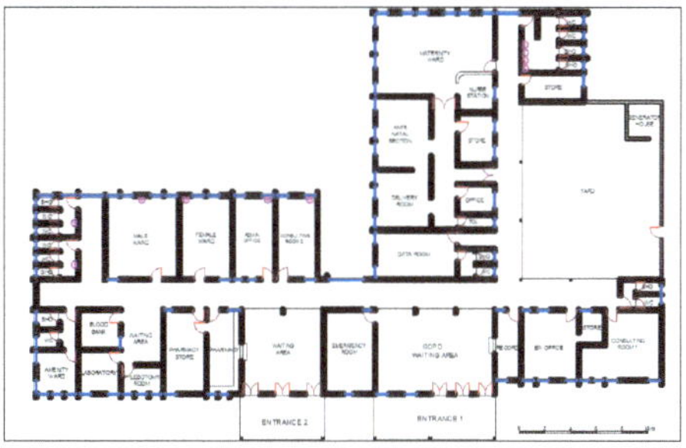

Figure 13. Comprehensive Health Centre floor plan.

CASE STUDY 6: COTTAGE HOSPITAL

Classification: Secondary health care facility.
Facility documented: Adewole Cottage Hospital, Ilorin.
Location: Adewole, Ilorin West Local Government.
Date commissioned: 1980, Upgraded 1996.
Architect: S. A. Adetoro (Kwara State Housing Corporation).

As a secondary health care facility, the Cottage Hospital goes beyond the level of the comprehensive health centre, essentially because they provide surgical services. Owned by the state government, the one documented serves a half of Ilorin, the capital of Kwara State. Although it was also originally called a basic health centre, further understanding of its function and upgrading led to its subsequent re-classification.

The facility has a waiting area for the general out-patients department (GOPD) which is used for health talks and has the pharmacy, revenue collection room and records room around it. The GOPD room is the space used for injections, dressing and checking of vital signs like temperature, pulse and blood pressure. The facility has two consulting rooms, one of which is used also as the ultrasound room. The maternity section has a first stage labour room, a delivery room, a post-natal ward and a nurses' room which doubles as ante-natal room. As expected, the operating room is near the maternity section and it is used for surgical procedures like caesarean section, appendectomy, glaucoma, circumcision. The Centre has an emergency room, male and female wards and what was designated as an amenity ward but is only used as a store. Its pharmacy has a store and pharmacist's office, the laboratory has a phlebotomy bay, office and store/blood bank (Figure 14-15).

CASE STUDY 7: GENERAL HOSPITAL

Classification: Secondary health care facility.
Facility documented: General Hospital, Omu Aran.
Location: Omu Aran, Irepodun Local Government Area.
Date commissioned: 1973, Remodelled 2013.
Architect: Designer not known but remodelled by P.S. Consultants Limited.

The general hospital typology is a secondary health care facility owned by the state government. The one documented is located in Omu-Aran, Kwara State but it serves the entire region. The expansion and remodelling included the construction of an accident and emergency building. There are several variants of this typology so that although the design may not be the same as that of others, the facilities provided are typical of the general hospitals in Nigeria. The facility is a complex of 9 buildings, 8 of which are connected with covered walkways, the mortuary being the only stand-alone building. The main building has the general out-patients department (GOPD), records, consulting rooms, operating theatre, delivery room and 5 wards. The wards are male, female, maternity, paediatric and eye wards. The accident and emergency, pharmacy, laundry, laboratories, radiology, family planning clinic and administration are in other buildings linked to one another and the main building by covered walkways. All the wards are open wards; there are no private wards or amenity wards in the hospital. Glazed ceramic tiles are used to finish the walls of the operating room and the delivery room walls. Mobile operating lamps are provided for the operating room which has two operating tables. Table top sterilizers, autoclaves and suction machines are provided for the operating room. The laboratory also has table top equipment in addition to test strips and an inverter is installed to provide back-up power especially for the blood bank. The Pharmacy has adopted drug counselling instead of window dispensing of drugs and this is reflected in the partitioning created for the purpose. There are 2 x-ray rooms but only one

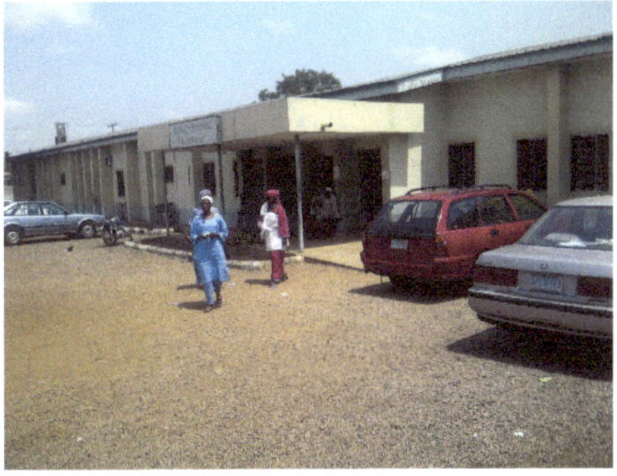

Figure 14. Cottage Hospital.

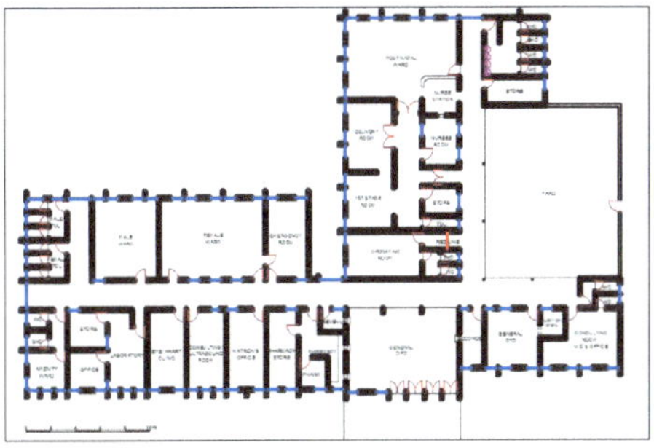

Figure 15. Cottage Hospital floor plan.

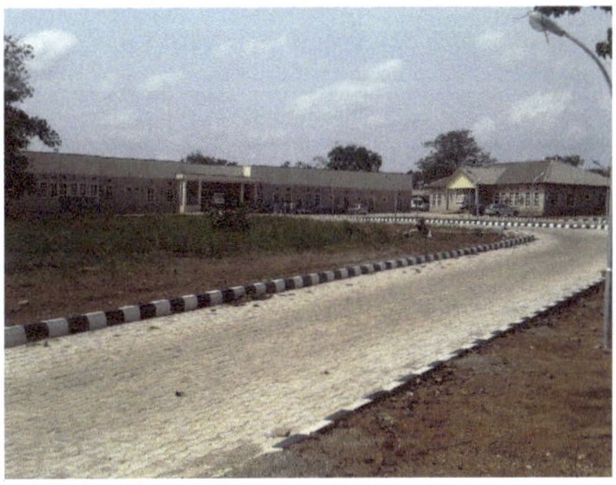

Figure 16. General Hospital.

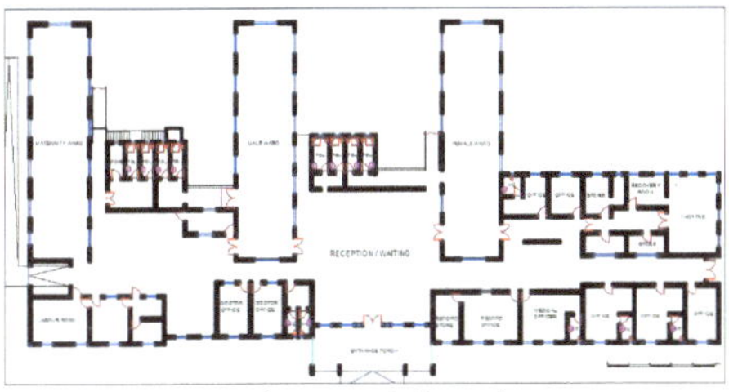

Figure 17. General Hospital floor plan.

machine is installed. A movable lead screen is provided for the radiographer but the walls and openings of the rooms are not lead lined. Washing machines have been installed as part of the remodelling to replace the manual washing previously done (Figure 16-17).

CASE STUDY 8: TEACHING HOSPITAL

Classification: Tertiary health care facility.
Facility documented: University of Ilorin Teaching Hospital, Ilorin.
Location: Ilorin.
Date commissioned: 2007.
Designer: Pearson International and Tomikimi Design Company.

The Teaching Hospital is a tertiary health care facility serving as a referral centre as well as providing for the training of specialists in the various fields of medical science. The facility documented, University of Ilorin Teaching Hospital, is one of the second generation teaching hospitals in the country. Owned by the federal government, the main hospital according to the initial design is a complex of 11 interconnected buildings housing the different units on 4 floors although no building has more than 3 floors. Designed as a 500 bed hospital, it also had two detached buildings which are the laundry and workshops (Figure 18-19).

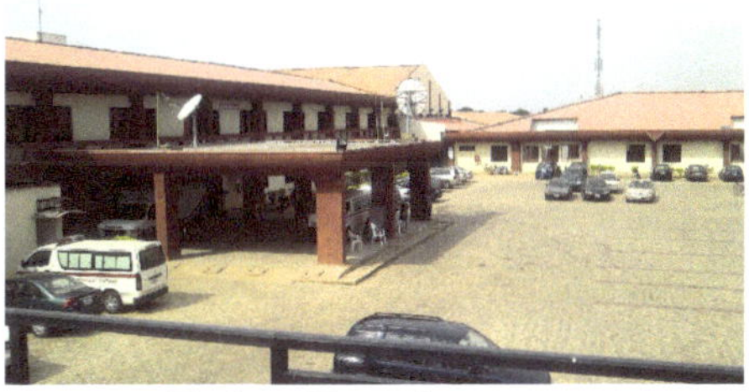

Figure 18. Teaching Hospital.

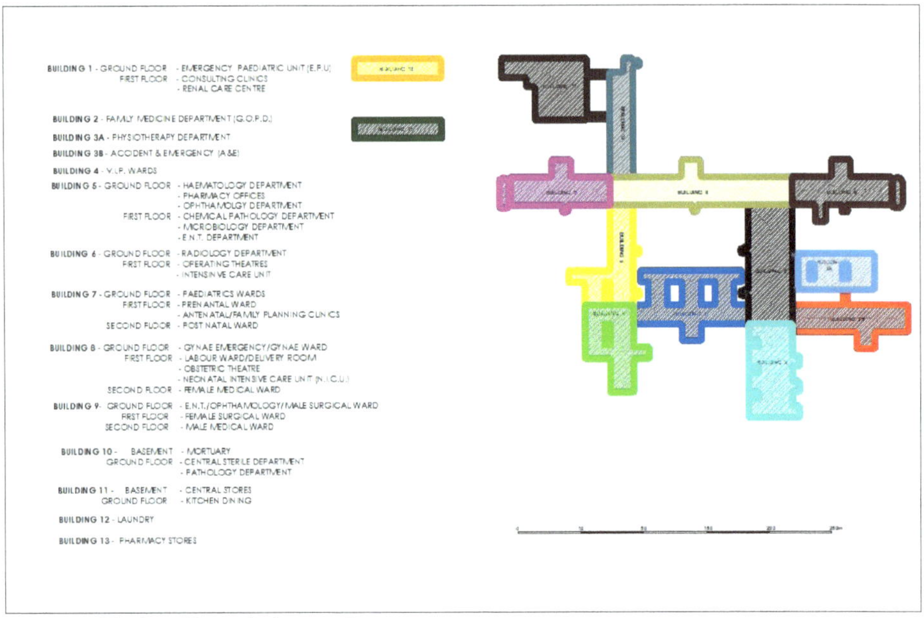

Figure 19. Teaching Hospital schematic layout.

CASE STUDY 9: DIAGNOSTIC CENTRE

Classification: Tertiary health care facility.
Facility documented: Kwara Advanced Diagnostic Centre, Ilorin.
Location: Ilorin.
Date commissioned: 2012.
Designer: Tunji Kusa and Partners.

The Kwara Advanced Diagnostic Centre, Ilorin, is one of the emerging trends in public health care facilities in Nigeria.

Although a tertiary health care facility, it is solely owned by the Kwara State Government and managed by Medequip Medical Services, an international healthcare company with headquarters in the USA. It is a modern state-of-the-art health care facility with the mission of consistently providing reliable comprehensive diagnostic and allied health care services.

The main building has the diagnostic facilities on the ground floor and the administration on the first floor. The ground floor has two wings on either side of the lounge. The left wing is for laboratory investigations while the right is for radiological investigations. The spaces for the laboratory investigations include the main haematology and biochemistry laboratory, immunology laboratory, microbiology laboratory and histopathology laboratory as well as sample collection rooms. The radiological investigations wing has spaces and equipment for magnetic resonance imaging (MRI), digital X-ray, 64-slice and 16-slice computed tomography (CT scan), ultrasound scanning with colour doppler, fluoroscopy, mammography, and echocardiography (ECG) with cardiac stress tests. The first floor has offices for the medical director, accountant, other senior administrative staff and utility rooms (Figure 20-21).

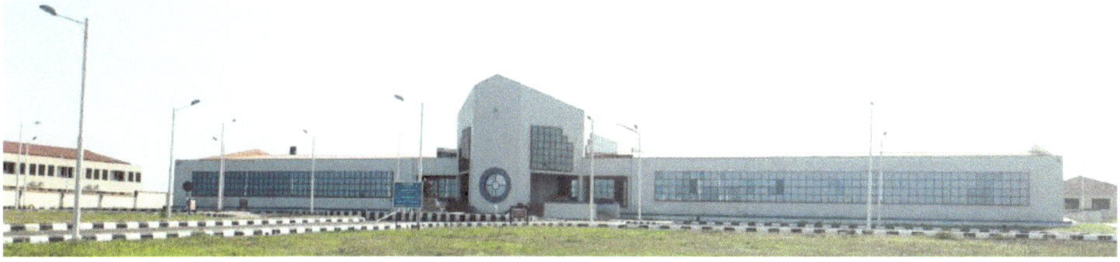

Figure 20. Diagnostic Centre.

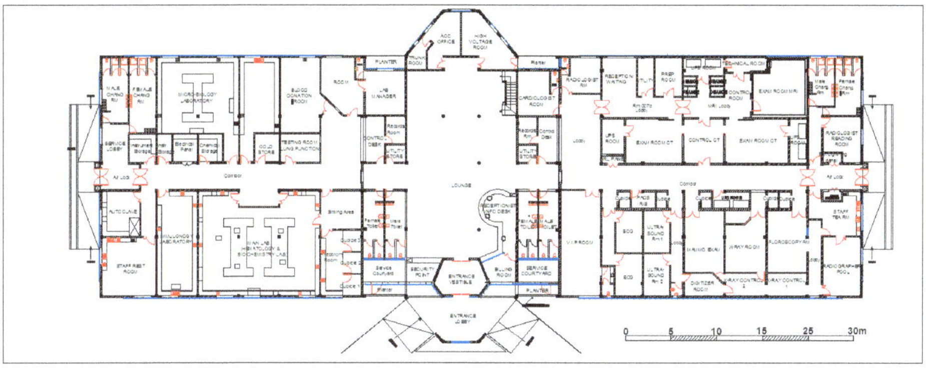

Figure 21. Diagnostic Centre ground floor plan.

Recommendations and Conclusion

This study has led to a number of recommendations. Primary health care facilities do not need many spaces as the spaces can be multifunctional. This helps to keep construction and maintenance costs low and ensures optimal use of space in the facility.

Primary health care facilities can be at different levels, with slightly higher levels overseeing or serving as referral centres for a few basic or smaller ones thereby leading to economies in building, manpower, logistics and equipment.

Governments, health planners and architects can initiate physical development programmes for health care facilities to accelerate the attainment of set goals or milestones like the areas where they are lacking in the Millennium Development Goals.

Appropriate technology applicable to the situation should be employed for the provision of required services especially at the secondary health care level considering regional constraints e.g. power.

In the light of new discoveries always arising in medicine with respect to new disease conditions or new methods of management, public health care facilities should always be designed for flexibility of use.

The design of public health care facilities should always be to the scale of the population it serves, considering their peculiar medical needs.

Bearing in mind the changing realities of the present world, the design of public health care facilities should always leave room for expansion and improvement.

In designing public health care facilities, attention should be given to patient convenience so that required or related services are put in the same location to reduce the need to move back and forth from one part of the hospital to another which often leads to patient dissatisfaction.

Governments, health planners and architects should be open to bring required healthcare facilities and equipment to meet the needs of their populace even if it be on a regional basis. Collaborations like that with Vamed Engineering of Austria and Medequip of USA which were employed in the two tertiary health care facilities documented.

The design and documentation of public health care facilities planning and design is indeed very instructive as it aids in better output for future projects.

References

Adeyemo, DO., 2005. Local government and health care delivery in Nigeria: A case study, *Journal of Human Ecology*, vol. 18, no. 2, pp. 149-160.

Akande, TM., 2004. Referral system in Nigeria: Study of a tertiary health facility, *Annals of African Medicine*, Vol. 3, No. 3, pp. 130 – 133.

Akpomuvie, OB., 2010. Poverty, access to health care services and human capital development in Nigeria, *African Research Review*, Vol. 4, no. 3a, pp. 41-55.

Becker, B et al., 1994-2012. Case Studies. Writing @CSU', Colorado State University, viewed 20 January 2014.

Federal Ministry of Health, 2009. *The National Strategic Health Development Plan Framework (2009-2015)*, FMOH, Abuja.

Federal Ministry of Health, 2010. *National Health Policy*, FMOH, Abuja.

Federal Ministry of Health, 2010. *National Strategic Health Development Plan (2010-2015)*, FMOH, Abuja

Iliyasu Z et al., 2010. Patients' satisfaction with services obtained from Aminu Kano teaching hospital, Kano, Northern Nigeria, *Nigerian Journal of Clinical Practice*, Vol. 13, no. 4, pp. 371-378.

Kwara Advanced Diagnostic Centre website, 2014. Viewed 13 March 2014.

National Agency for Control of HIV/AIDS (NACA), 2011. National baseline survey of primary health care services and utilization in Nigeria survey report, NACA, Abuja.

Wikimedia, 2014. *Nigeria political map*, viewed 12 March 2014.

Wikipedia, 2014. *Demographics of Nigeria*, viewed 12 March 2014.

World Health Organization, 1987. *Alma Ata Conference 1978 Report*, WHO, Geneva.

Beyond Design: Transforming Health Care Infrastructure into Development Strategies

Garret Gantner

garret.gantner@gmail.com
University of the Witwatersrand, South Africa

Typical views of architecture and public health see little relationship between the two, other than buildings as containers for health care delivery. This approach minimizes the potential impact of design and construction processes to one that is diagnostic (identifying needs and responding), rather than one that is preventive (developing strategies for economic development and understanding of health care provisions), thereby creating only a partial result in the ultimate goal of improved public health. The role of architecture may be expanded in a more holistic vision of this goal, through principles of resource effectiveness, labour upturning, and infrastructure maximisation. A case study of the design and construction of Butaro Hospital in Burera District, Rwanda, illustrates some of these concepts in a real scenario, with results that are anecdotally successful but require further study. Ultimately, the most effective design solutions to health care problems can be analysed as a means to further the design profession's ability to contribute to such an important cause.

Keywords: *architecture and development, social impact, health care design.*

Introduction

The premise behind this paper requires a willingness to cast aside the standard boundaries of the role of the architectural profession and embrace an expanded expertise capable of creating or facilitating positive change in communities, particularly in the developing world, and particularly in the interrelated fields of public health and economic development. It considers architects not only as designers, but as strategy-makers for a more holistic health improvement that goes beyond the building(s).

The World Health Organization (WHO) explicitly states that "the lack of resources allocated to health is not the only obstacle to the effective implementation of pro-poor health policies, but it is a major, and inescapable, part of the problem" (WHO OECD 2003), making the discipline of architecture (or at least that of building) a player in the provision of health care. The building(s) it/themselves are where most would draw the line between the fields of architecture, health, and development. This paper questions whether the clear delineation of these boundaries is the best method of achieving ultimate development goals, and hypothesizes strategies for greater impact. To bring the discussion out of a purely theoretical forum, a single case study of a project adopting many of these hypotheses is explored and analysed.

The Link Between Health, Development, and Architecture

There is an abundance of data which suggests a positive correlation, at the macro-scale, between income levels (up to a certain extent) and health indicators. Recent evidence suggests that the traditional wisdom that wealth produces overall health may be flawed, and that there is significant evidence that the converse may be true: that health produces overall wealth – or at minimum there is a co-dependence of the two. Some studies have found a roughly equal percentage and correlated increase between adult survival rates and GDP (Bhargava et al. 1991); others find an even greater increase in labour productivity levels (Brown & Canning 2005).

Architecture, too, has a role in health care delivery, as the provision of health care facilities is a necessary component to the overall functioning of the delivery system. Whether architects recognize it or not, architecture for health care falls within the spectrum of responsibility for public health. The widely held vision – typical of the way in which architecture is practiced and buildings are built – is that architecture's role is purely a diagnostic one: it assesses the needs of a target population and creates a physical response which will be used when people happen to require care. This approach, however, reduces the effectiveness of design and limits the role of architecture to a reactive one. This limitation is an artificial creation of the architectural discipline; when design is approached not as the production of a physical result but as a strategy for further development, this traditional limitation begins to evaporate. Since the objective of a health care facility is to play the most effective role it can in a health care delivery model, with public health being the ultimate goal, viewing architecture as having a diagnostic role is too narrow a view to reach the ultimate goals. As public health is largely based on preventive care, an architectural project supporting this goal needs also to consider how the design and implementation of health care architecture can be part of a holistic, preventive care deliverable. Rather than designing only to house people who are sick (a diagnostic method), architects may expand their role in planning and design to development strategies that may help prevent the target population from becoming sick (a preventive method).

Design Avenues to Promote Development

Identified here are three concepts of strategic thinking with design implications that may become catalysts for development, if properly applied. These are not intended to be comprehensive, and remain largely theoretical at this point. Specific approaches using these concepts would have to be carefully constructed to operate within the context of specific projects, as there will never be a prescriptive method for linking design to development given the vast array of possible differences between projects. Nonetheless, they represent a starting point as strategies to work through an architectural design.

Resource effectiveness

First and foremost is the resource effectiveness of the facilities themselves. Although this falls within the realm of what may be considered the normal realm of architecture – i.e. the design and detailing of buildings – it is important not just to cover the basic programmatic requirements. Health care facilities require very specific performance criteria, particularly in infection control measures, to prevent them from becoming breeding grounds for disease. Infection control measures may encompass a wide range of design strategies (ventilation, surface materials, patient flow patterns, etc.), for which there may be numerous potential solutions. Resource effectiveness is about using means of meeting performance criteria which allow for (or, at minimum, do not prohibit) maximum investment in other development strategies.

Labour upturning

Similar in principle is a concept I will call labour upturning. This has several tenets, all of them particularly impactful in low income countries or non-industrial economies; in Africa, in particular, construction labour is often the first job opportunity of migrants from rural areas to towns (ILO 2000), and within rural areas themselves. Primarily, labour upturning is about investing in the target population that the health facility is intended to serve, aligning construction practices with health care delivery goals outlined by the World Health Organization. Because of the correlation between income levels and health indicators, utilizing project expenditures to produce income for that population by employing them directly in the project construction is a direct means of investment, and directly supports the WHO's goal of creating more meaningful community participation in the health care delivery process (Oakely 1989, WHO OECD 2003).
While there is of course a concern of a lack of applicable skills, this is a reduced concern in much of the developing world (especially in rural areas), where the cost of engaging large (often foreign) professional contractors in non-urban areas is high and the cost of rural labour low. This investment in the community that the facility serves has several subsets.

Infrastructure maximisation

A third central concept to expanding the impact of architecture on health care and development may be termed infrastructure maximisation. This is most relevant in both urban and rural, underdeveloped areas of lower income countries. Health care buildings are very large consumers of water and electricity, large producers of waste, and therefore require relatively large infrastructural interventions. A typical design approach would be to size infrastructural requirements to serve only the building(s); but as hospitals and clinics are chiefly diagnostic facilities, not preventative ones, this approach covers only the smaller of the two efforts to promote public health. While incorporating new infrastructure to serve a new facility is often an expensive undertaking, sizing services for a higher capacity than needed for the building(s) alone is necessarily a commensurate increase in cost –

and when analysed against public health outcomes, may actually lead to long-term savings. A health care facility in the midst of a densely urban informal settlement without adequate drinking water supply or sanitation, for example, may be able to provide clean and safe drinking water and sewage treatment for a population larger than that of the hospital staff and patient load as a means of promoting daily public health practices, without an enormous increase in infrastructure cost relative to the returns. In rural outposts, the provision of electricity to facilities of un-electrified areas may have a positive impact on economic development for similar reasons – especially considering that indoor air pollution from cooking fires of wood, dung or biomass are a serious detriment to human health and productivity (Bloom & Canning 2000).

PRINCIPLES IN ACTION: THE CASE OF BUTARO HOSPITAL, RWANDA

It is worth exploring how these design as development strategies have been implemented in practice, and a useful example of this is Butaro Hospital in the Burera District of Rwanda, with an official target population (the District) of 336,455, though the actual catchment area is likely larger than that. The background of Butaro Hospital is a unique confluence of partnering organizations and entities: it is managed by the Rwanda Ministry of Health; construction was funded by Inshuti Mu Buzima (IMB), the Rwanda arm of the international NGO Partners in Health (PIH), which also acted as the contractor on the project.

The design was done by MASS Design Group, in collaboration with PIH and Ministry officials; I was a designer and Project Manager for construction administration on the project (Figure 1). Completed in 2011, the impacts are still being researched and investigated.

It is important to note that the hospital was implemented prior to the development of this paper, and was not in the image of the specific framework outlined here. Nevertheless, many of the principles are the same, and can be at least partially evaluated.

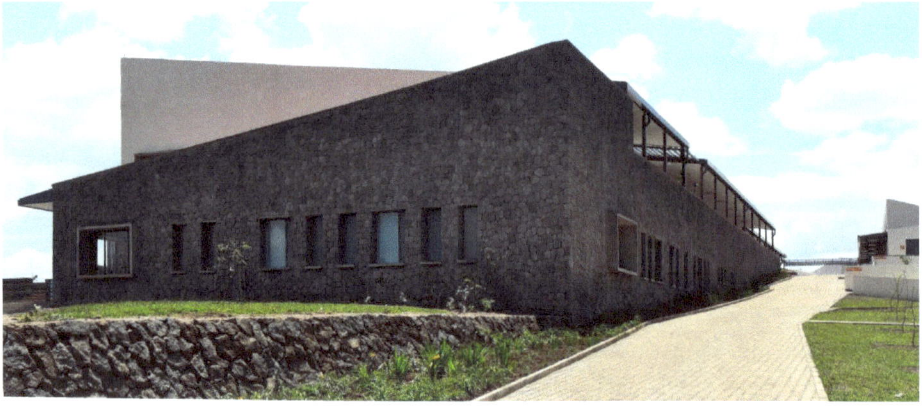

Figure 1. Butaro Hospital just before opening in 2011, Burera District, Rwanda. Photo by the author.

Resource Effectiveness in the Design of Butaro Hospital

Numerous design decisions were made to maximize resource effectiveness at Butaro Hospital. Since construction was done off the grid (prior to electrification of the area), low-energy and passive techniques were used as strategies for infection control. Rwanda's mild, pleasant climate allowed waiting areas and circulation spaces (some of the most dangerous areas from an infection control standpoint) to be kept on the exterior, maximising ventilation without adding cost. For interior spaces, a mixed-mode ventilation system was employed, relying on natural ventilation principles as a primary strategy, and a system of high-volume low-speed fans and germicidal UV lights as an additional safeguard (Figure 2). These fixtures use far less electricity than the robust mechanical system which would otherwise be required to meet international standards for airborne infection control. Airflow testing done during the construction indicate that ventilation rates meet WHO recommendations in the wards, (Almas Syed 2010) but these tests were very limited in scope and sample size so cannot be taken as definitive. Further research on the resource effectiveness (particularly, the functioning of airborne infection control methods) and general design strategies on work performance is ongoing, and data is not yet available.

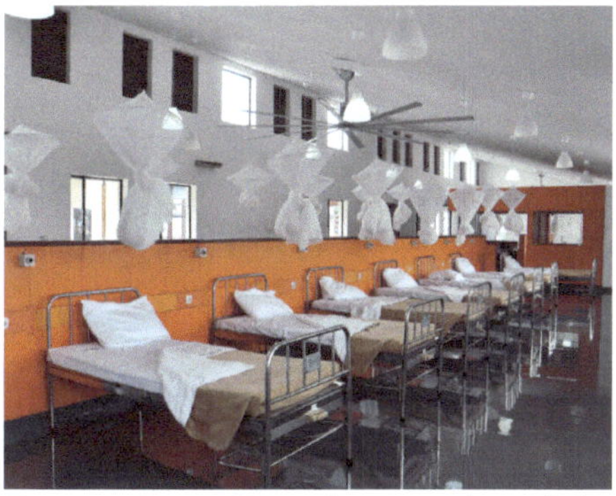

Figure 2. Butaro Hospital open ward, just before opening in 2011. Operable windows and upper clerestory windows provide a natural cross-ventilation system, a high-volume low-speed fan aids in passing air over an upper air 'kill zone' radiated with germicidal ultraviolet light from fixtures visible on the back wall. Photo by the author.

Butaro's labour upturning

From the beginning, IMB approached the construction of the hospital as a development initiative. The vast majority of labour was drawn from within Burera District, totalling (at the time of project completion) 3,898 skilled labour jobs and over 12,000 total employees through the duration of the construction. Some of this achievement may be attributed to the decision to employ people of this rural district and build primarily by hand, rather than rent expensive heavy machinery. The decision from the upstart to build by hand has obvious design implications, placing (beneficial) constraints on the design and detailing done by the MASS team – thus using an architectural approach to a development strategy. It also expanded the employment opportunities which – backbreaking labour though it was – were in high demand in a location where, by the District's own reporting, "the private sector is almost non-existent" (Burera District 2013). Wherever possible, manual labour was used in place of machinery – not always the most immediately cost-efficient method, but representing a longer term investment in the financial well-being of participants.

To achieve the extraordinary number of over 12,000 people being employed on the project, Inshuti Mu Buzima instituted a rotating casual labour employment policy. Under this, most unskilled workers were employed for a set period of time, and upon expiry of the contracts others were given an opportunity. While this method had an obvious drawback of being a very limited, short-term source of income for these individuals, it did have two main advantages (Figure 3).

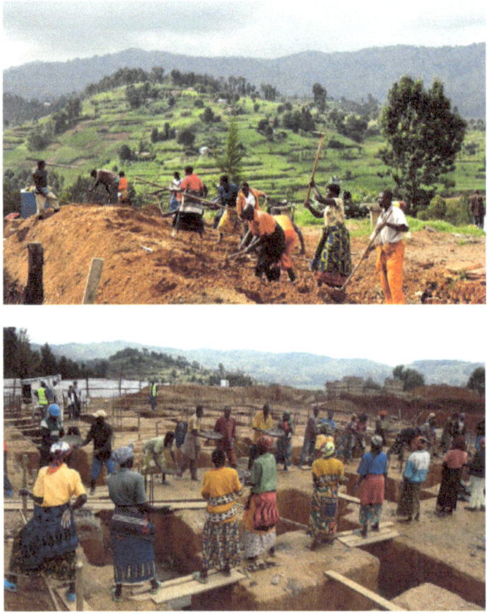

Figure 3. To maximize labour upturning, employees form the community were used in place of heavy machinery wherever possible. Excavation was done much by hand (top), and distribution lines were formed during concrete pours in place of pumps, hoses and mixing trucks (below). Photos by James Cody Birkey of MASS Design Group.

First, it greatly expanded the number of people receiving wages, albeit temporarily, which helps to build community interest and investment in the project as major stakeholders and reduces suspicions of preferential treatment by the organization towards particular individuals in the community. The message that was communicated was that the community as a whole was needed and considered valuable. Second, it allowed access to otherwise rare income-generating employment without an enormous opportunity cost for work at home. Since more than 80% of residents in Burera District are subsistence farmers (Burera District 2013), time away from household and agricultural work could have a significant negative impact on the primary source of family livelihood. Using the rotational contracts helped to reduce or eliminate these potential negative effects, making the employment a net positive gain where it otherwise may not be – showing a well-calculated sensitivity to the local conditions.

One hundred percent of the construction labourers were residents of Rwanda (the team included citizens of the DR Congo, Burundi, and Uganda, who were residents in the area), something that may sound trivial but is fairly rare on large construction projects in a country where the construction industry is still developing, and large projects are often gobbled up by firms from elsewhere in East Africa or China.

An important analysis of the effectiveness of this approach as a larger development model is, as described, whether the skills gained are transferrable into regular productive employment. Evidence of this remains anecdotal and is not (yet) backed by definitive data, but there is evidence to suggest some progress in this regard. Masons who worked on the hospital's distinctive volcanic stone walls (sometimes colloquially known as 'Butaro stone') have gone on to market their skills for use in other projects, including additional work to support the expansion of the hospital through housing and other services, and private homes in the capital Kigali – all of which may be in some way ascribed to the architectural design decision to use this local stone and express it in a particular way (Figure 4). Another group from the site crew on the Butaro Hospital construction has formed a tradecraft cooperative in Rwinkwavu, Eastern Province, which offers training in carpentry, welding, masonry and tailoring to new recruits, then offering them on-site experience as the co-op lands construction job (Hategekimana 2013). This co-op was contracted on the construction of another health facility funded by Inshuti Mu Buzima and UNICEF in Rwinkwavu: a neonatal and maternal surgery unit also designed by MASS, for which I was the lead designer and Project Manager (Figure 5-6).

Regarding the re-investment of this newfound income within the community, greater study is needed. It is difficult to trace the source of economic development, and proving causality may be all but impossible. Anecdotally, it is observed that new businesses have opened, including a branch of the Bank of Kigali, something that might have been previously restricted to much larger cities and towns.

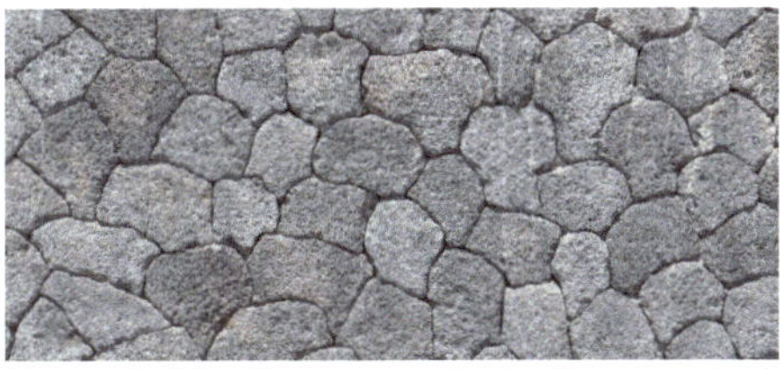

Figure 4. The 'Butaro stone;' a locally sourced volcanic stone used in construction for both architectural and skill-building purposes. Photo by the author.

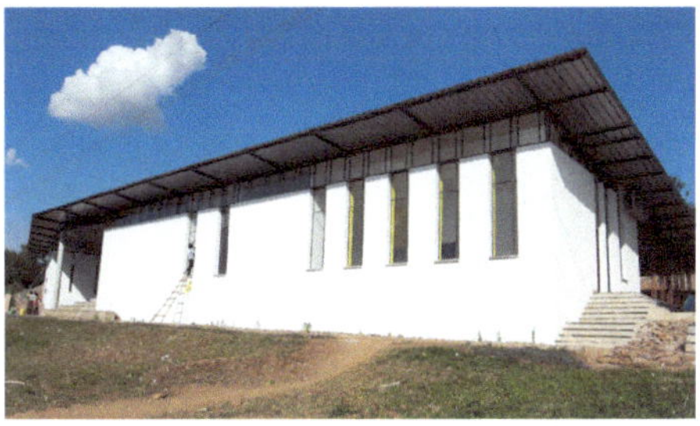

Figure 5. The Rwinkwavu neonatal & maternal surgery building in construction, designed by MASS, built by IMB using labour from a co-op formed by site workers on the Butaro Hospital project. Photo by Amelie Ntigulirwa of MASS Design Group.

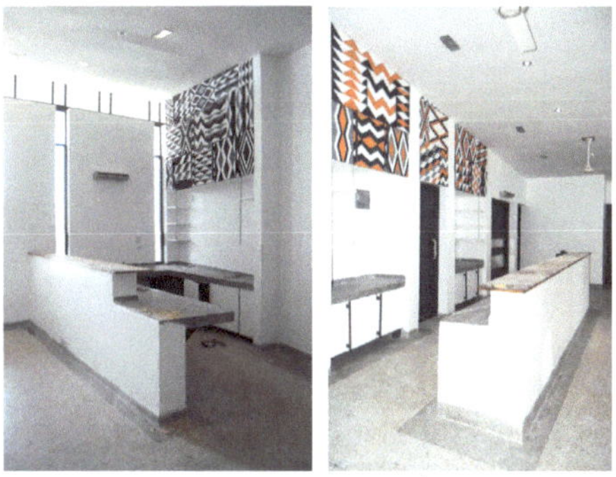

Figure 6. Rwinkwavu neonatal & maternity surgery building in construction. Local artists were engaged in the production of cabinetry panelling. Photos by Amelie Ntigulirwa of MASS Design Group.

BUTARO'S INFRASTRUCTURE MAXIMIZATION

While the Butaro Hospital project itself did not explicitly oversize it's supporting infrastructure to benefit the target population outside the hospital campus, it did increase the pressure to complete a hydroelectric power plant being constructed in the town a few kilometres away by the Ministry of Infrastructure. The dam and power plant had been in construction before construction of the hospital began, and were completed about 2 months after the hospital opened, bringing electricity to this rural area for the first time.

Conclusions

Macro-scale evidence suggests that there are strong linkages between public health and economic development, and as health infrastructure expands, the architects' role in larger development strategies must be analysed and expanded to focus on holistic health outcomes. Strategies for developing this approach include enhancing resource effectiveness of building projects, which helps ensure that resources are devoted to the maximally effective procedures for improving public health; labour upturning, which, through design, invests in the target population intended to be served by the health care facility; and infrastructure maximization, which seeks to find a point of maximum return on health and development indicators without major cost increases over the bare essentials.

References

Baird, M & Shetty, S., 2003. Getting there: How to accelerate progress toward the millennium development goals, *Health and development: Why investing in health is critical for achieving economic development goals*, International Monetary Fund, Washington, DC.

Bhargava et al., 1991. Modeling the effects of health on economic growth, *GPE Discussion Paper Series*, no. 33, WHO, Geneva.

Bloom, DE & Canning, D., 2000. The health and wealth of nations, *Science*, vol. 287, no. 5456, pp. 1207-1209.

Bloom, DE & Canning, D., 2005. Health and economic growth: Reconciling the micro and macro evidence, *CDDRL Working Papers, Center on Democracy, Development and the Rule of Law*, Stanford Institute on International Studies, Stanford, CA.

Burera District, 2013. *District Development Plan, 2013-2018*, Republic of Rwanda.

International Labour Organization (ILO), 2001. *The construction industry in the Twenty-First century: It's image, employment prospects and skill requirements*, International Labour Office, Geneva.

Kahssay, HM, Taylor, ME & Berman, PA., 1998. Community health workers: The way forward, *Public Health in Action*, no. 4, WHO, Geneva.

Oakley, P., 1989. Community involvement in health development: An examination of the critical issues, in HM Kahssay & P Oakley (eds), *Community involvement in health development. A review of the concept and practice*, WHO, Geneva.

Syme, LS & Ritterman, ML., 2009. The importance of community development for health and well-being, *Community Development Investment Review*, vol. 5, no. 3, Federal Reserve Bank of San Francisco, San Francisco, CA.

WHO, *Organisation for Economic Co-operation and Development (OECD), 2003. Poverty and health, DAC guidelines and reference series*, OECD, Paris.

Zeba, AS., 2010. *Butaro airflow experiment final report, Prepared for MASS Design Group*, 10 August 2010.

A Promise Fulfilled: Healthcare at the Grass Roots Level
The Declaration of Alma-Ata in Valenzuela City, Philippines

Prosperidad Luis[1], Elda Shina Samoza[2], Dana Angela Bantigue[3]

luis_associates@yahoo.com
[1]Principal of Luis and Associates, Philippines
[2]Associate Architect of Luis and Associates, Philippines
[3]Senior Architect of Luis and Associates, Philippines

The International Conference on Primary Health Care held in Alma-Ata, USSR in 1978 produced a most enduring declaration that up to this time, three and a half decades later, still resounds with its truth and values for communities all over the world. Health, it declared, is a fundamental human right, and primary health care is a key to its attainment. Primary health care is essential care that is practical and scientific, accessible and affordable, and located as close as possible to where people live and work.

With the best of intentions, without even having heard of Alma Ata, a young and energetic politician campaigned on these values as one of his platforms, to become the Mayor of Valenzuela City, and won overwhelmingly. If elected, one of his promises was to upgrade the services and facilities of the Barangay Health Stations (BHS) during the first 100 days of his term of office. Even before the vigorous campaign period that preceded election, he commissioned a study of all 46 of them.

The BHS delivers primary health services in general medicine, paediatrics, obstetrics and non-surgical gynaecology; family planning; dental medicine; and tuberculosis monitoring.

The study delivered a compendium of information on the site conditions of each BHS, population served, services delivered, physical spaces and conditions; and analysed them against standards of the Department of Health. The analysis resulted to specific recommendations on what to do with each BHS:

1. *"retain" – spaces are adequate, merely improve on site;*
2. *"extend" – spaces are inadequate, expand on available space on site;*
3. *"relocate" – available site is inadequate, build in another site.*

This paper will describe the study in detail and the implementation of the "promise" during the first 100 days and beyond, of the Mayor's term of office.

Keywords: *grassroots, Alma Ata, primary health.*

INTRODUCTION

Primary health care is essential care that is practical and scientific, accessible and affordable, and located as close as possible to where people live and work.

With the best of intentions, without even having heard of Alma Ata, a young and energetic politician campaigned on these values as one of his platforms, to become the Mayor of Valenzuela City, Philippines, and won overwhelmingly. If elected, one of his promises was to look at primary health care and upgrade the services and facilities of the Barangay Health Stations (BHS) during the first 100 days of his term of office. Even before the vigorous campaign period that preceded election, he commissioned a study of all 46 of them.

The BHS delivers primary health services in general medicine, paediatrics, obstetrics and non-surgical gynaecology; family planning; dental medicine; and tuberculosis monitoring. There are 46 BHSs in Valenzuela City and all 46 of them have to be evaluated to determine how best to upgrade them within their individual circumstances.

Apart from the existing 46 BHSs, Valenzuela City also has hospitals run by the government and the private sector. The government hospitals are the Valenzuela City Emergency Hospital run by the city and the Valenzuela City General Hospital run by the national government. The privately-owned hospitals are the Calalang General Hospital, the Sanctissimo Rosario General Hospital and the Fatima University Medical Center. There are plans to construct another hospital and initial actions are being undertaken to acquire the necessary site for the hospital. However, even while this was occurring, the priority remained to be the improvement of the physical facilities at grass-roots level; and so, the BHSs were given immediate attention.

THE CITY OF VALENZUELA

The City of Valenzuela is one of the cities of the Republic of the Philippines and one of the 16 cities plus a municipality that compose Metropolitan Manila. Located 7.9 miles north of the City of Manila, it is categorized as a highly urbanized and first class city based on income classification and number of population. It has an area of 44.59 square kilometres and a population of around 600,000 and as such, is considered the 13th most populous city in the Philippines. Valenzuela City has two congressional districts each represented by a congressman in the Philippine Legislature. It has 33 barangays, 23 of which are in District 1 and 10 of which are in District 2. The barangay is the smallest administrative division in the Philippines. It is a Filipino term for a village or a ward. There are a total of 42,028 barangays in the Philippines.

EVALUATION OF THE EXISTING BARANGAY HEALTH STATIONS

Valenzuela City has a total of 46 Barangay Health Stations distributed in its 2 Districts and serving populations in the available areas of their physical facilities.
Malinta serves the biggest population at 42,040 in its available 92.63 square meters of facilities, while Polo serves

only 1,254 in its available large area of 97.46 square meters. On the other hand, Marulas Puericulture has the biggest area at 149.41 square meters and serves a population of 11,724, while Mabolo has the smallest facility at 21.27 square meters, serving an equivalent small population at 1,617.

The target population versus the number of BHS ratio is 1-BHS per 10,000 population and so, Valenzuela City has underprovided and over-provided barangays and a rationalization must somehow be undertaken.
A total of 18 additional BHS should be constructed. It was decided that additional new BHSs would be constructed after the upgrading of the existing BHSs.

The physical configuration of the layouts of the BHSs varies. Most are regular rectangular shapes, but there are some that are thin long strips, trapezoids, etc., indicating that these specific BHSs were fitted into available spaces. There are some sites where available spaces are so small that their waiting spaces had to be on sidewalks, protected from the elements by a tent, usually donated by local individuals, government officials or firms (Figure 1-8).

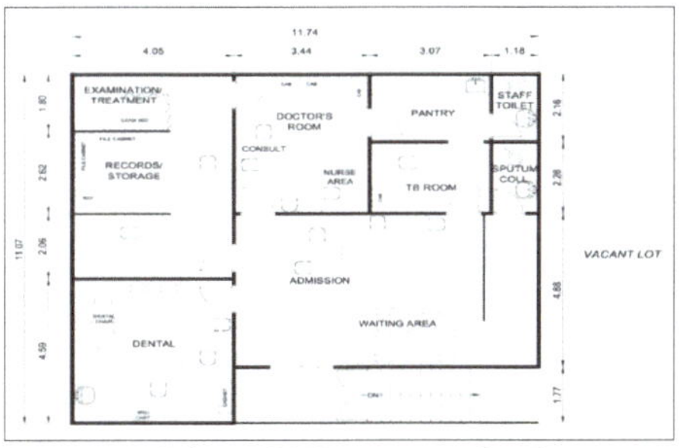

Figure 1. Coloong BHS – rectangular, large, complete spaces per DOH, located at 2nd floor.

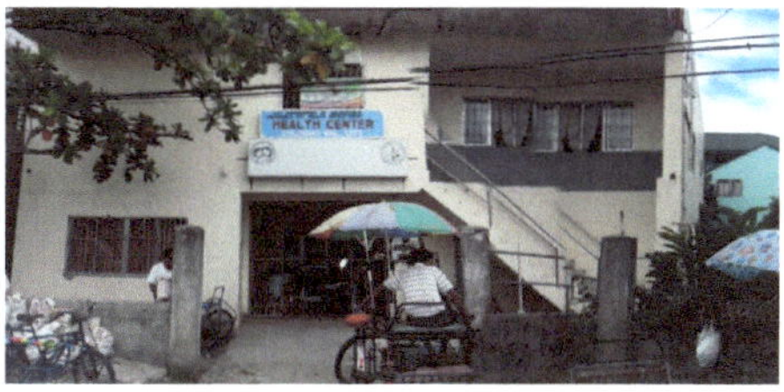

Figure 2. Coloong BHS – façade showing stairs that lead to 2nd floor.

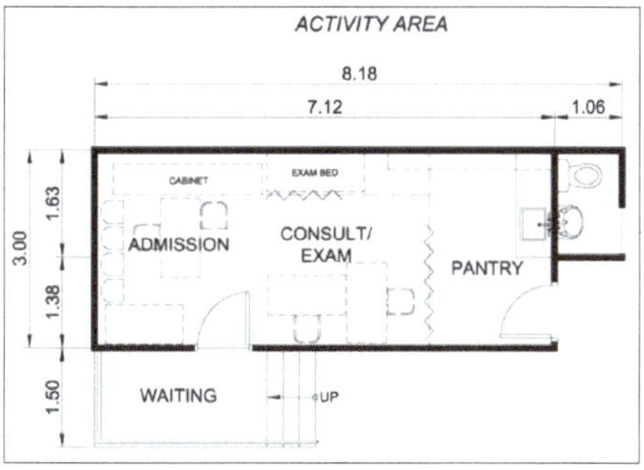

Figure 3. Mabolo BHS – thin long strip, smallest area at 21.27 sm.

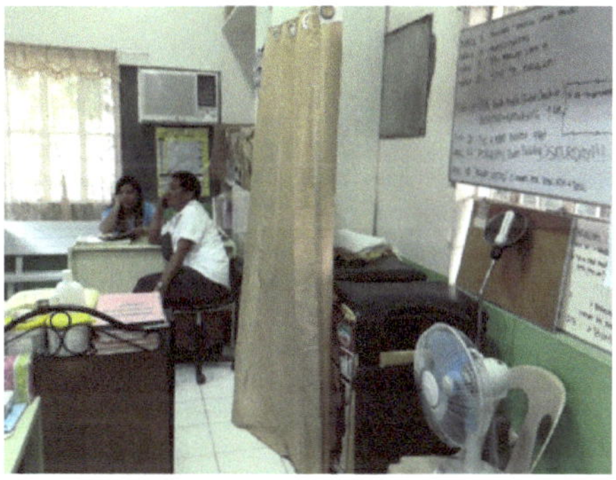

Figure 4. Mabolo BHS – examination room, cramped, with curtain cover.

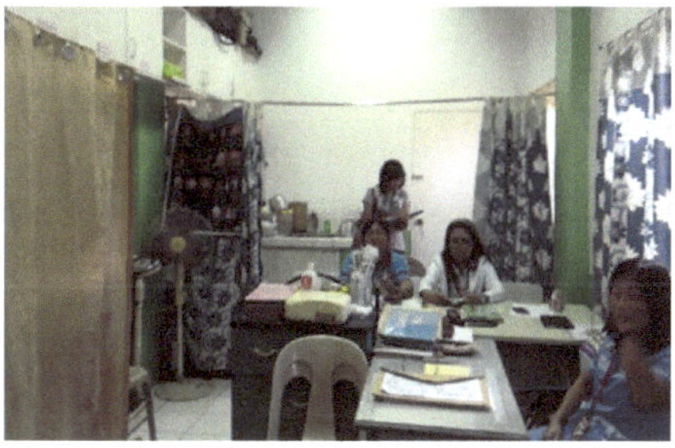

Figure 5. Mabolo BHS – very small consultation area, at left is curtained examination room.

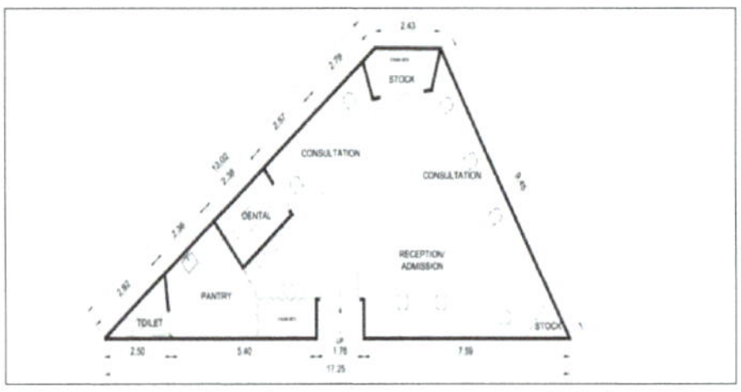

Figure 6. Balangkas BHS – trapezoidal shape.

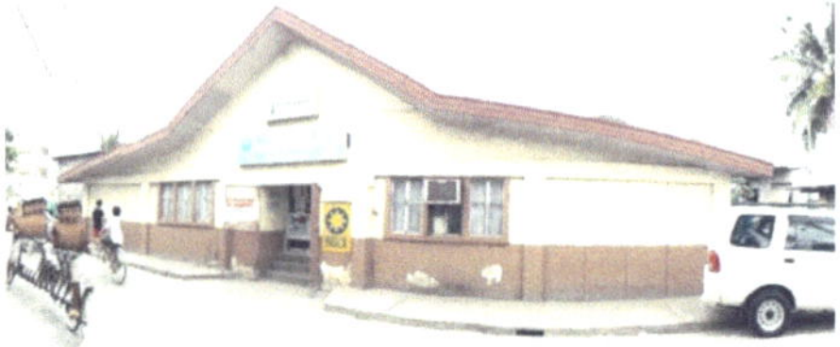
Figure 7. Balangkas BHS: - façade of the single-storey structure.

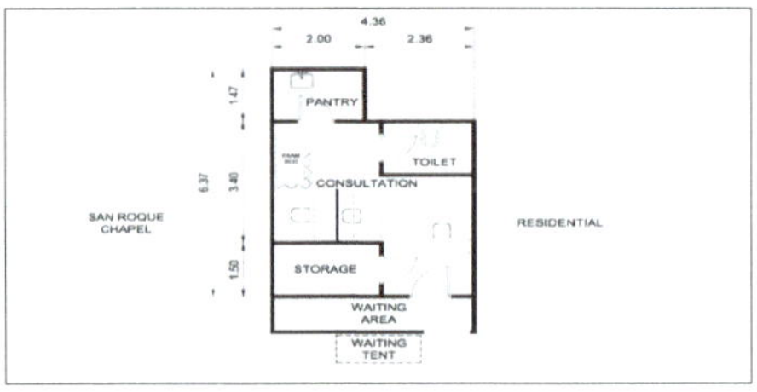

Figure 8. Kabatuhan BHS – small area at 24.30sm, waiting area under a tent on sidewalk.

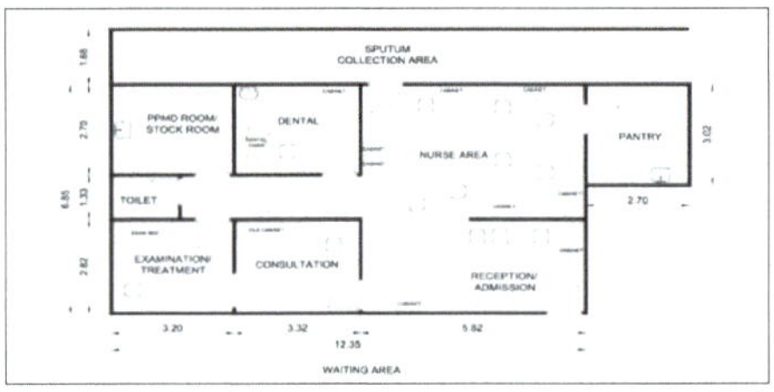

Figure 9. Malinta BHS – TB DOTS sputum collection in a balcony hall.

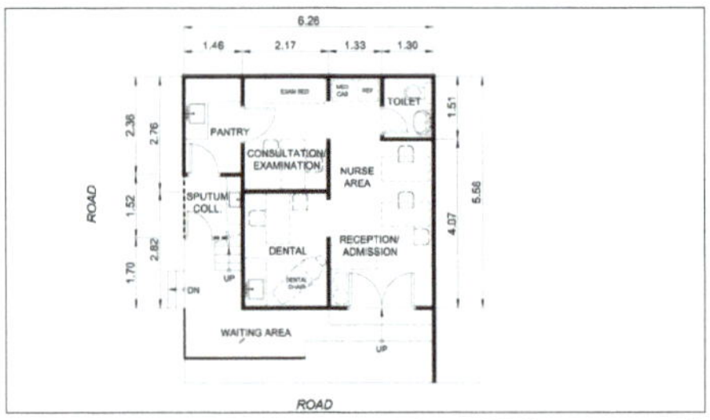

Figure 10. Punturin BHS – TB DOTS sputum collection at waiting area adjacent to pantry.

Most BHSs have provided the minimum spaces required by the Department of Health, namely: a reception-admission, consultation-examination, dental, toilet, pantry and storage. But what is dangerous and unhealthy is the delivery of TB-DOTS (TB Directly Observed Treatment, Short-Course) by BHSs that do not have dedicated spaces for such service. As such, collection of sputum is done in the toilet which is usually closely connected with the pantry, or in public balcony halls and waiting areas; and the service for a communicable disease is merged with other services. A majority, 33 out of 46 BHSs do not have a separate and dedicated area for TB consultation-examination and specimen collection (Figure 9-10).

It was therefore decided that upgrading for all BHSs would include the provision of TB-DOTS spaces and a clinical laboratory for immediate analysis of specimens.

To provide for the standard minimum requirements of the DOH for a BHS and to add TB-DOTS spaces and a clinical laboratory, it is estimated that an area of 60-80 square meters is needed. It is along this range that the total area of each BHS was checked for adequacy or inadequacy. A BHS should have an area of at least 60 square meters to accommodate all the space requirements of an updated and upgraded BHS. When evaluated, it was found out that the BHSs can be categorized according to the adequacy or inadequacy of available spaces as follows:

Category 1: Retain

These BHSs have more than adequate space within their building envelope and so may be upgraded on site through repartitioning; repainting; repair of various parts such as ceilings and walls; repair of sanitary, electrical and mechanical systems; and the replacement of worn-out fixtures and furnishings.

Category 2: Extend

These BHSs have inadequate space within their building envelope but there are adjoining exterior spaces available unto which the BHSs may expand and extend on site. The same description of work will be undertaken as Category 1, but additional new construction work will also be undertaken on the expansion space.

Category 3: Relocate

These BHSs have inadequate space within their building envelope and there are no adjoining exterior spaces available unto which the BHSs may expand and extend on site.
The spaces within the existing BHSs being grossly inadequate for the upgrading, there is no recourse but to look for another site and relocate the BHSs. This is the most difficult of the categories because it entails the search, selection and acquisition of a new site.

GUIDELINES FOR DESIGN

The following design guidelines of the Department of Health will be complied with as much as possible:
- Natural lighting and ventilation;
- Typhoon resistance;
- Flood resistance;
- Fire resistance;
- Non-slip and heavy duty flooring;
- Compliance with codes;
- Compliance with Accessibility Law;
- Emergency electrical, power and water supply;
- Parking area for emergency transport.

One of the most important brief from the Valenzuela City government is for the design of all BHS to have a common architectural character, and a colour scheme that is the same for all so that the BHSs would be easily recognizable by the citizens of the city.

According to a study, the most important changes the citizens of Valenzuela City would like to see in their Health Centres are the following:
- better services (prompt, more courteous and more competent);
- additional free medicines;
- better, more equipped and more beautiful health centres;
- more doctors and healthcare providers for more days and longer hours;
- more health education and information dissemination programs.

IMPLEMENTATION

After all of the BHSs, had been evaluated and assessed, design was undertaken after which local, small contracting firms were invited to bid. Several firms were awarded contracts and each firm was assigned several BHSs, thus making construction activities simultaneous to shorten the time required to complete construction.

The BHSs under Categories 1 and 2 were prioritized. "Before" and "After" images are illustrated in Figures 11-14.

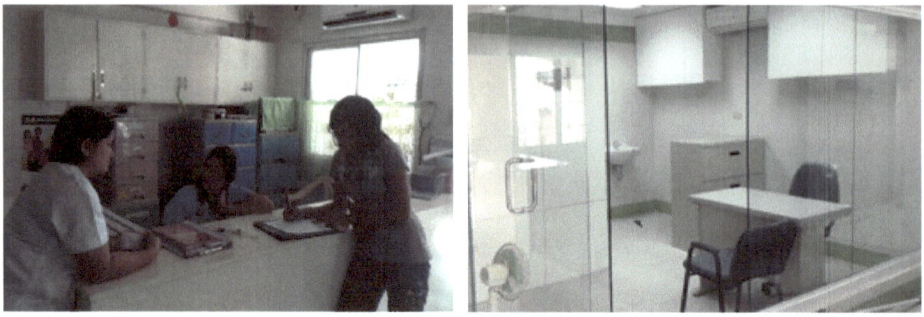

Figure 11. Palasan BHS: old nurse station/examination area (left) and new airy and light interior atmosphere (right).

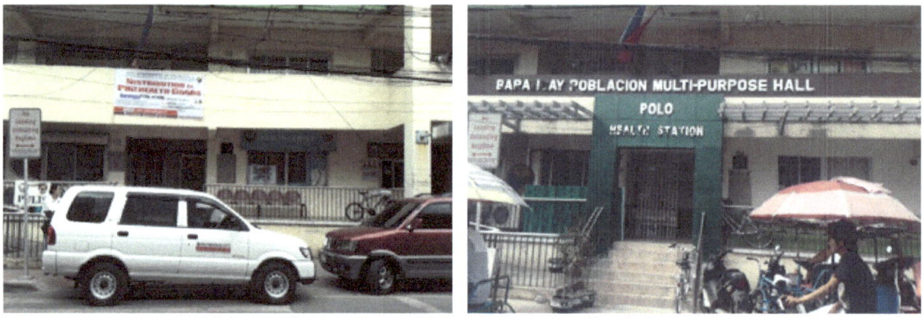

Figure 12. Polo BHS: old façade (left) and new façade with standard arch feature (right).

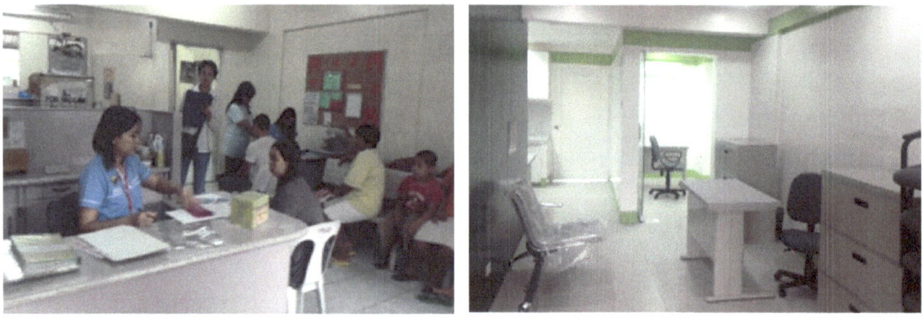

Figure 13. Polo BHS: old waiting/admission area (left) and new light atmosphere, new furniture (right).

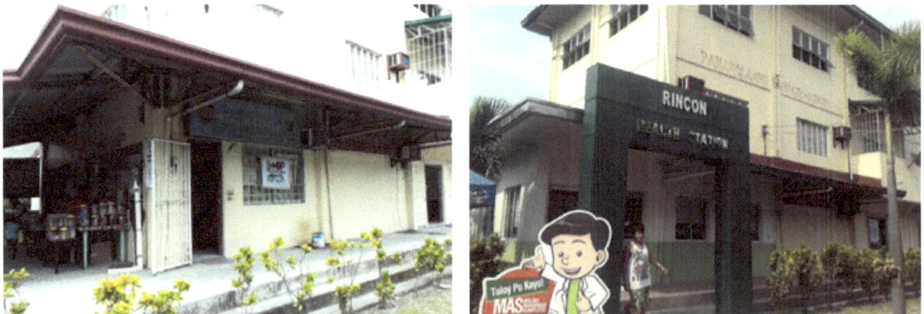

Figure 14. Rincon BHS: old façade and entrance (left) and new façade with standardized entry arch (right).

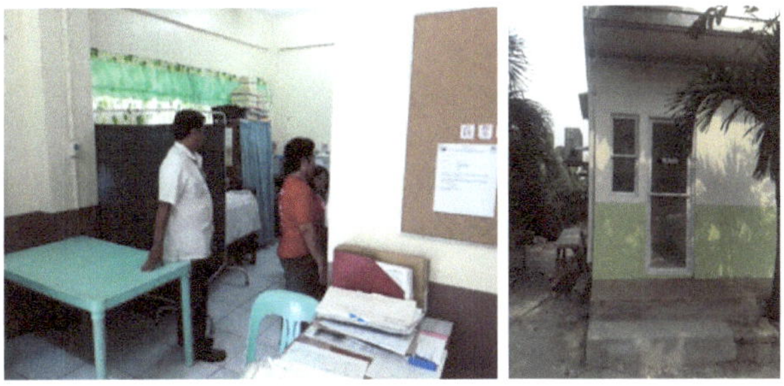

Figure 15. Rincon BHS: old examination area (left) and New dedicated TB-DOTS area with separate entrance (right).

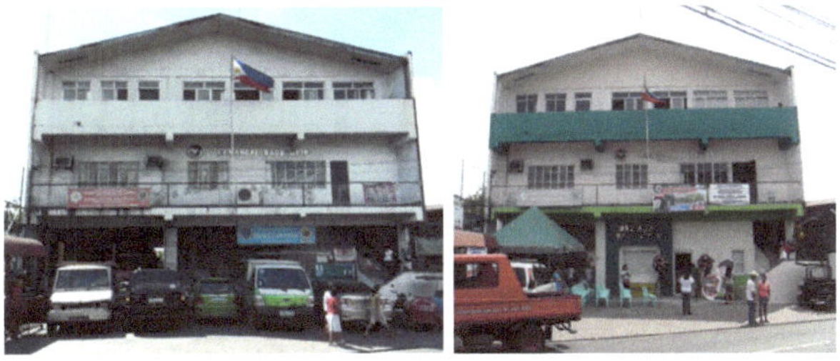

Figure 16. Bagbaguin BHS: old façade (left) and new façade in standard color and entry arch on inauguration day (right).

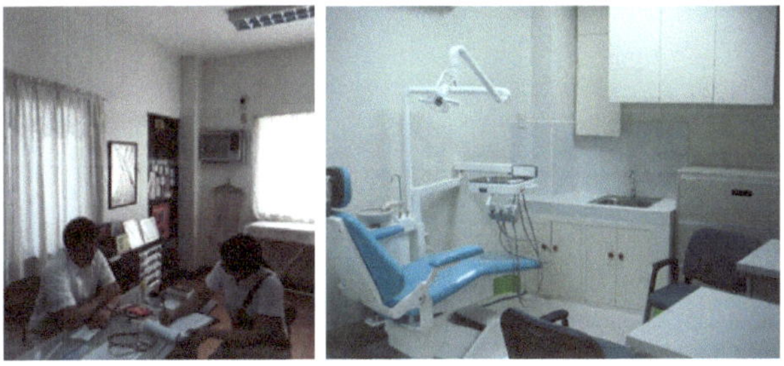

Figure 17. Bagbaguin BHS: old consultation room (left) and new dental room with new equipment (right).

Corollary to physical facilities standardization and upgrade, the city administration had undertaken the following complementary actions to upgrade the services in the BHS:

a. additional budget for operations and maintenance;

b. additional medical equipment;

c. additional manpower, to include clerks to support medical staff and utility staff to oversee cleanliness;

d. assignment of a person from the Engineering Office to overlook and monitor the BHSs to ensure proper maintenance;

e. inclusion of budget increase for health programs in the City Investment Plan;

f. per directive of the Mayor, all aspects that would complete the primary health care services in the BHSs were augmented.

A Continuing Project

There is a next phase to this project – the construction of new BHSs in their new relocation sites. This endeavour is a greater challenge to the incumbent city administration because new sites have yet to be selected and obtained. However, the Mayor of the City, during the almost daily inauguration of the 21 completed BHSs, reiterated his commitment to the prioritization of primary health care in his city.

Conclusions

The best way to evaluate the Project is to ask and answer ten questions derived from the principles of the Declaration of Alma Ata:

1. Would it help attain health, a fundamental human right of the people of Valenzuela City? YES!
2. Would it help bring equality in health status among the people? YES!
3. Will it contribute to economic and social development? YES!
4. Will it contribute to the participation of the people in the planning and implementation of their health care? YES!
5. Will it contribute to attaining a high level of health through primary health care? YES!
6. Will it provide essential health that is both practical and scientific? YES!
7. Will it promote maximum community and individual self-reliance through primary health care? YES!
8. Is it an indication of the intention and the plan of the city government to integrate primary health care in their comprehensive health system? YES!
9. Is it an indication that the City of Valenzuela is cooperating in the world-wide effort to attain primary health care? YES!
10. Is it an example of good use of resources to attain an acceptable level of health for the people? YES!

At this point in time, the "YES" answers denote the good intentions of the city government. At some future time, these questions should be asked again, this time, in terms of how successful the implementation had been. At any rate, Valenzuela City is a model, a good example to emulate and follow in its grass roots approach to community health, the Alma-Ata way.

References

Cabral, Esperanza I., 2012. *Health Care Needs Assessment for Valenzuela City*. An unpublished research paper, Quezon City.

Luis and Associates, 2013. *Assessment of Existing Barangay Health Stations in Valenzuela City*, Books No. 1: Compendium of Information on All Barangays. An unpublished project report, Quezon City.

Luis and Associates, 2013. *Assessment of Existing Barangay Health Stations in Valenzuela City*, Book No. 2: Analysis and Recommendations. An unpublished project report, Quezon City.

Valenzuela City Website. http://valenzuela.gov.ph.

World Health Organization Website. *Health Services Development: Information on Primary Health Care*.

Wikipedia. Information on the Alma Ata Declaration, Barangays and Valenzuela City.

Extracting the Principles of Sustainability From the Architecture of Colonial Hospitals in Malaysia: Appreciating Past Wisdom as Best Practice

Norwina Mohd Nawawi, Abdul Razak Sapian, Srazali Aripin, Noor Hanita Abdul Majid, Zuraini Denan, Aliyah Nur Zafirah

norwina19@gmail.com, arazaks@iium.edu.my, srazali88@yahoo.com, hanita@iium.edu.my, zdenan@iium.edu.my, aliyah@iium.edu.my
International Islamic University Malaysia, Malaysia

Malaysia's sturdy hospital buildings built by the colonial government throughout the country are still in use today. These hospitals withstood years of operation and contributed, together with the current hospital buildings, in improving the health and well-being of Malaysians today. Hospitals are both expensive to build and to maintain. The quest for sustainable design includes the evaluation of the performance of both old and modern hospitals buildings for future guidance. This paper focuses on the performance of selected colonial hospital buildings in Malaysia currently in-use. The objective is to learn, understand and extract the good values and wisdom from the past planning and design legacies as best practice. Qualitative approaches adopted for this study include a content analysis of relevant literature; fieldwork survey; random interviews and observations. The study analysed the hospital locations, its site planning, building massing, building attributes and environmental performance on thermal comfort, visual, day-lighting and ventilation. Findings of the study provide practical recommendations on criteria for site selection, site planning, building configuration, building depths and widths, and openings for ventilation and day-lighting. Limitations include the duration and number of buildings studied within the stipulated time frame, as well as permission to access the site. The significance of this study is the collection of past best practices on hospital design physical, sustainable attributes that are evergreen before they slowly disappear.

Keywords: *sustainable, design, colonial hospitals.*

Hospital	Batu Gajah	Kampar
Site	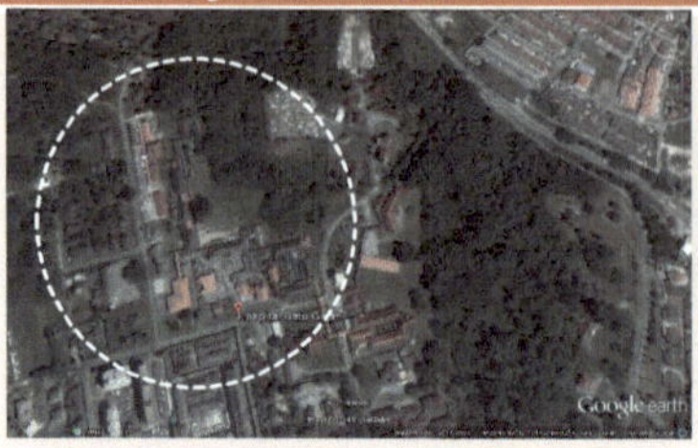	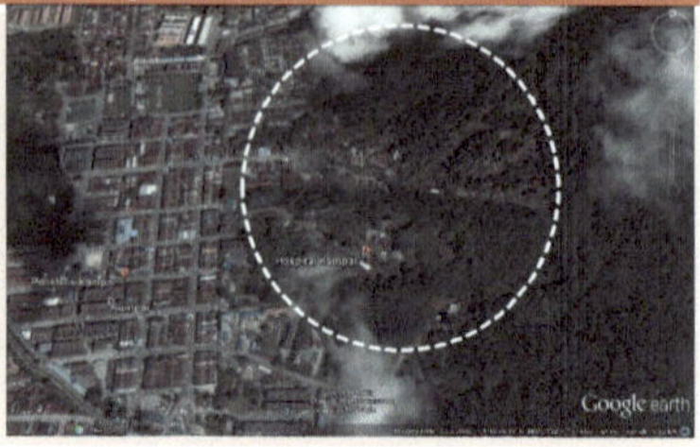
Description	The hospital is situated on top of a hill with other administrative and government buildings as part of the town plan.	Snugly on the side of the hill near Kampar town away from the mining area at the flat land. Away from flood waters with view of the town
Analysis	On the hill with other institutional building	On the hill on its own

Choice of the site.

Hospital	Batu Gajah	Kampar
Building layout	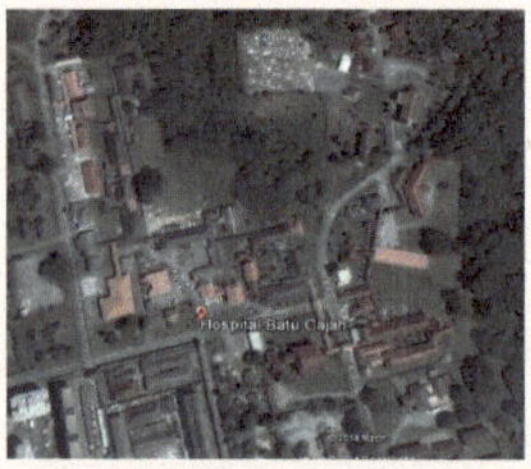	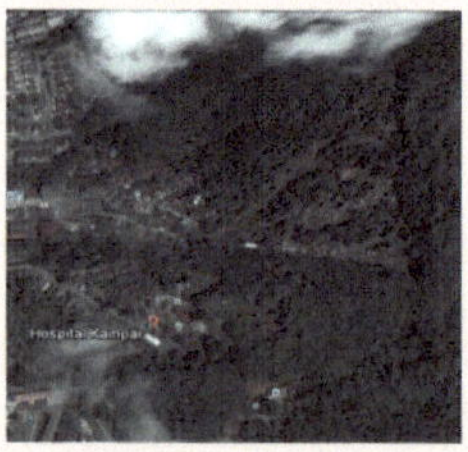
Description	The layout of the hospital was quite open, although there were limited physical barriers between other buildings. There was a open field in front of the ward, next to a therapeutic garden.	The male ward is not connected to other wards, but the design was similar.
Analysis	Individual rectangular, square or T shape block or pavilion by function linked by covered corridors Linear pattern	Rectangular but small pavilions linked by covered corridors where possible. Terrace pattern

Hospital configuration.

Hospital	Batu Gajah	Kampar
Ward orientation	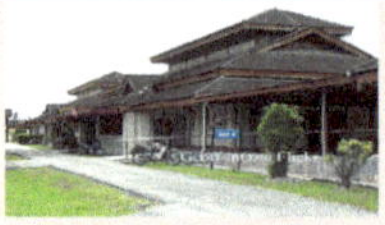 Source: flickr	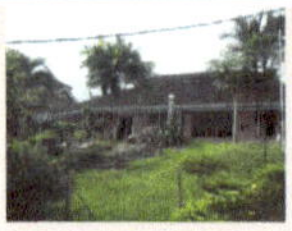 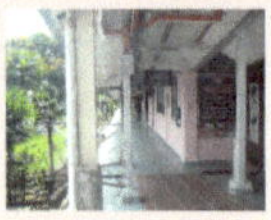
Analysis	The wards is on West and East window orientation	The wards are following the hill terrace with view of the town

Ward orientation.

De-Hospitalization & Mini-Hospitals: Study of a New Frontier to Design Healthcare Buildings

Walkiria Tamar de Morais Erse

wwerse@terra.com.br
Associated Member of UIA-PHG – Public Health Group, Representative of ABDEH for International Relations (Associação Brasileira para Desenvolvimento do Edificio Hospitalar), Representative of IPH for International Relations (Instituto de Pesquisas Hospitalares - arq Jarbas Karman)

Demand for hospital beds in Brazil is gigantic. De-hospitalization is one of the ways used to increase hospital beds. The process of de-hospitalizing follows the traditional way of promoting anticipated discharges of patients based on medical criteria and continuing recovery care at another healthcare facility. Since 1990, Brazil has adopted a new way of releasing hospital beds, no longer de-hospitalizing but to avoid hospitalizing patients of low and medium complexity surgery in big hospitals. Day hospitals were built for that role. Over time, day hospitals have assumed to give assistance to specialized issues of clinical care such as TB, HIV, oncology, better performed procedures of low and medium complexity. Again the demand for more hospital beds has become less assisted. Answering the demand for more hospital beds, the private market for healthcare has created a new kind of facility to act as a vector for attending ambulatory surgeries. The new facility called, for effects of this paper, mini-hospital has different qualities and technical performances and is separated from day hospitals by a frontier line which this study now investigates. Mini hospitals are facilities designed to promote healthy and scientific spaces capable of giving prompt answers to patients and the staff. They welcome patients into cozy shelters of homelike spaces where they receive proceedings of healing and are close to their physicians. Homelike spaces as proposed in the architecture program means being known to patients without losing their scientific mission. Mini hospitals are healthy and scientific buildings.

Keywords: *small hospital, de-hospitalization, mini-hospital, healthcare architecture.*

Architecture is a legitimate therapeutic modality. It can release stress, promote wellbeing, create that good first impression and, in the words of Derek Parker, offer clues that, inside that room, somebody takes care of you.

Imagine a man lying on a stretcher on the way to the operating room far from his family members, naked of his clothes, glasses, dental prosthesis and wedding ring.

When inside, he can see only "pairs of eyes", the unique parts of people wearing uniforms, masks, aprons, gloves and caps. He certainly asks himself what will happen to his body, which scars will remain. That scene defines the most crucial moments of a man in a hospital (Figure 1).

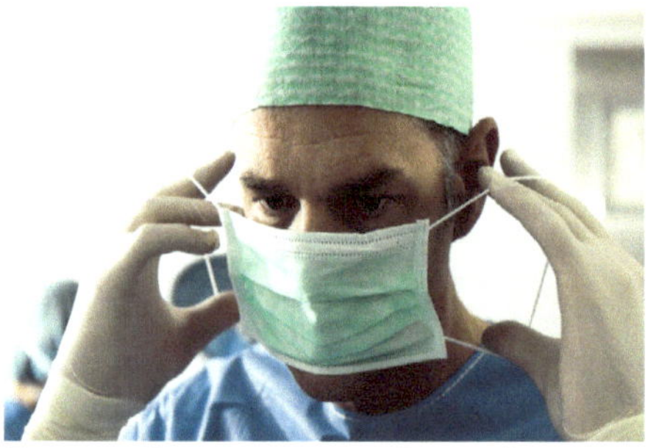

Figure 1. Patient perspective: "pairs of eyes".

In my experience as resident architect working for Hospital Pérola Byington I have occasionally observed these crucial moments. Most of the time I was called to the surgical center to improve climatization, illumination and qualities of rooms, I have never been called to upgrade well being to a patient about to be invaded by a surgical procedure. Those pre-operating moments show how fragile patient become and how desperately they look for clues showing that somebody, inside that room, cares about him.
To give additional clues to patient architects must go beyond the frontier of healthcare architecture diving into medicine and public health, studying medical procedures and human reactions, designing spaces in which patient is the element of great importance.
In Frank Lloyd Wright words patient must be treated inside rooms that do not show the "paraphernalia of abnormality" of hospitals. Wright reinforces saying that hospitals must be smaller, more numerous and homelike.
In southern Brazil access to a hospital bed is a constant struggle due to the great lack of beds.

Brazil is a gigantic country with an estimated population 202 million habitants. It is a young country when compared to Europeans countries and, in South America is a mature leader. Mature, with the joy of youth and sometimes with flashes of adolescent - mainly in Carnival.
Public Healthcare in Brazil - SUS – offers free and universal assistance to all citizens, since the primary care to the high complexity procedures such as transplants and heart, head and neck surgeries (Figure 2).

Despite of being the seventh economy in the world Brazil is responsible only for 46% of total investments in healthcare assistance. The other 54% come from private investments (Figure 3).
Only 8.9 % of annual budget goes to Health while international average is 11.7 %. Health is the fifth participant on the Brazilian annual budget (Figure 4).
For the last years Brazil has been living a development period when industry, agriculture and production of goods and services have increased. The number of new jobs raised and private health insurance takes care of 51 million of lives, 56.7 % more than 10 years ago (Figure 5).
SUS takes care of the other 151 million habitants.
Brazilian hospitals suffer from consequences of those unbalanced bills.
There are almost 470 thousand hospital beds to attend 202 million habitants. That makes 2.45 beds/ 1.000 habitants.
If we consider only beds for surgery, as declared in our statistics, situation is more dramatic. In southern region, the richest and most crowded of the country, there is less than one bed/1000 habitants.

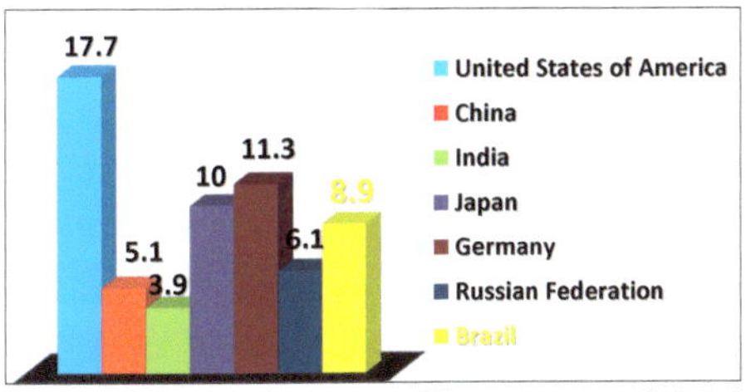

Figure 2. Brazil- % Health Expenses of GDP seventh largest GDP-2011 in the world. Source: WHO, World Healt Statistics - 2014; World Bank, 2011 International Comparison Program (ICP) published in 2014 - Note: GDP ranking in PPP(Purchasing Power Parity) based.

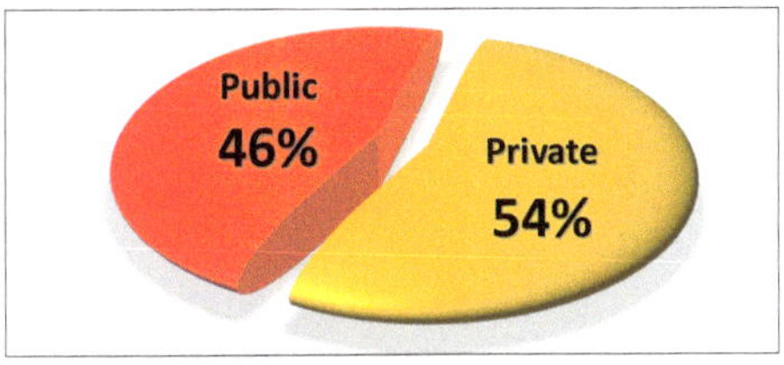

Figure 3. % Brazil Total Health Expenses - 2011. Source: WHO, World Health Statistics - 2014.

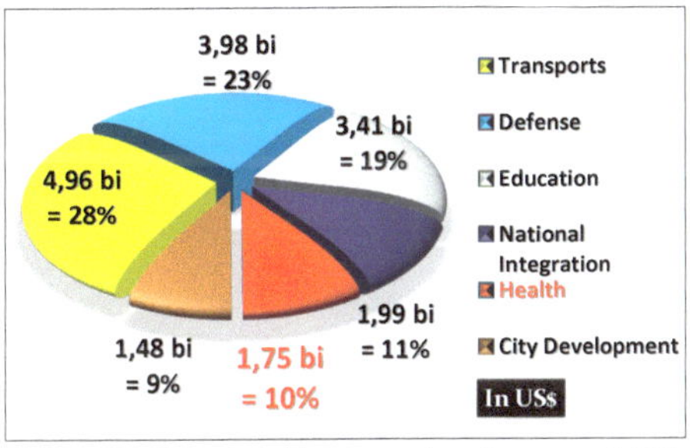

Figure 4. Brazil – Expenses by Sectors - 2013. DATA Source: SIAFI (Integrated Financial Management System) - Federal Government.

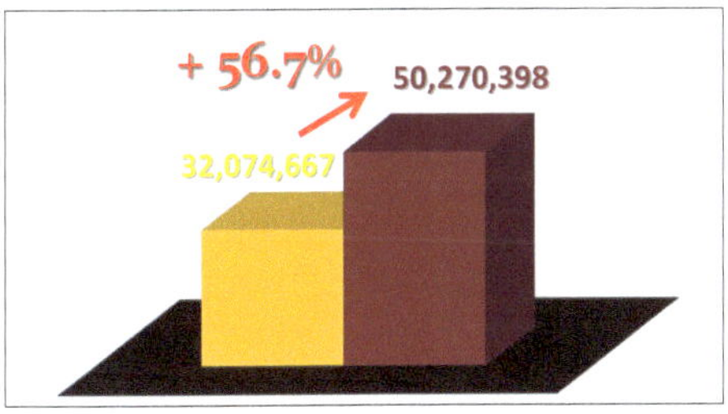

Figure 5. Beneficiaries of private health plan 2003 – 2013. Source: Beneficiaries Information System/ ANS/BR Ministery of Health, 12/2013.

The chart of surgeries organized by complexity shows that ambulatory + low and medium complexity surgeries are 68.2% of total surgeries.

High complexity and special surgeries are 31.8%.

So hospitals beds are occupied in majority by patients of ambulatory + low and medium complexity surgical procedures (Figure 6).

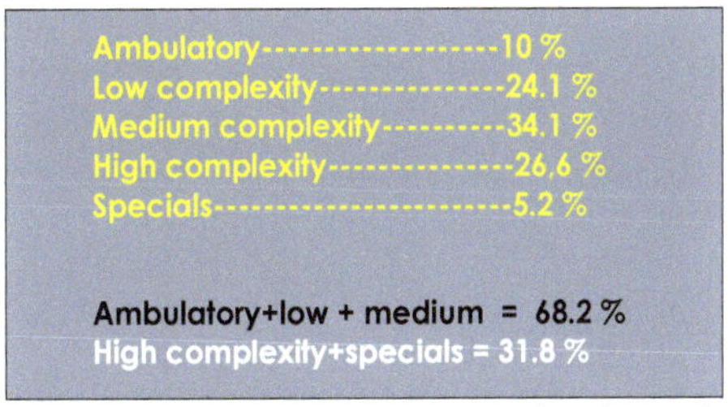

Figure 6. Chart of surgeries in Brazilian hospitals. Datasus-tabnet-2012.

Some tries were adopted to solve the lack of beds in Hospitals. To anticipate discharges was one of them.

Anticipated discharges, here denominated de-hospitalization, happen under severe medical criteria and with the allowance of patient's family.

Families are taken as partners for the recovering treatment, following instructions of doctors.

Experiences of de-hospitalization became possible due to advances of medicine that turned surgeries less invasive and safer.

Surgical procedures, impacted by development of new medicines to anesthesia, technologies and medical equipment, demanded sometimes no admission in a hospital but just a post operatory rest.

Private system has started to build small hospitals dedicated to do low and medium complexity surgeries, fasten attending the demand and consequently liberating beds in big hospitals.

Small hospitals need ICU. Price of space and staff appropriated to ICU could turn prohibitive the survival of small hospitals in financial terms. Solution to that came through a contract with a back office hospital with guarantee of having an ICU bed anytime it was necessary.

Design a small hospital was a huge and enjoyable challenge for us. We had to design a 4 beds hospital, less than 500 m^2 and, there was no land for its construction (Figure 7-8).

First challenge, the lack of land was solved by taking off an existing roof, reinforcing local structure and, encrusting the Mini-Hospital.

Our team classified the ideal values to the project: designing a sane and scientific building.

The most important scientific conditions turn to be:

- Qualify the surgical center with two operating rooms. Like in an airplane, where there are always two devices to the same task, a hospital, even Mini, cannot depend on a single room for surgery.
- Add a mini sterilization system with soiled, preparation, sterilization and, sterile materials rooms.

Reminding that crucial moment of a man on the way to the surgical center we offered some clues showing that architects were there to take care of him providing:

- colorful picture on the ceiling to offer an escape of that terrible situation;
- TV screen close to him to show peaceful images;
- music of his choice reported on his medical records.

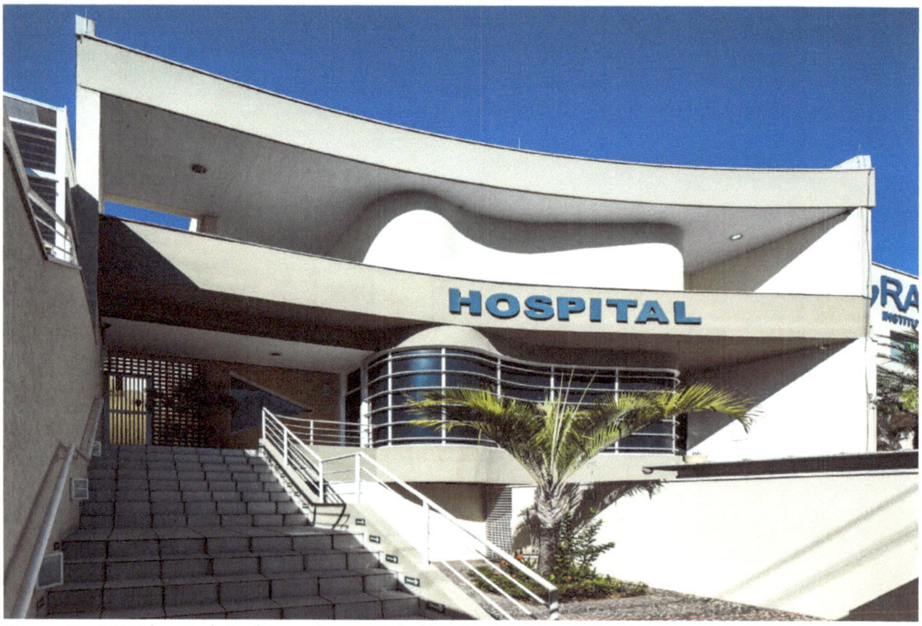

Figure 7. Mini hospital: Radium - Instituto de Oncologia – Hospital.

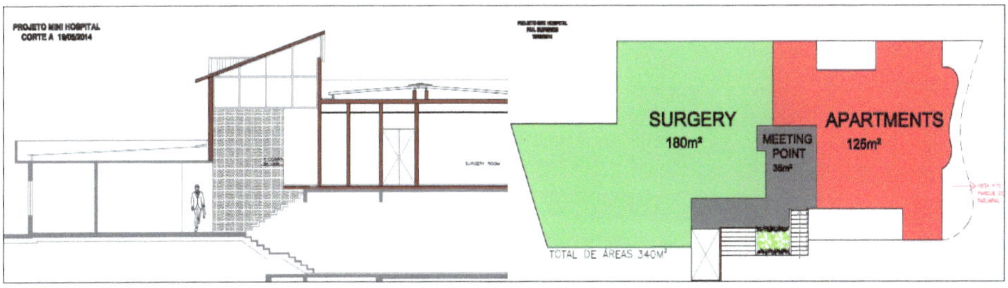

Figure 8. Project, section and plan.

Unfortunately none of these suggestions have been accepted at first sight by my client.

The good news is that recently he called us to talk about adding values to the operating theater and to admission room, focusing on patient. When built we can measure results by post occupancy evaluation which will be part of this ongoing study.

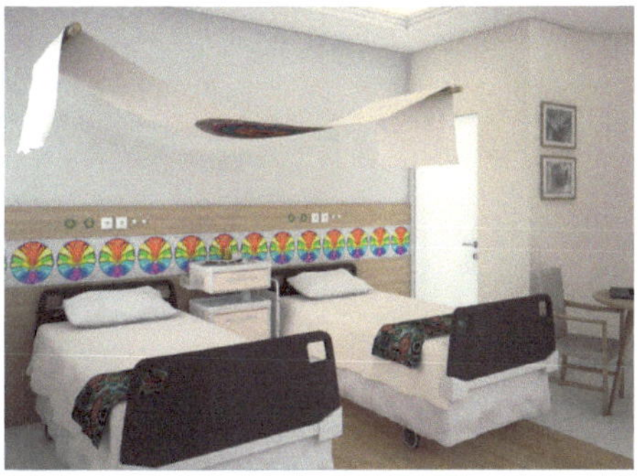

Figure 9. Patient room.

For the admission area we borrowed from TV some cultural icons of patients everyday life linked to his imaginary. A great part of Brazilians follow soap operas on TV, talking about it as if it was a national issue or a famous movie.

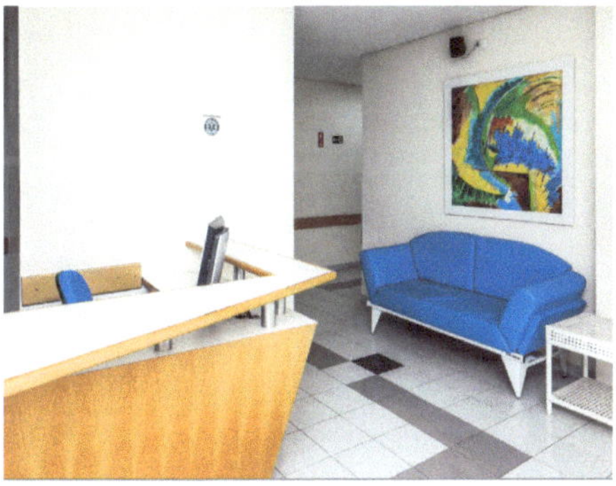

Figure 10. Meeting point.

Besides, we adopted values of "pousadas de charme", a kind of hostelry existing by the beaches and mountainsl, with cozy interior and expensive rates, not always accessible to beneficiaries of health plans. Due to the short time inside the room we provided the apartment with impact objects.

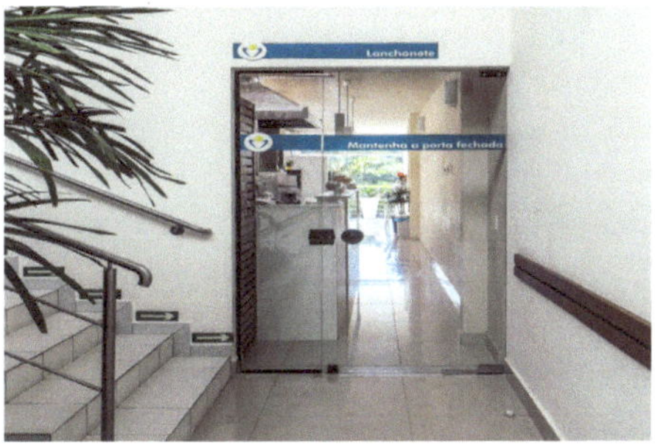

Figure 11. Cafeteria.

For example two identical beds for patient and companion, crowned with a schematic canopy. The amazing canopy, reminding royal beds, aims to open a special time in the middle of that conflicting pre-surgical period (Figure 9).

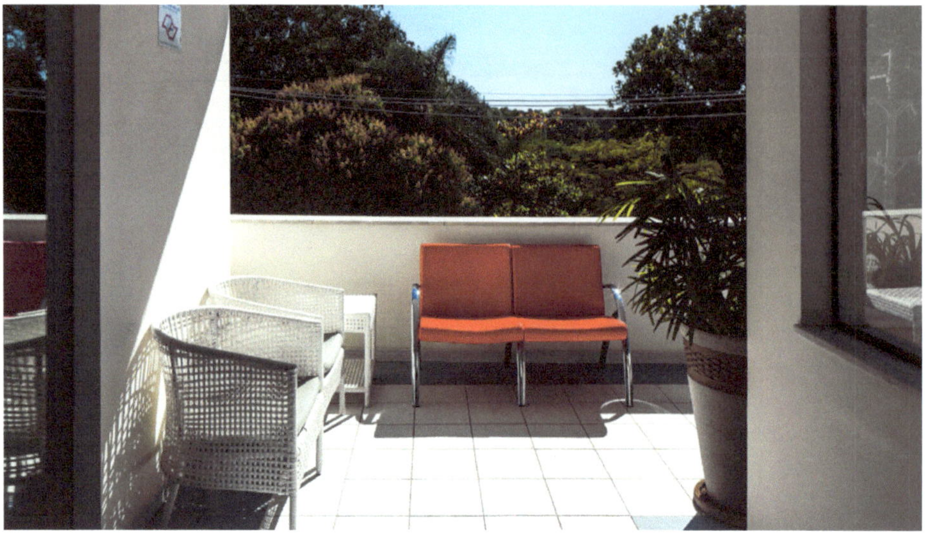

Figure 12. Waiting room for companions.

A large mirror hanged on the wall acts as a tool of appropriation of the space. In western culture the sense of eye-sight is historically regarded as the noblest of the senses (Juhani Palaasmaa, "Skin's eyes"). Seeing himself inside that room through the mirror can make the patient realize that he is the owner of that space.

A comfortable armchair can fascinate the doctor to remain a few minutes more in the room during round. There is a frequent contradictory situation witnessed by me in hospitals: patient expects to meet the doctor while the doctor prefers not to meet him. The doctor's visit makes him think, with good humor, that the doctor is "the runaway groom".
A small meeting point, between the apartments and surgery center entrance-exit, reinforces possibility of patients to meet doctors.
A nice waiting room and a small cafeteria, as dressing the project, are options for the companions (Figure 10-12).

CONCLUSIONS

To design a new building such as a Mini-Hospital, architects must go beyond architecture and dive into medicine and public healthcare.
In Brazil, healthcare architecture must always be designed with the proposal to provide inputs to the sustainability of public health system. Mini-Hospital shows good conditions to be inserted in urban environments of big cities as well as in small neighborhoods and favelas.
Architecture struggled to give competent solutions by:

- making itself compact enough to respond to functional destinations
- being integrative enough to promote a meeting point to doctors and patient
- and bringing positive impact, positive enough to releave crucial moments.

And, by the way, be one of 4 patients of the day in a hospital is a privilege, an honor!

An Adaptive Approach to Primary Healthcare Facility Design in the Western Cape

Ulrike Kuscke

Ulrike.Kuschke@westerncape.gov.za
Western Cape Government, Department of Transport and Public Works, South Africa

The Western Cape Government Department of Transport and Public Works is responsible for the design and construction of new public health facilities, as well as extending and upgrading existing facilities.
We identified the need to develop appropriate primary healthcare outpatient facility design guidelines that are relevant to the current South African context. By assessing the available literature on primary healthcare facilities, analysing our recently completed facilities, and interviewing patients, clinical, and administrative staff, we have been able to test our findings. These have included a series of interactive workshops with the Department of Health.
At the initial workshop we presented a 'Lego' building block approach to primary healthcare design with 'generic' units and components. This was then further developed into a toolkit for a wide range of varied applications. A series of prototypes has been applied and evaluated with the results continuously fed back into the design process.
This approach has promoted design integration and knowledge transfer between disciplines within the public and the private sector and provides an excellent training opportunity for new built environment professionals entering the specialised world of health facility design. It also questions the traditional workflow processes adopted by clinical staff, and reflects the need to continuously evaluate patterns of use. A structured 'Post-Occupancy Evaluation' tool, developed in conjunction with a research organisation, is carried out 18 months after the commissioning of each facility.
The toolkit methodology has since been applied to a wide range of project types, including new facilities, upgrades, extensions, temporary and re-locatable facilities, and maintenance to existing facilities. Having advanced the design process in this manner, our challenge now is:

> *How do we deliver exemplary, adaptable facilities faster and for less money invested across the project life cycle, whilst improving and supporting social and environmental sustainability?*

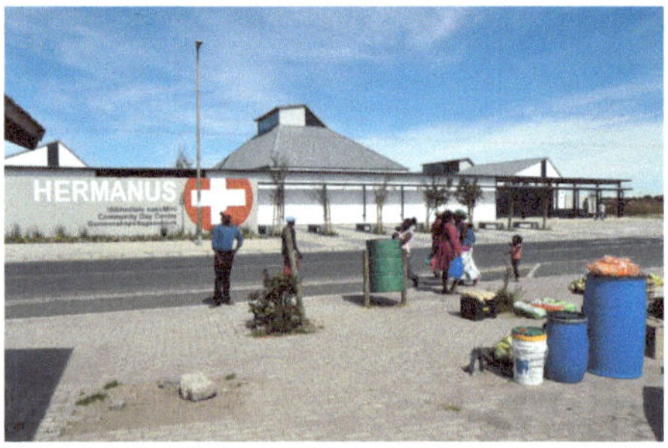

Main entrance to the Hermanus Community Day Centre. Consultant Architect: Gallagher Lourens Architects. Image: Gallagher Lourens Architects.

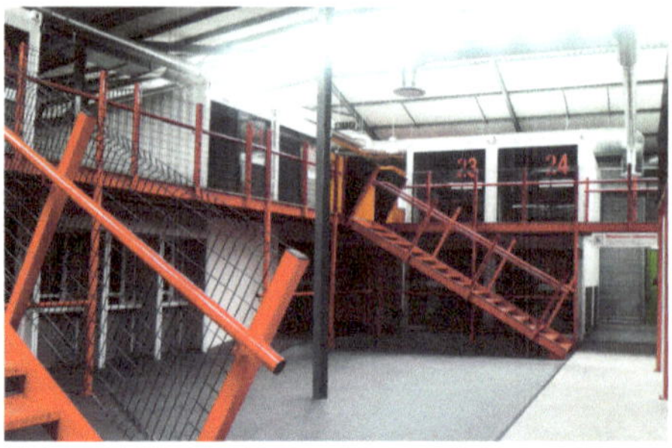

Internal Atrium at Du Noon Temporary Clinic. Consultant Architect: Revel Fox & Partners. Image: Revel Fox & Partners.

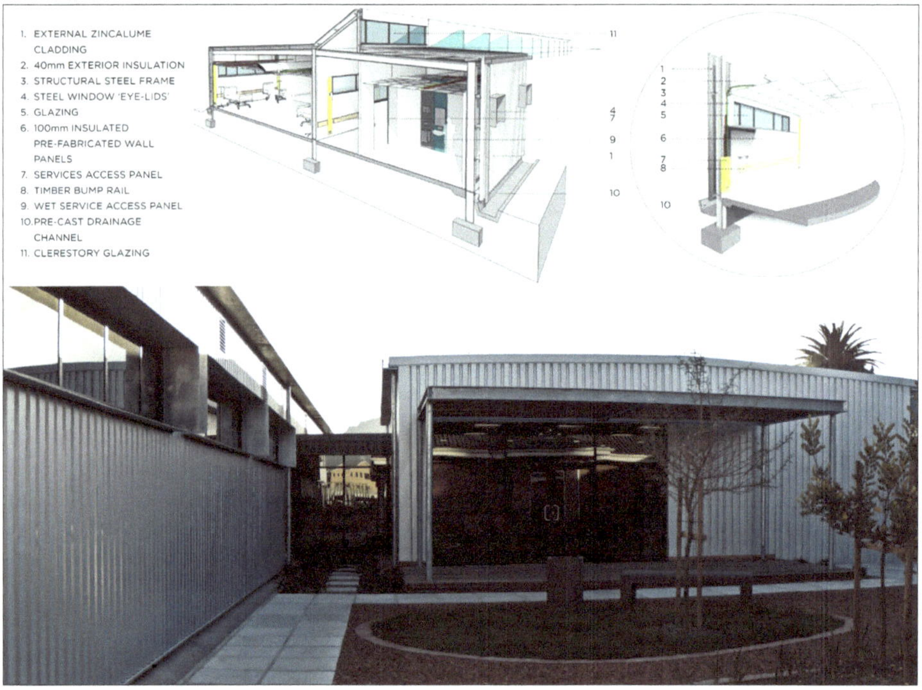

Construction and material study at Heideveld Temporary Emergency Centre. Consultant Architect: Workshop 6 Architecture. Image: Workshop 6 Architecture & Charlton Botha.

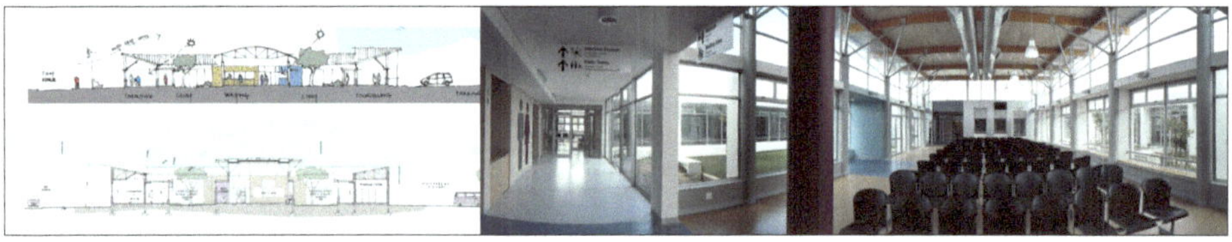

Sectional development study at Grassy Park Clinic. Consultant Architect: Amanda Katz Architects. Image: Amanda Katz Architects.

ANNEXES

International Union of Architects Public Health Group PHG at UIA 2014 Durban Congress

Pre-Congress Cape Town Tour: 30 July - 1 August 2014

A short tour of recent primary health care facilities in Cape Town provided an opportunity for PHG members to visit an integrated set of facilities designed to improve the quality of primary health care services to the extensive and rapidly growing Cape Flats communities in Cape Town. Recent planning emphasised the need to improve first level district services to provide service opportunities closer to the communities requiring services and to reduce the load on existing secondary and tertiary level facilities. All facilities visited were completed during the last four years.

Improving services through upgrading, expanding and adding new facilities while retaining and improving access to all levels of service is a complex task requiring innovation, compromise and some lateral thinking. Services, for instance, to the fast growing community in Du Noon were provided in a rapidly deployed temporary clinic while a more comprehensive new community health centre (CHC) was being designed and built. The tour started with a visit to the existing **Du Noon Temporary Clinic** where Duncan Rendall of the Western Cape Department of Health, on behalf of Dr Laura Angelletti du Toit Chief Director at the Department of Health, Western Cape Government, provided a brief overview of the planning of healthcare services and infrastructure focussing on services in the Cape Peninsula and Cape Town Metropolitan area (Figure 1).

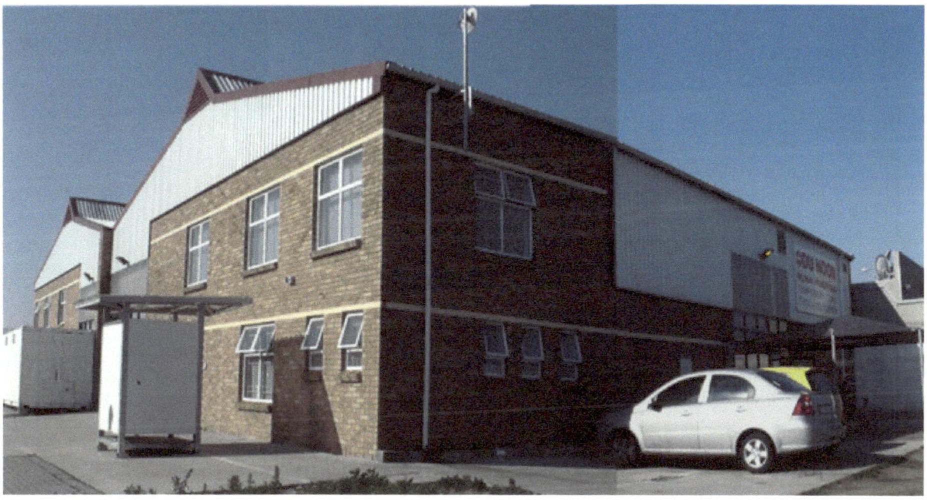

Figure 1. Du Noon temporary clinic – the modest rented warehouse is home to a set of 28 converted shipping containers.

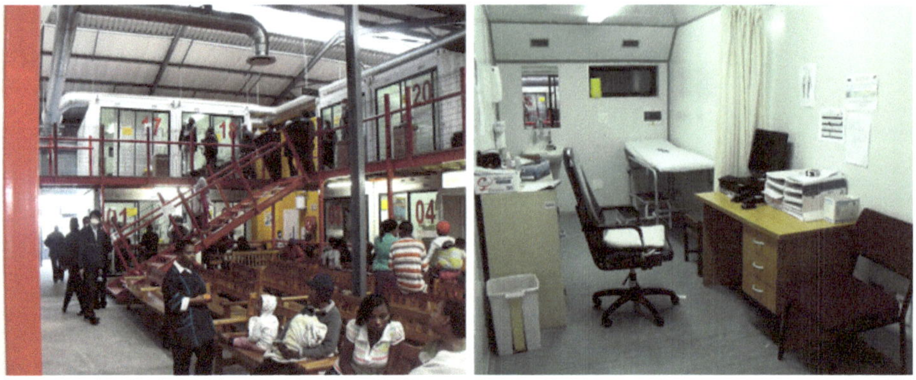

Figure 2. Du Noon temporary clinic – inside the stacked containers form a square round a double volume waiting area with industrial stair and walkways provide access to the clearly numbered set of consulting rooms.

Once the new Du Noon centre is operational the temporary clinic would be closed and the containers and walkways moved to the new Mfuleni multi-purpose community hall to serve again as a temporary clinic while the new permanent Mfuleni health centre is built (Figure 2).

The new **Du Noon Community Health Centre** was nearing completion when visited and will provide a full range of PHC day services and will include a 24 hour emergency and midwifery unit. The 5140m2 facility is built round a series of courtyards providing public gathering and visual relief spaces to the formal clinical areas. The building echoes the industrial motif of the area with the raised roofs providing light and ventilation to the public areas (Figure 3).

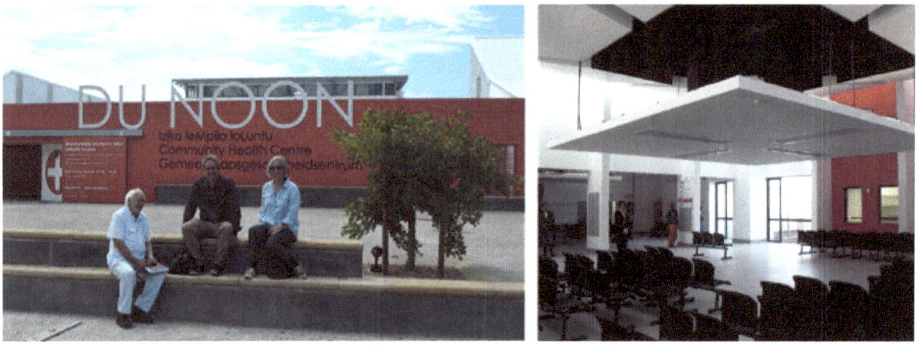

Figure 3. New Du Noon Community Health Centre – Main entrance façade and main waiting area (nearing completion).

Overcrowding in formal and informal settlements contribute to the high burden of TB and drug-resistant TB in the Cape Flats. The new Drug-resistant treatment centre at the **Brooklyn Chest Hospital** visited by the group is designed to reduce the possibility of cross-infection between patients through the provision of permanently ventilated single rooms for long stay patients (Figure 4).

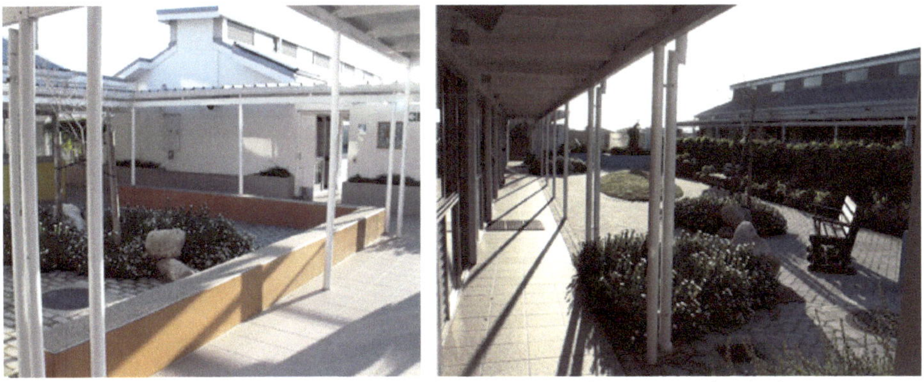

Figure 4. Drug-resistant TB Centre at the Brooklyn Chest Hospital – open corridors lead to patient wings with banks of ridge ventilated single rooms opening onto landscaped courtyards encouraging contact in open areas where the risk of cross infection is reduced.

The **Heideveld Emergency Centre** is another temporary facility bridging a critical service gap while the nearby GF Jooste District Hospital is decommissioned and rebuilt on its existing site. The portal shed structure is clad inside and out with cold room panels and was planned, designed and built in seventeen months primarily using components prefabricated off site. The structure is largely demountable and can mostly be reused elsewhere once the new hospital is completed (Figure 5).

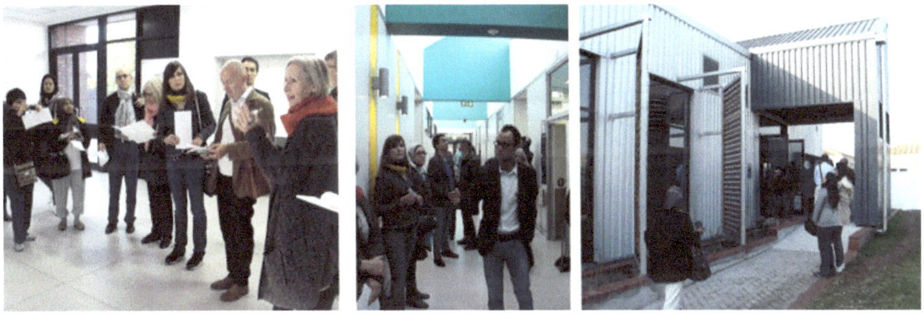

Figure 5. Heideveld Emergency Centre – Provincial Hospitals Architect Ulrike Kushke provides project background to the PHG tour group, central rooflit corridor and end façade of building with shading to windows looking out towards Table Mountain.

Gassy Park Community Day Centre (CDC) provides core PHC services and acts as a first point of call for the immediate community. The facility fills the available site and is inward looking into two courtyards flanking the open primary waiting area. Consulting areas open off circulation and waiting areas looking out into the landscaped courtyards (Figure 6).

The new **Delft Community Day Centre**, nearing completion when visited, offers a different design solution with clinic areas radiating out from a central admission core and large courtyard which also provides civic and public meeting spaces for the rapidly growing community. The project includes an extensive community arts initiative with mosaics integral with the organic design (Figure 7).

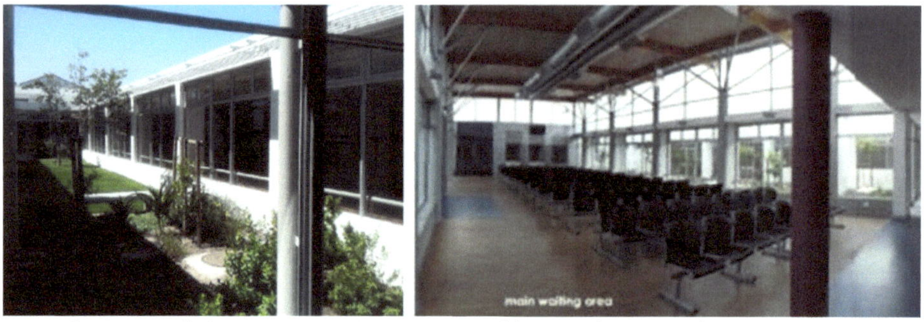

Figure 6. Grassy Park Community Day Centre – courtyard from circulation corridor and main waiting area.

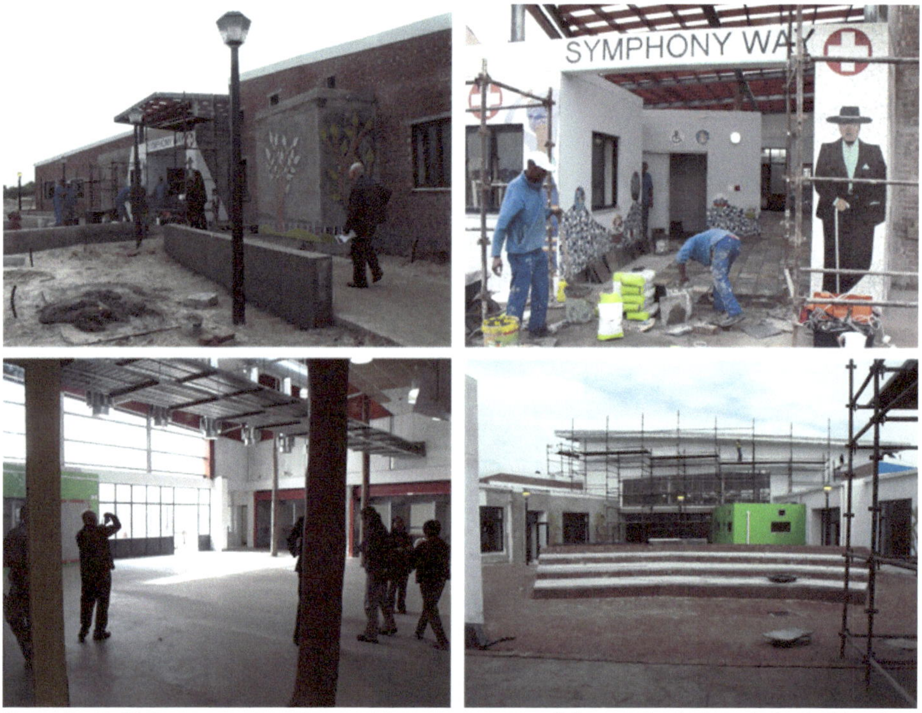

Figure 7. Delft Community Day Centre – The main entrance off the street leads through the double volume waiting, reception and public meeting area out into the large internal courtyard around which the clinic areas are clustered.

The group also visited two new District Hospitals which provide referral services for the network of CDC's and CHC's. The hospitals, built from essentially the same brief, provide substantially different design solutions. Both have 230 beds and offer a full range of district hospital services including out-patients, emergency, radiology with CT scanner, level 1 inpatient and day surgery, obstetrics, inpatient and rehabilitation services.

Khayelitsha District Hospital, the first to be completed (January 2012) is a 3 storey complex on an open central urban site. Security is a key concern and while access is carefully managed the entrance areas are open and inviting with landscaping and artwork playing important roles. Natural lighting and ventilation and key concerns with open courtyards providing constant links to the exterior. The front block is primarily two storey with admission, outpatients, emergency and obstetric services on the ground floor and administration and surgery on the first floor. The block is linked by a central spine corridor to the three storey ward block and support and industrial services blocks (Figure 8).

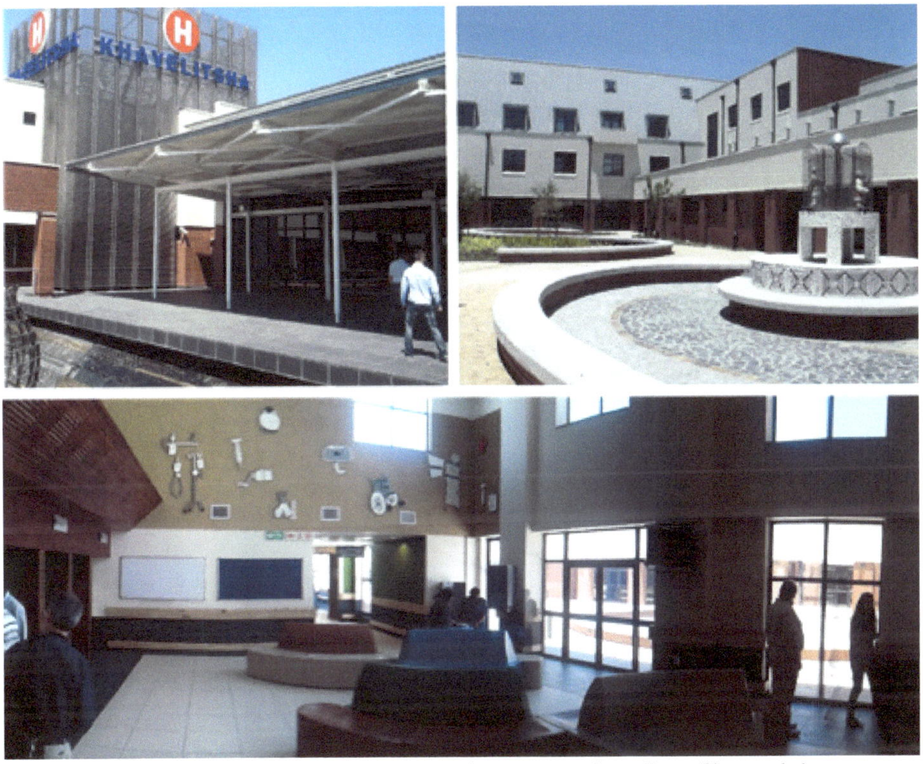

Figure 8. Khyalitsha District Hospital – entrance marking, courtyards, rooflit staff base and pharmacy waiting area.

Mitchells Plain Hospital in contrast is built on an ecologically sensitive site and the footprint was kept to a minimum to preserve as much of the unique Sandveld fynbos site as possible. The facility was built towards the back of the site on ground that had already been disturbed leaving the roadside portion largely undisturbed. Plants and animals in areas that were disturbed were moved to a nursery and holding area and replaced once building operations were completed. A number of community empowerment initiatives were implemented during construction creating a sense of pride and local ownership (Figure 9).

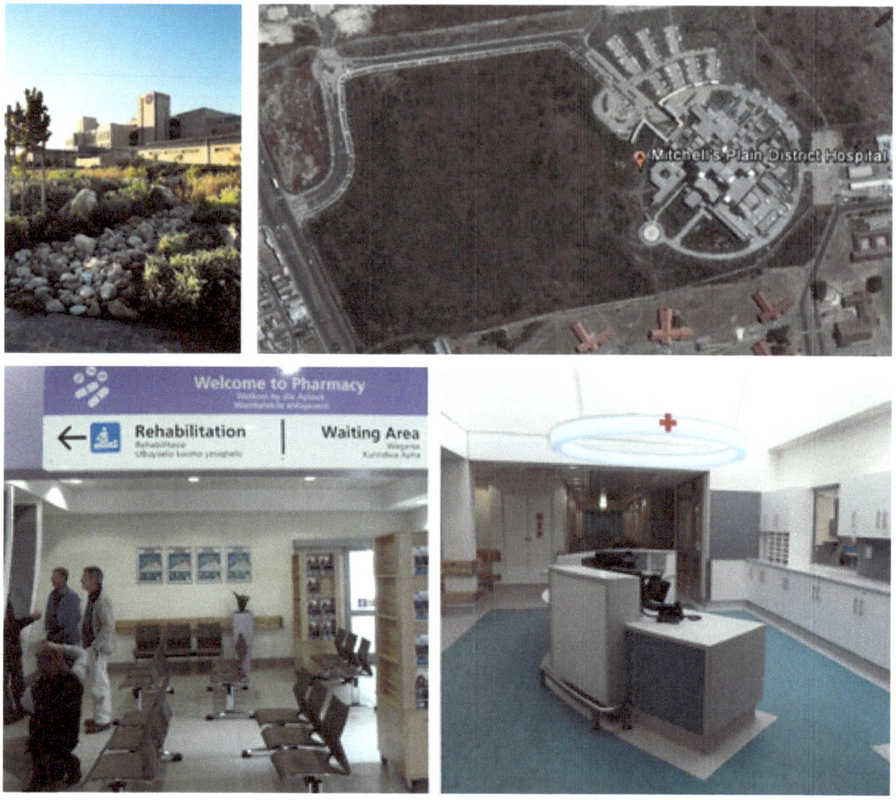

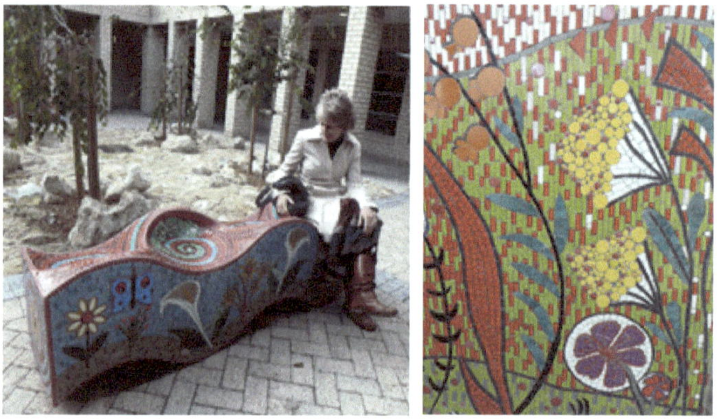

Figure 9. Mitchells Plain District Hospital – the design preserves local fauna and flora and community based artists created mosaics and objects such as the seating in the entrance courtyard are widely used and reinforce the environmental and community themes.

Special thanks to Dr Laura Angeletti du Toit, Chief Director Infrastructure and Technical Management, Department of Health, Western Cape Government and to Ulrike Kuschke, Chief Architect Health Directorate, Department of Transport and Public Works, Western Cape Government and their staff for support in facilitating visits and accompanying the Public Health Group.

Optional Pre-Congress Tour: Sunday 3 August 2014

One of the most pressing problems facing health care service in South Africa generally is a high level of TB and drug-resistant TB, a highly transmissable airborne disease, coupled with high levels in the immunocompromised community of people living with HIV and AIDS. To provide some insight into these challenges, how they are affected by and influence the local built environment response, the International Union of Architects Public Health Group hosted an optional tour to selected healthcare services and facilities in the Durban metropolis ahead of the 2014 UIA Congress on Sunday 3 August 2014.

The tour began with a half-day visit to the KwaZulu-Natal Research Unit for Tuberculosis and HIV (KRITH), followed by traditional Durban lunch of "bunny chow" and an afternoon at the Cyril Zulu Infectious Diseases Clinic and Warwick Junction. The choice of facilities was poignant as representing diversity in design approach and investment in South Africa today. KRITH is a sophisticated, technological-advanced laboratory and research facility associated with the University of KwaZulu-Natal Medical School: Cyril Zulu Infectious Diseases Clinic is a clinic, run by eThekwini Municipality, which serves both a local community as well as the community moving daily through the Warwick Junction.

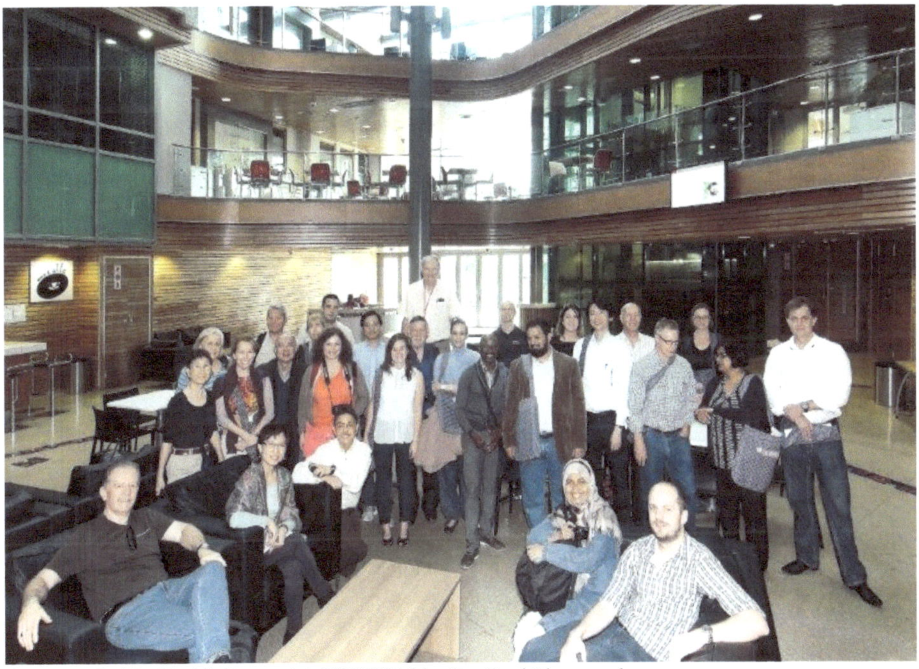

Figure 1. Public Health Group visit KRITH lobby. Roy Reed Photography.

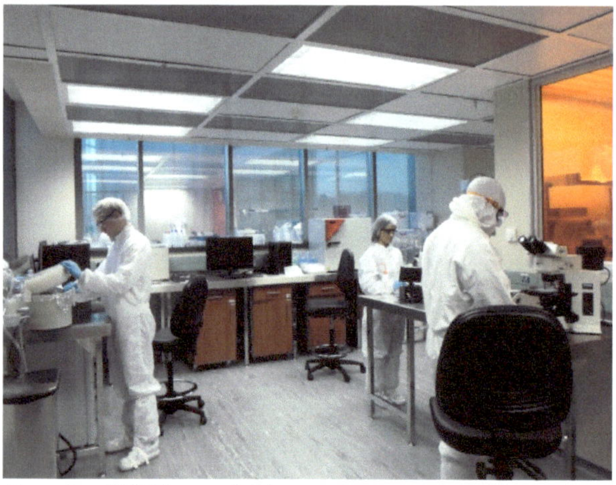

Figure 2. KRITH research laboratory.

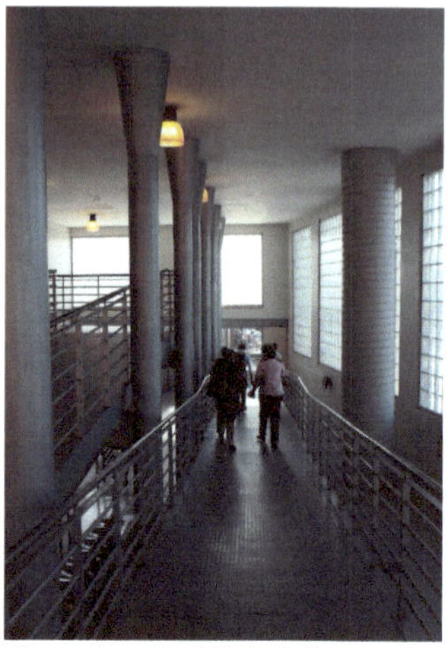

Figure 3. Cyril Zulu Infectious Diseases Clinic, Jako Nice photo.

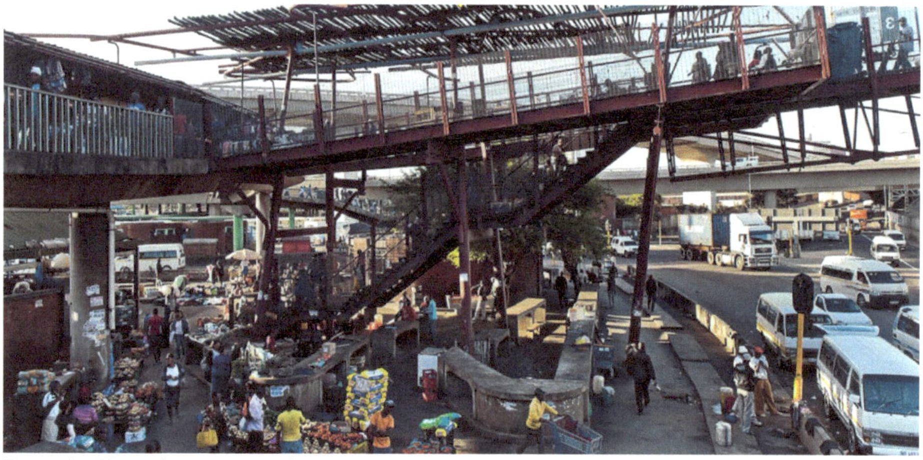

Figure 4. Warwick Junction market.

Warwick Junction is a major transport node and commercial hub in the Durban area, housing a number of traditional and informal markets. Warwick Junction is also of interest as the site of both the main UIA 2014 Durban Congress Student Competition as well as the PHG Healthcare Otherwhere Student Competition site. Delegates on the tour were accompanied by the architects and engineers of the facility, facilities managers, officials from eThekwini Health Department and local business owners who explained the design rationale and answered questions.

Special thanks to Dr Andrew Robinson, Kevin Bingham, James Trinder, Bryan Mc-Master, Tiligavath Chinappa, Ayo Olowolagba, Santosh Hansraj, Sindy Ngobese, Vasie Pillay, Nosipo Hlophe, John Royal and Richard.

Geoff Abbott, Public Health Group UIA

UIA 2014 HEALTHCARE OTHERWHERE INTERNATIONAL STUDENT COMPETITION

anOTHER International Student Competition

As part of promoting healthcare as a subspecialist discipline, a 'Healthcare Otherwhere' International Student Competition was created as a feature in the International Union of Architects Public Health Group (UIA-PHG) activities during the Durban 2014 UIA Congress. The competition was prepared in announced in early 2014 and distributed via UIA-PHG and GUPHA member networks. The competition invited students to propose architectural interventions explicitly used to address local public health issues. In doing so, they were encouraged to consider collaboration between various professions, communities, government and developers; explore medical and public health practise; reconcile traditional and alternative and western medicine; and reflect how hostile aspects of urban environment can be sustainably transformed into healthy human habitat to enhance human health and wellbeing through architectural design. The competition site was Warwick Junction, Durban, and the immediate surrounding area including the Central Durban Cemetery edge.

As South Africa was host nation, CSIR Built Environment Unit provided the local organising committee for the UIA-PHG track at the International Congress, including initiating, coordinating and administering the International Student Competition. This team consisted of Jako Nice, Roekshana Benjamin, Claire du Trevou, Nsindiso Hlatshwayo, Geoff Abbott and Peta de Jager.

Healthcare Otherwhere Competition Jury

Warren Kerr, presiding Director of the UIA-PHG convened a competition jury comprising a very prestigious group of selected healthcare architects and academics representing all the UIA PHG regions (Western Europe, Eastern Europe, Americas, Asia and Oceania and Africa). The adjudication process was a complete blind assessment and conforming to UNESCO-UIA rules for international architecture and town planning competitions.

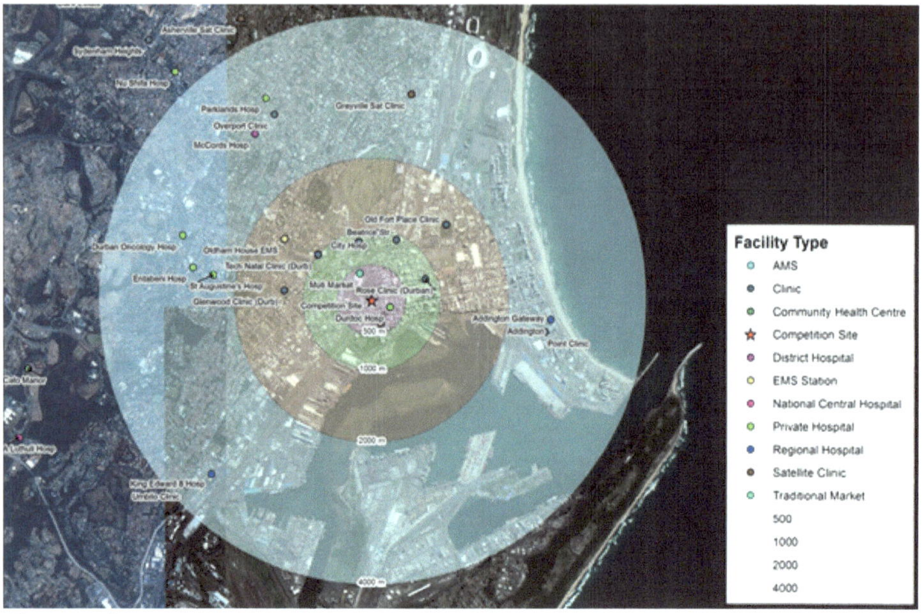

Figure 1. Competition site.

MIKE NIGHTINGALE
Jury Convenor
United Kingdom – UIA Region I (Western Europe)

Mike is an internationally recognised healthcare architect and the founder of Nightingale Associates. He is devoted to raising the standard of architecture in healthcare and the public sector. He is also the Chairman of the Mike Nightingale Fellowship, a UK registered charity focussing on changing lives through sustainable development in South Africa Mike has played a pivotal role in promoting quality of healthcare architecture. He was the author of 'Better by Design', the design guide published by the National Health Service, was a founder committee member for Architects for Health and the RIBA Health Client Forum. He is a member of the NHS Estates Knowledge Network Group for Building Design and was the External Examiner for the MARU MSc in Planning Buildings for Health. He regularly reviews healthcare projects as a member of the NHS Design Review Panel. Mike is on the International and Editorial Review Panels of the International Academy of Design & Health. He is also a Fellow of the Royal Society of Arts. Mike was born in South Africa and has lived in India and Canada, and believes in a global approach to the design of healthcare buildings. Subsequently he provides guidance on key forms of procurement such as PFI, in the UK and abroad. Mike travels the world as a key-note speaker for international conferences. He also inspires young talent by guest lecturing at universities. Mike is a member of the IBI Health Strategy Group, overseeing the future development of the co-ordinated IBI response to global healthcare markets.

SUSAN FRANCIS
United Kingdom – UIA Region I (Western Europe)

Susan is currently Programme Director for Architects for Health, an RIBA Linked Society and membership organization for design professionals in the UK. Our aim is to promote and campaign for better healthcare environments through bringing together organisations and individuals who share an interest in excellence in the planning and design of healthcare facilities. AfH has run for 7 years a successful Student Design Charette facilitating students to design for health in studio. Qualified as an architect, Susan has worked in practice and as an academic developing research, presentations, publications and post graduate training in this specialised field for 20 years.

FANI VAVILI-TSINIKA
Greece – UIA Region II (Eastern Europe and Middle East)

Professor Fani Vavili, MA, PhD, is teaching and practicing architectural design. She is teaching health care facilities design for over 30 years at the School of Architecture AUTh, Greece. Her work includes health care facilities planning & design and has published many articles, research results etc. Among them are the following books: Hospital Design at the beginning of the 21st Century (ed), Designing for the Elderly, Designing for Mental Health, Aspects of Healing Environments (ed), Arts in Health Care Buildings (ed), Teaching Architecture in Extreme Conditions. Professor Vavili is an executive member of UIA-PHG (International Union of Architects / Public Health Group) and co-founder of GUPHA (Global University Programs in Healthcare Architecture).

GEORGE MANN
USA – UIA Region III (Americas)

Professor George J.Mann, AIA, is The Ronald L. Skaggs, Endowed Professor of Health Facilities Design, at the College of Architecture, Texas A&M University. He was also the first holder of the Skaggs - Sprague Endowed Chair, - at the College of Architecture at Texas A&M University. He is the official liaison from the US - AIA / AAH (Academy of Architecture for Health) to the UIA-PHG (International Union of Architects / Public Health Group) which meets annually in a different country. From 2012 - 2013 he served as the Director of the UIA - PHG.

He and his students have undertaken over 700 "Architecture for Health" projects since he founded the "Architecture for Health" Program at Texas A&M University in 1966. He has taught over 4000 students at Texas A&M University many of whom are leaders in the field of "Architecture for Health" in firms, universities and health and hospital facilities and agencies and organizations around the globe.

Professor Mann is co-founder and former President of GUPHA (Global University Programs in Healthcare Architecture); Founder and Advisory Board Chairman of The RPD (Resource Planning and Development) Group.

Professor Mann has practiced, lectured, and written extensively on "Architecture for Health" projects all over the world through his teaching, research and practice. He was awarded the George H.W. Bush Service Award by President George H.W. Bush. Professor Mann also became the First Recipient of the prestigious Dean J. Thomas Regan Award for Interdisciplinary Teaching, Research, and Public Service.

PROSPERIDAD LUIS
Philippines – UIA Region IV (Asia and Oceania)

Prosperidad Luis is both an active practitioner of architecture, being the Principal of the firm Luis and Associates; and an architectural educator, having taught and served as Dean of the College of Architecture of the University of the Philippines. She obtained her B.S Architecture and Master of Architecture degrees from the University of the Philippines; and her Postgraduate Diploma in Health Facilities Planning from the Medical Architecture Research Unit then attached to the University of North London. She is an active member of the UIA Public Health Group (UIA-PHG) and the Global University Program in Healthcare Architecture (GUPHA). She is also an active member of architectural organizations, local and international; and has served as National President of the United Architects of the Philippines, Deputy Chair for Zone B of the Architects Regional Council Asia (ARCASIA) and Secretary General of the APEC Architect Project Central Council.

TUNDE OLUWA
Nigeria / South Africa – UIA Region V (Africa)

Tunde Oluwa is the founder of Odyssey Architects S.A. whose growing expertise in sustainable development is signalled by their O. R. Tambo Environmental Centre in Benoni. As technical advisor and jury member in several international and national competitions he has contributed to informing contemporary architectural discourse. Tunde believes in a symbiotic relationship between practice and academia and maintains a close relationship with a number of universities in South Africa.

LESLIE MUSIKAVANHU
Zimbabwe / South Africa – UIA Region V (Africa)

Leslie Musikavanhu is an architect and entrepreneur with 18 years of senior management experience both locally and internationally, having worked in the United States and widely across Africa. He is Managing Director of Sharp Shop Architects (Pty) Ltd, a practice with a wide range of activity in the health, education, commercial and retail sectors across Southern Africa, including work in South Africa, Zimbabwe, Angola, Botswana, Mocambique and Uganda. He is also Managing Director of Cre8 Design & Innovation. Leslie holds a Bachelor of Architecture (Summa Cum Laude) from Tuskegee University, USA and is a registered architect in South Africa and member the Gauteng Institute of Architects and of the SA Federation of Hospital Engineers. Leslie has lectured at the University of the Witwatersrand and acted as external examiner.

GEOFF ABBOTT
South Africa – UIA Region V (Africa)

Geoff Abbott is an architect who had been active in research for over 35 years. His life-long interest and involvement with healthcare facilities started as a young graduate in practice in Cape Town and continued as a research architect, research group leader, programme manager and, more recently, as consultant at the CSIR. His work has focussed on the development of planning and design guidelines for healthcare facilities, applied research in projects such as facilities for drug-resistant TB services, and immovable asset planning, management and maintenance. A particular area of interest is strategic planning for healthcare infrastructure. He holds a master's degree in architecture from the University of Natal and a bachelor's degree from the University of Pretoria. Geoff is an Honorary Life Member and is a past National President and Regional Chairman of the South African Federation of Hospital Engineering. He is an Executive Member of the Public Health Group of the UIA and has been a contributing member since 1985. Geoff has been actively involved with capacity development while contributing to and running courses in Health Facility Planning and Design at the University of KwaZulu-Natal and has been a contributing lecturer at the universities of Cape Town, Witwatersrand, Pretoria, Free State and Medunsa.

CRITERIA

The jury assessed the submission according to a framework with defined criteria as follows: Has understanding of the context been achieved? Does the student express an appreciation for the morphological [urban] landscape of Warwick in its unique Durban location? Does the student have an understanding of the context in terms of the user groups and agents that operate in the area, as well as the patterns of use of space - and have they articulated how this impacts on the design decision-making processes for the project? Have "hostile" aspects of the existing urban environment been transformed into healthy human habitats in ways which are plausibly argued to be sustainable? Have the unique health challenges of the Warwick Junction population been appreciated in the proposed ways to enhance human health and wellbeing? Does the submission convey an understanding of the UIA Congress themes OTHERWHERE and OTHER PRACTICE:

a. foster collaboration between the architectural profession, government, communities and relevant development partners;
b. explore OTHER – namely medical and public health – practice;
c. reconcile or counterpoise alternative, traditional, conventional and contemporary emerging disciplines in medicine and public health)? Is the project innovative in approach? Is it well presented and are the concepts graphically competent?

Jury members reported a high overall quality of the submissions received and commended the innovative and creative diversity of entries.

The competition attracted nineteen entries from twelve countries, representing all continents with a very rich variety of design responses. The participants were not categorised based on experience which led to 1st year students competing with postgraduate masters students. The outcome reflected originality and new solutions. Both undergraduate and postgraduate students were well represented in the top ten finalists.

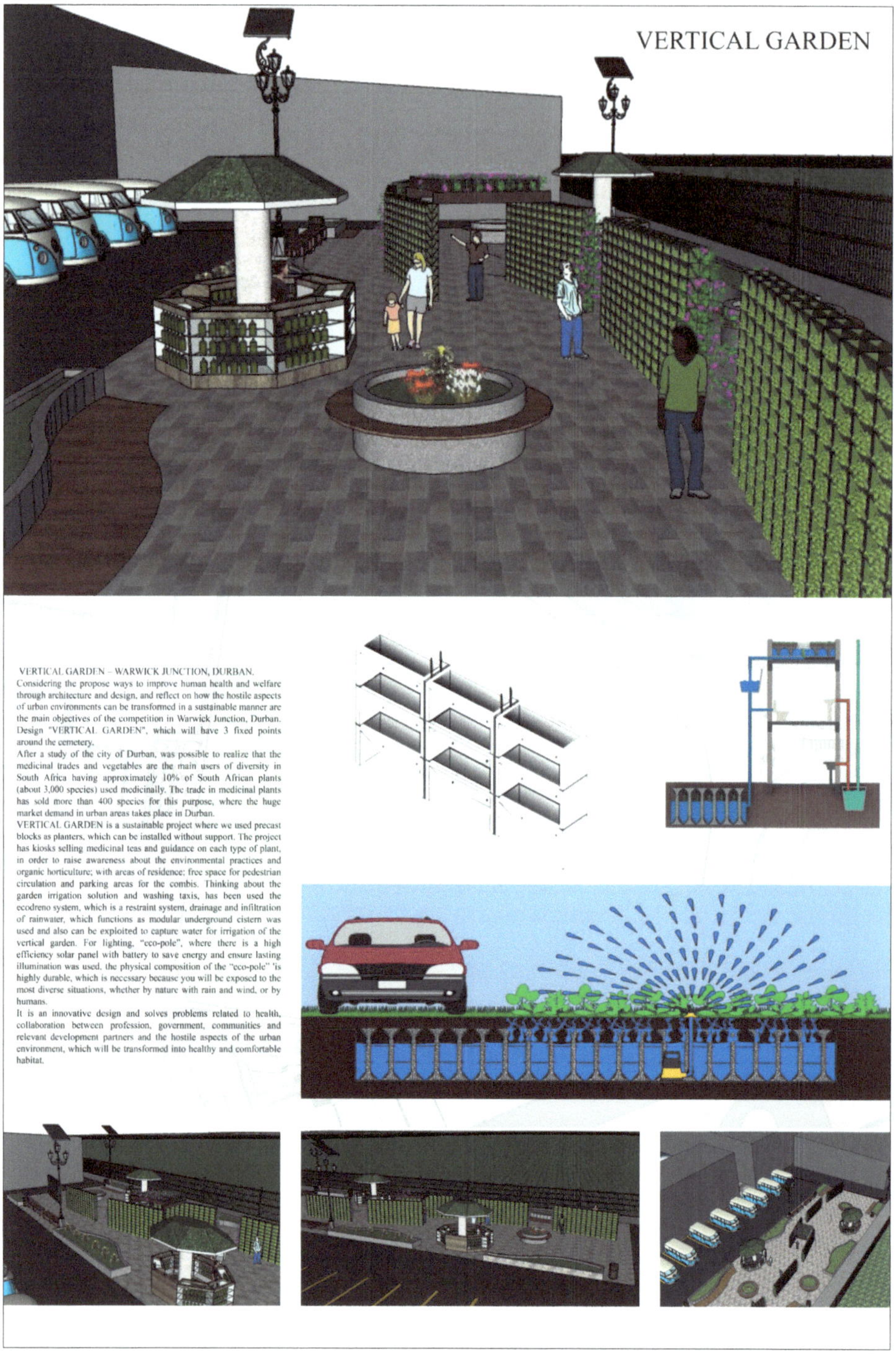

Figure 1. Commended: Lawane Barreto, Universidade Católica de Brasilia, Brazil.

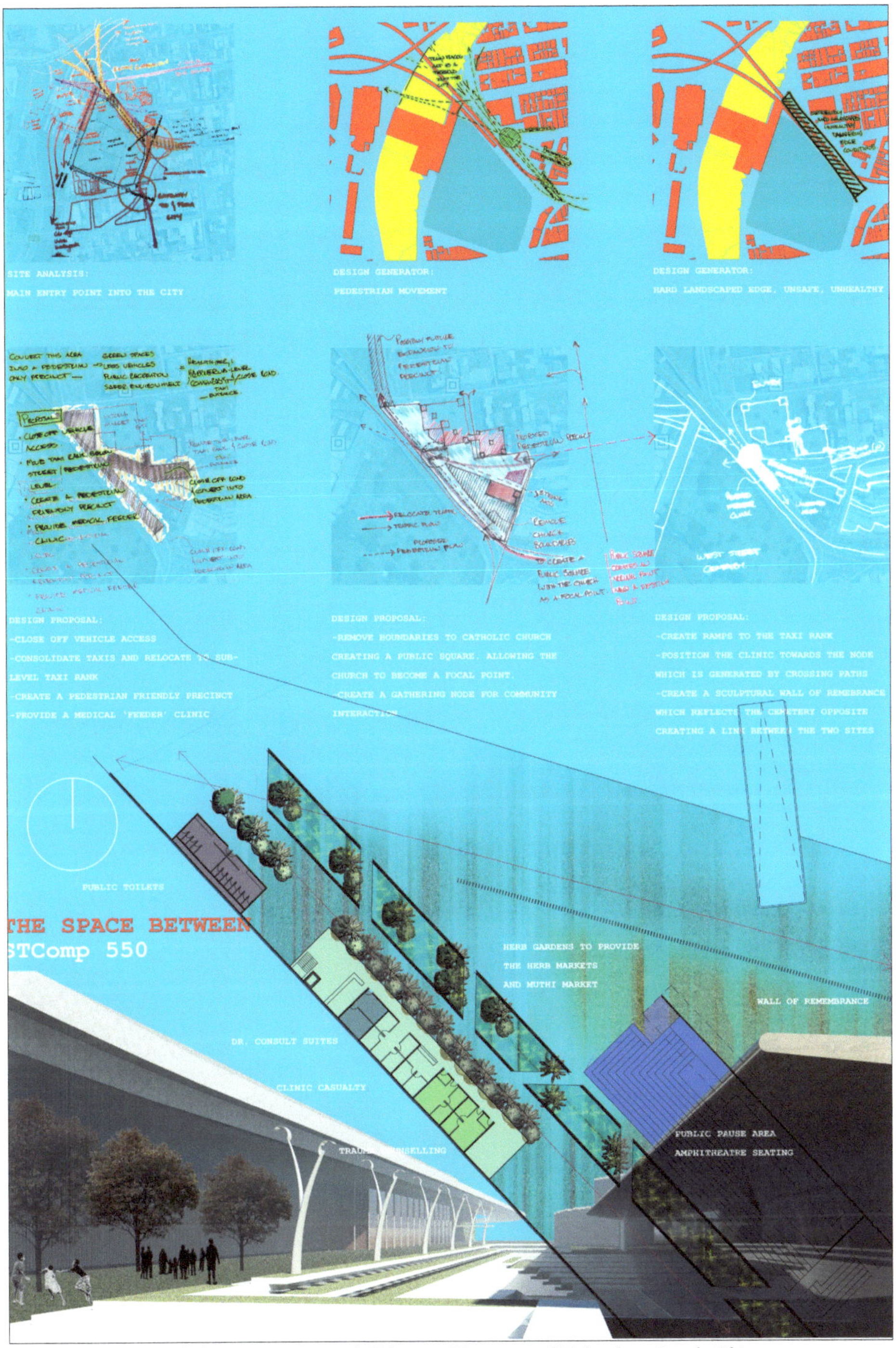

Figure 2. Commended: Greg Murgatroyd, Tshwane University of Technology, South Africa.

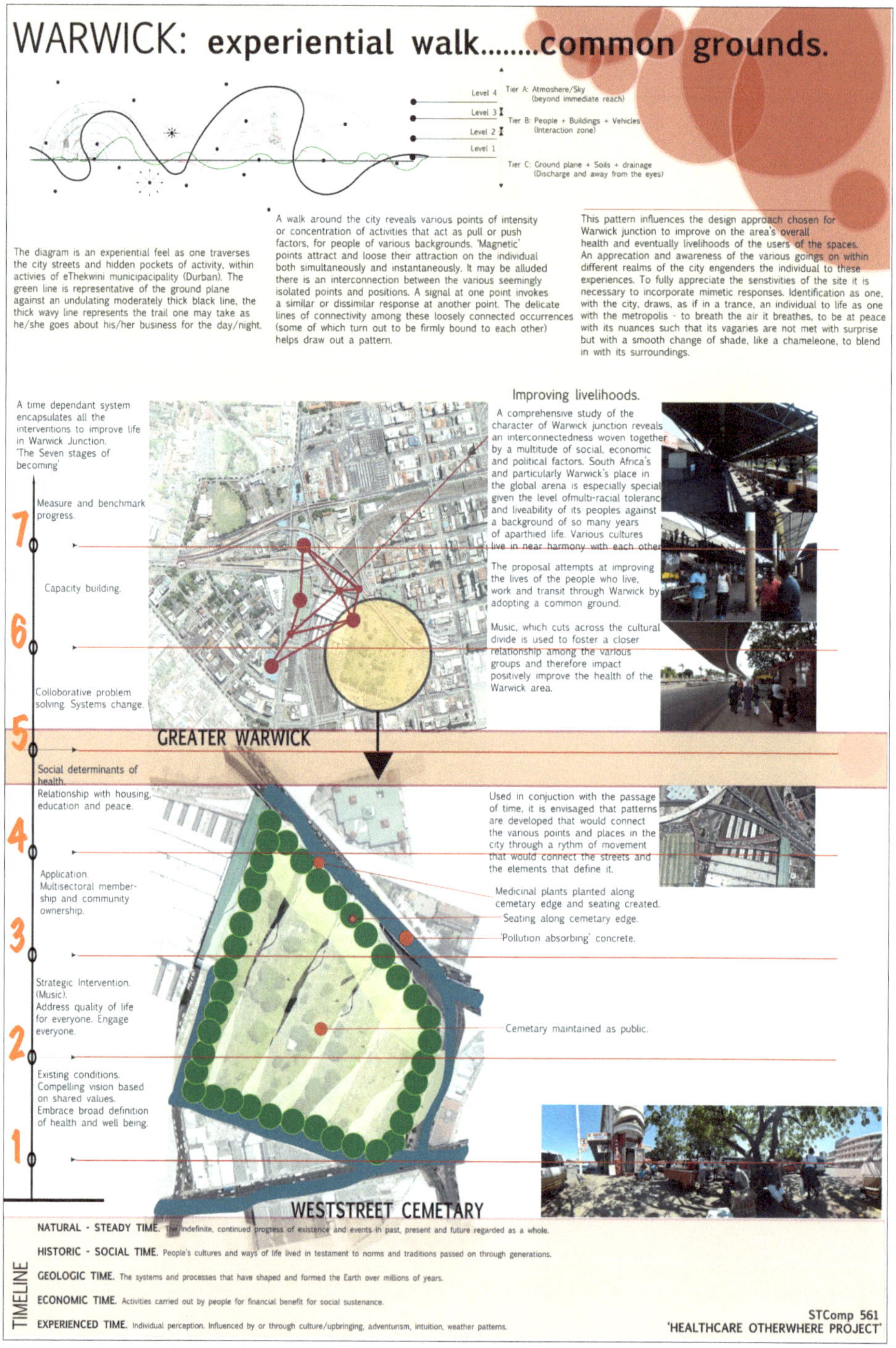

Figure 3. Commended: Herbert Candia Drazu, Uganda Martyrs University, Uganda.

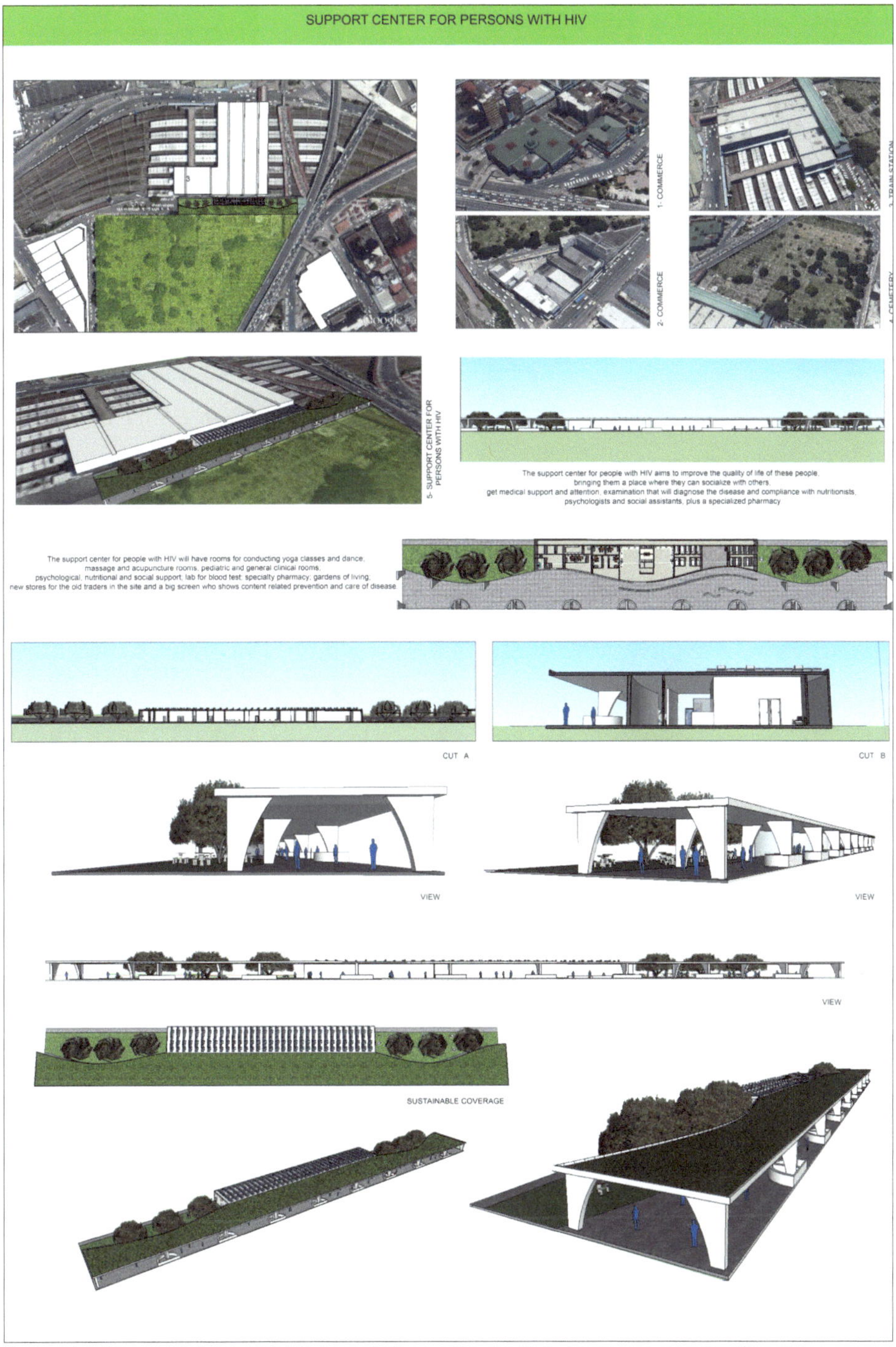

Figure 4. Commended: Manuela Cardoso de Faria, Universidade Católica de Brasilia, Brazil.

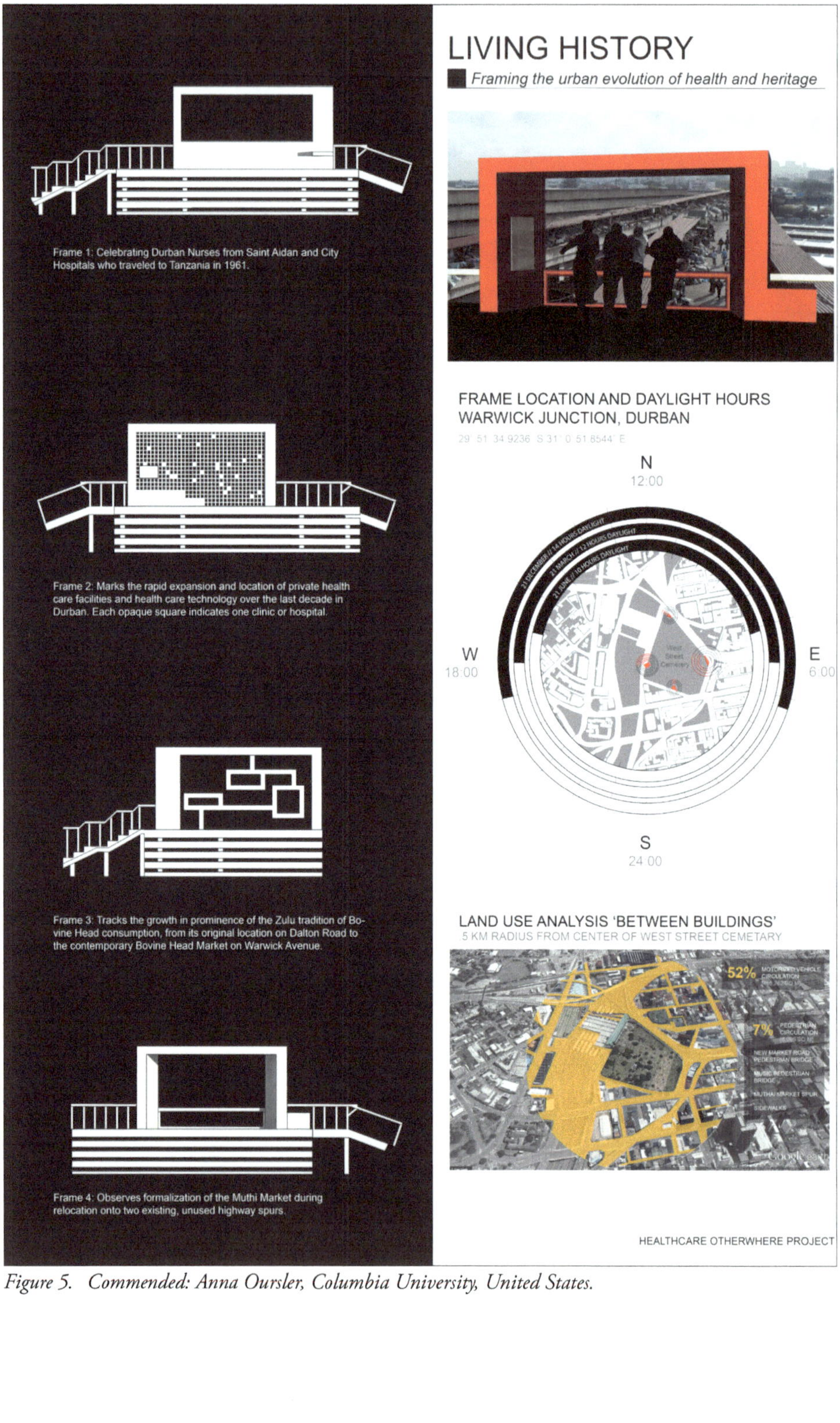

Figure 5. Commended: Anna Oursler, Columbia University, United States.

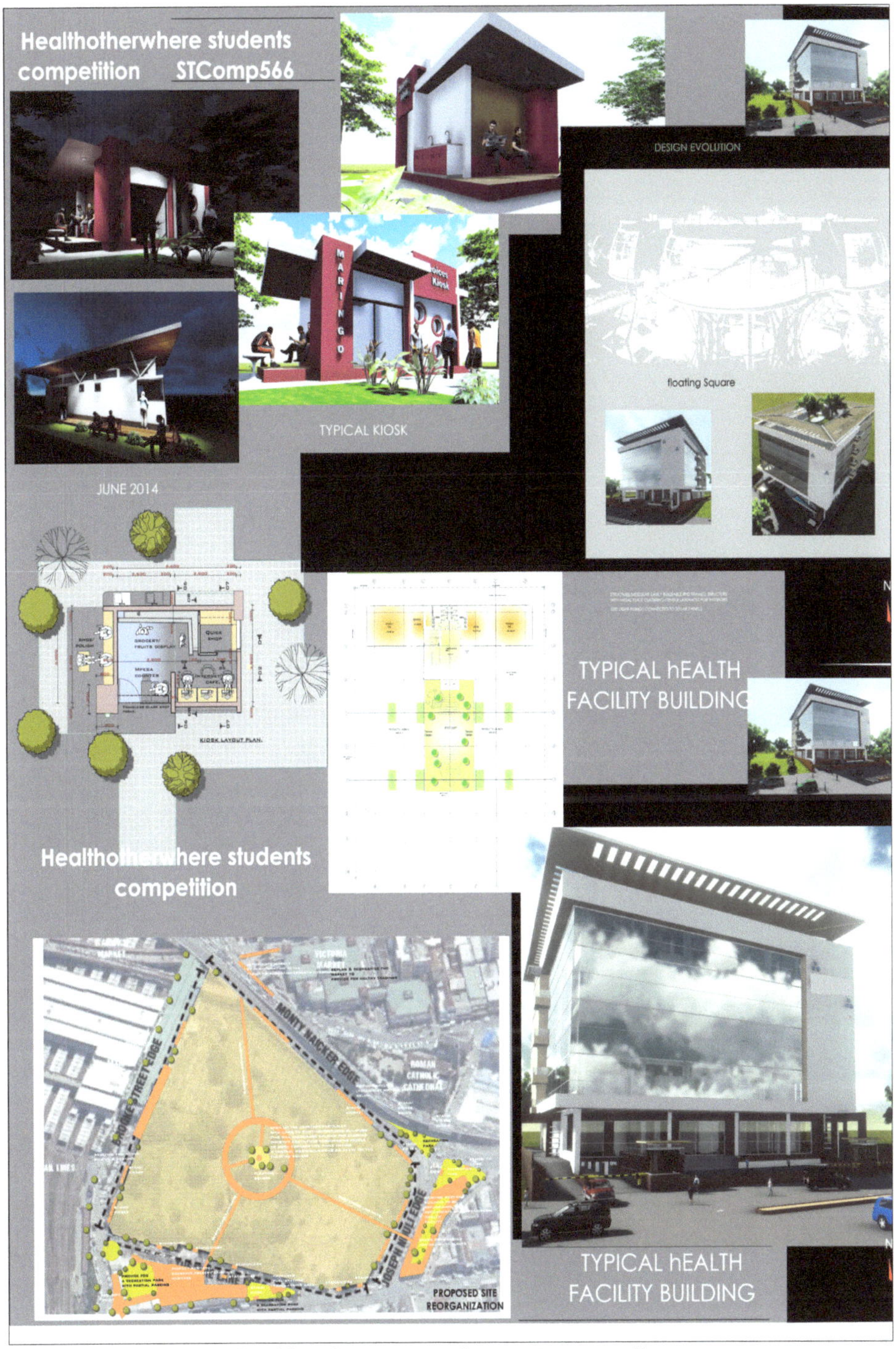

Figure 6. Commended: Bob Odihiambo Oyugi, Jomokenyatta University, Kenya.

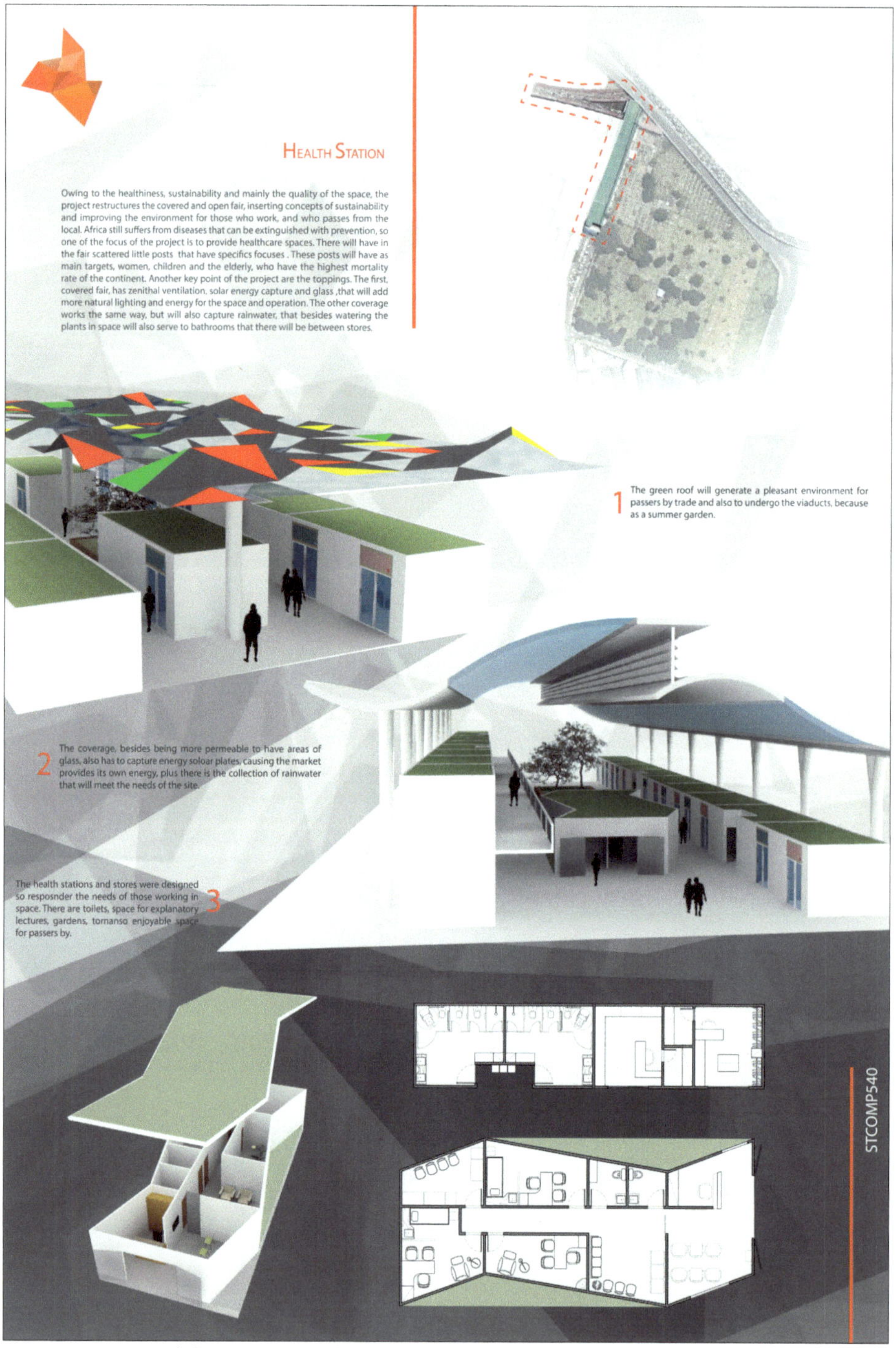

Figure 7. Commended: Livia Freire Falcao, Universidade Católica de Brasilia, Brazil.

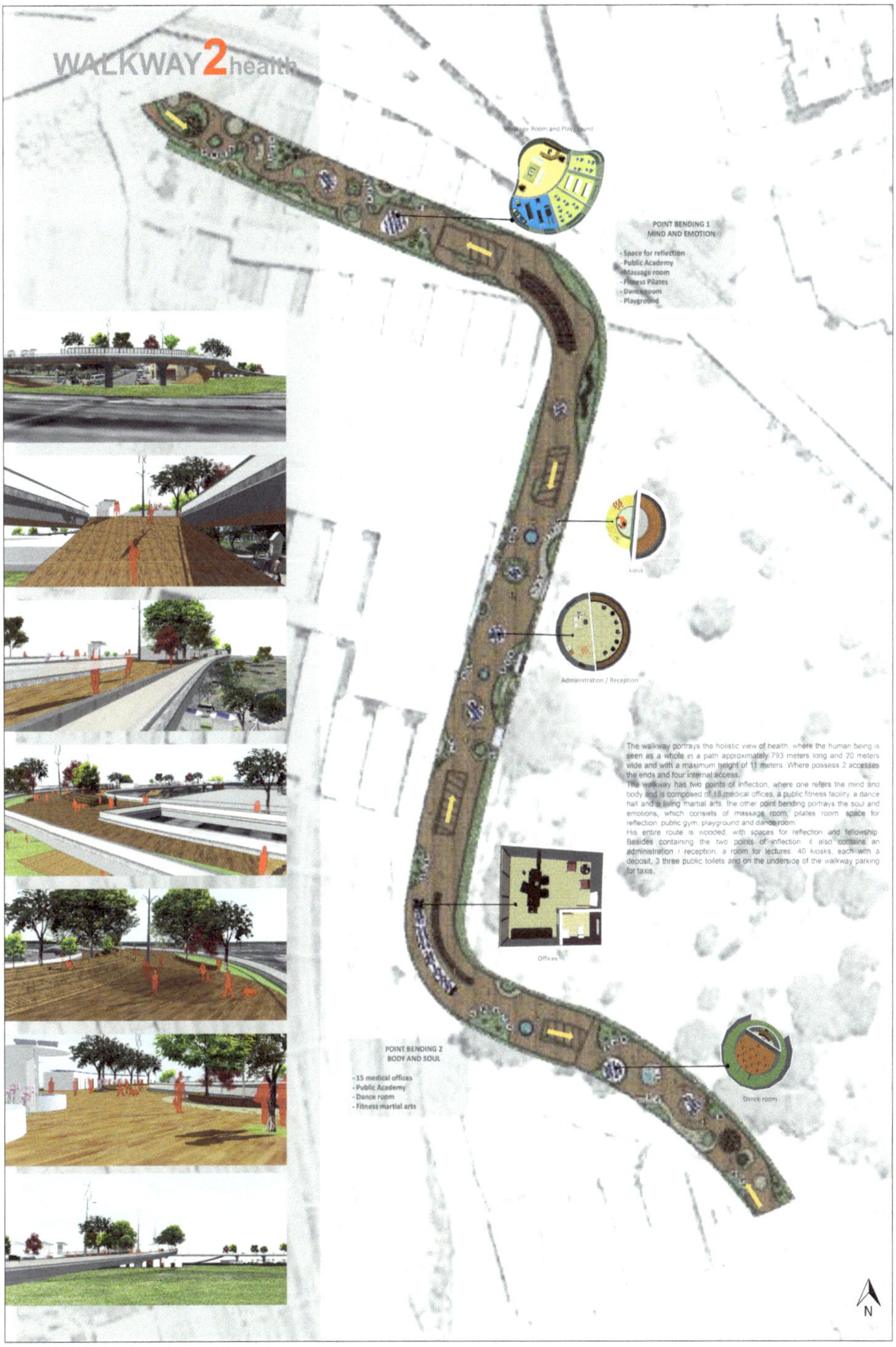

Figure 8. Commended: Lhoyranne Karollen Araujo Marques, Universidade Católica de Brasilia, Brazil.

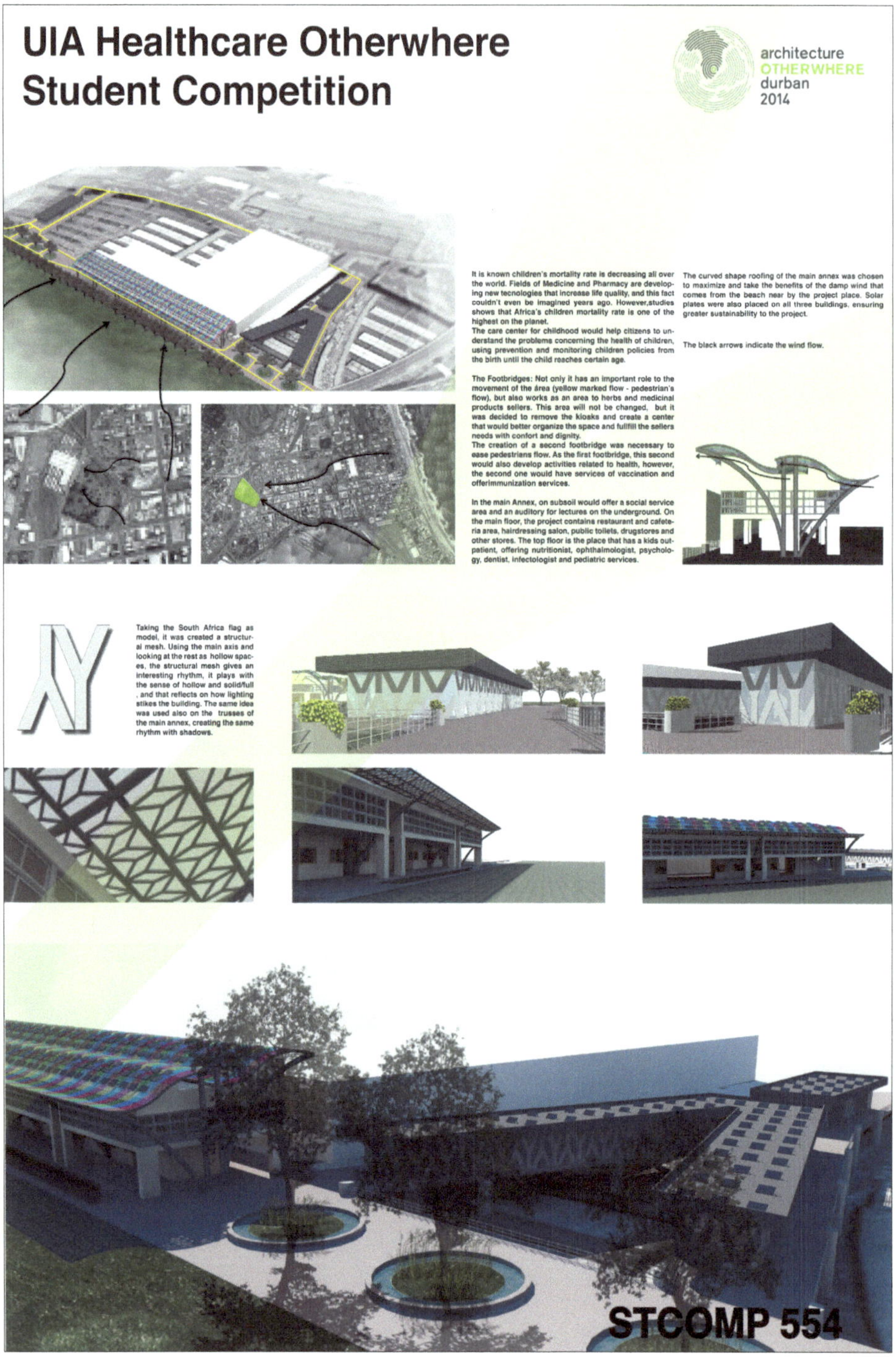

Figure 9. Top ten: Joyce Stival, Universidade Católica de Brasilia,Brazil.

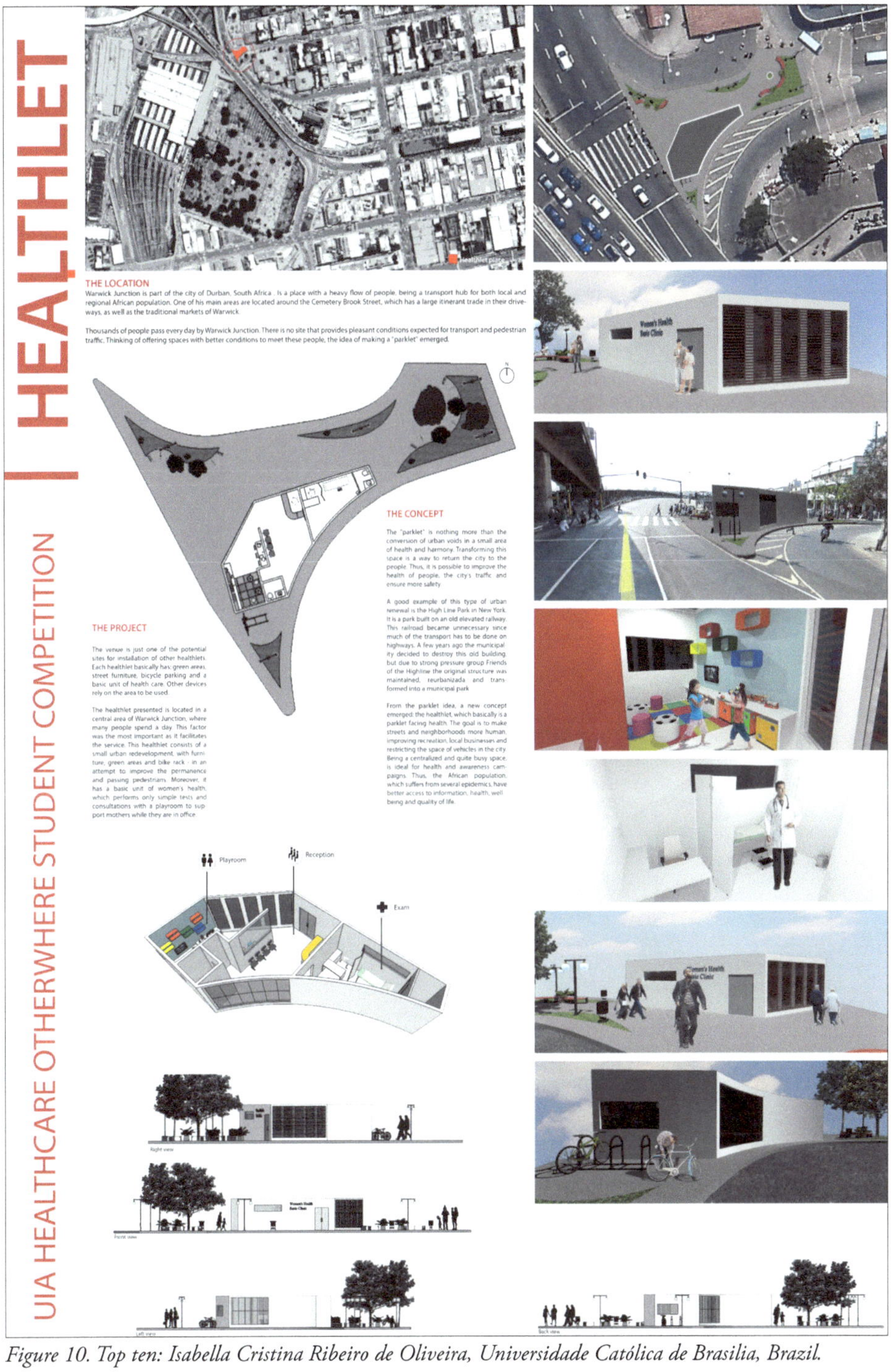

Figure 10. Top ten: Isabella Cristina Ribeiro de Oliveira, Universidade Católica de Brasilia, Brazil.

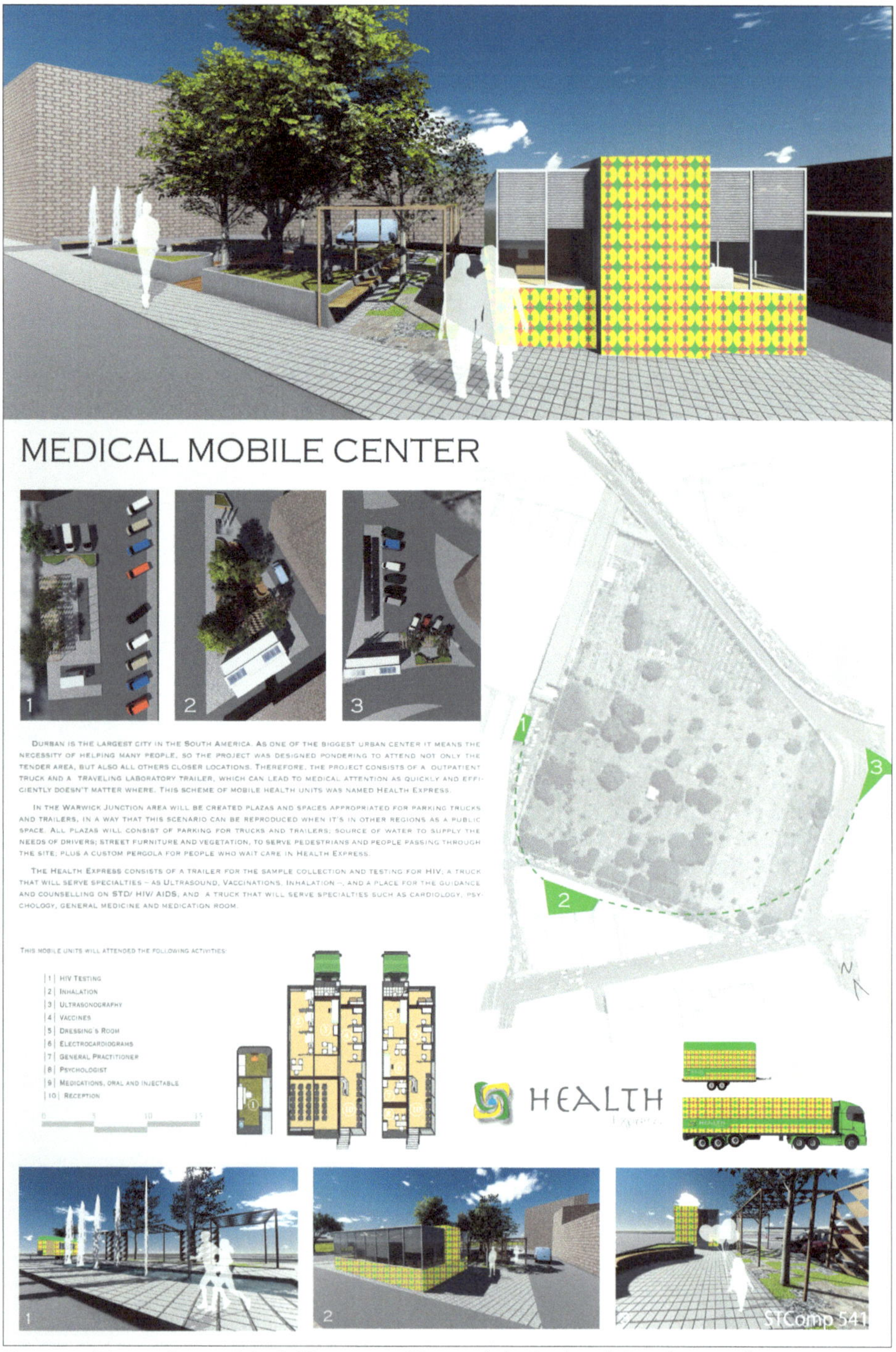

Figure 11. Top ten: Lorena Lelis do Nascimento, Universidade Católica de Brasilia, Brazil.

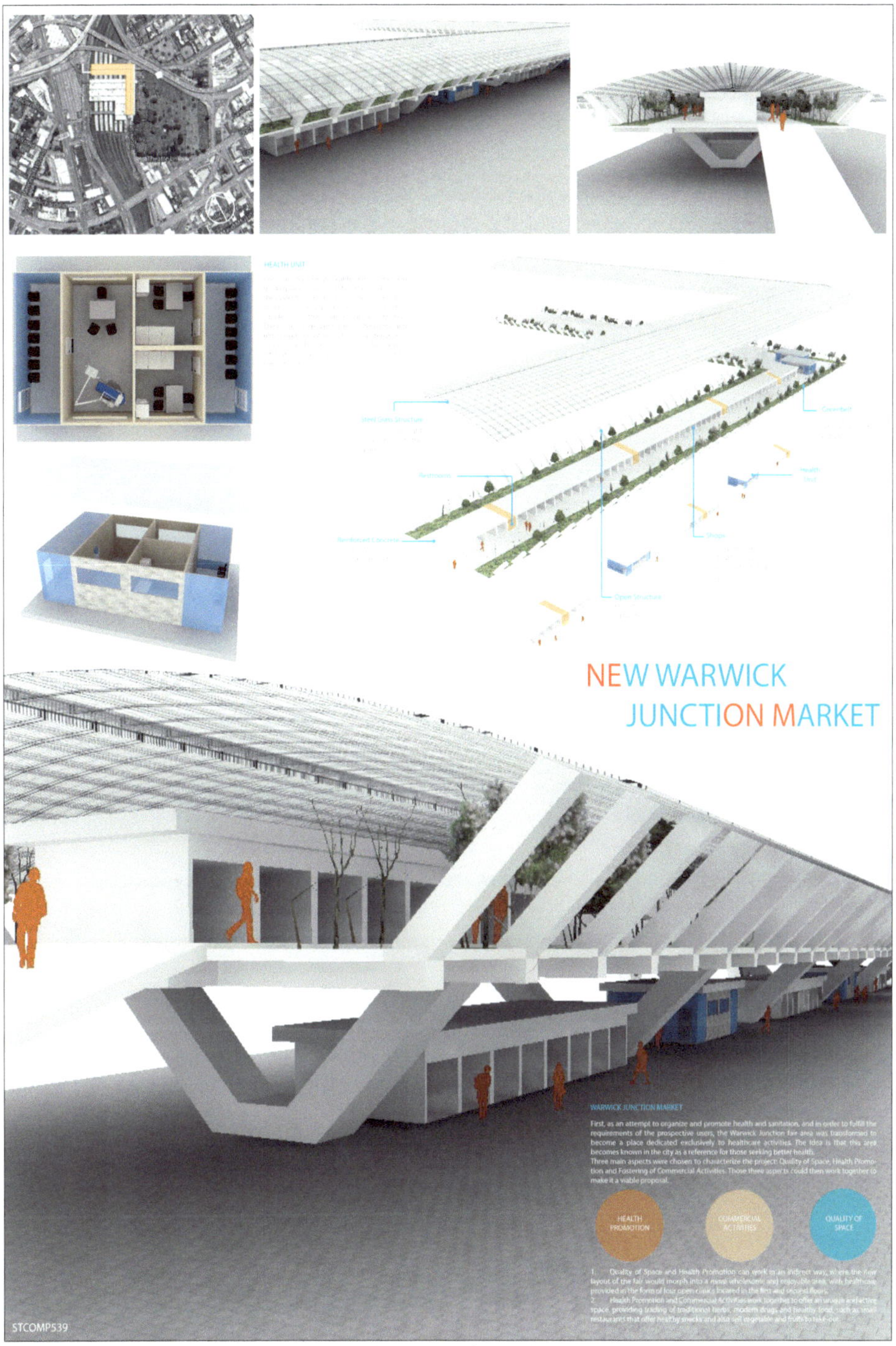

Figure 12. Top ten: Ruth Lopes, Universidade Católica de Brasilia, Brazil.

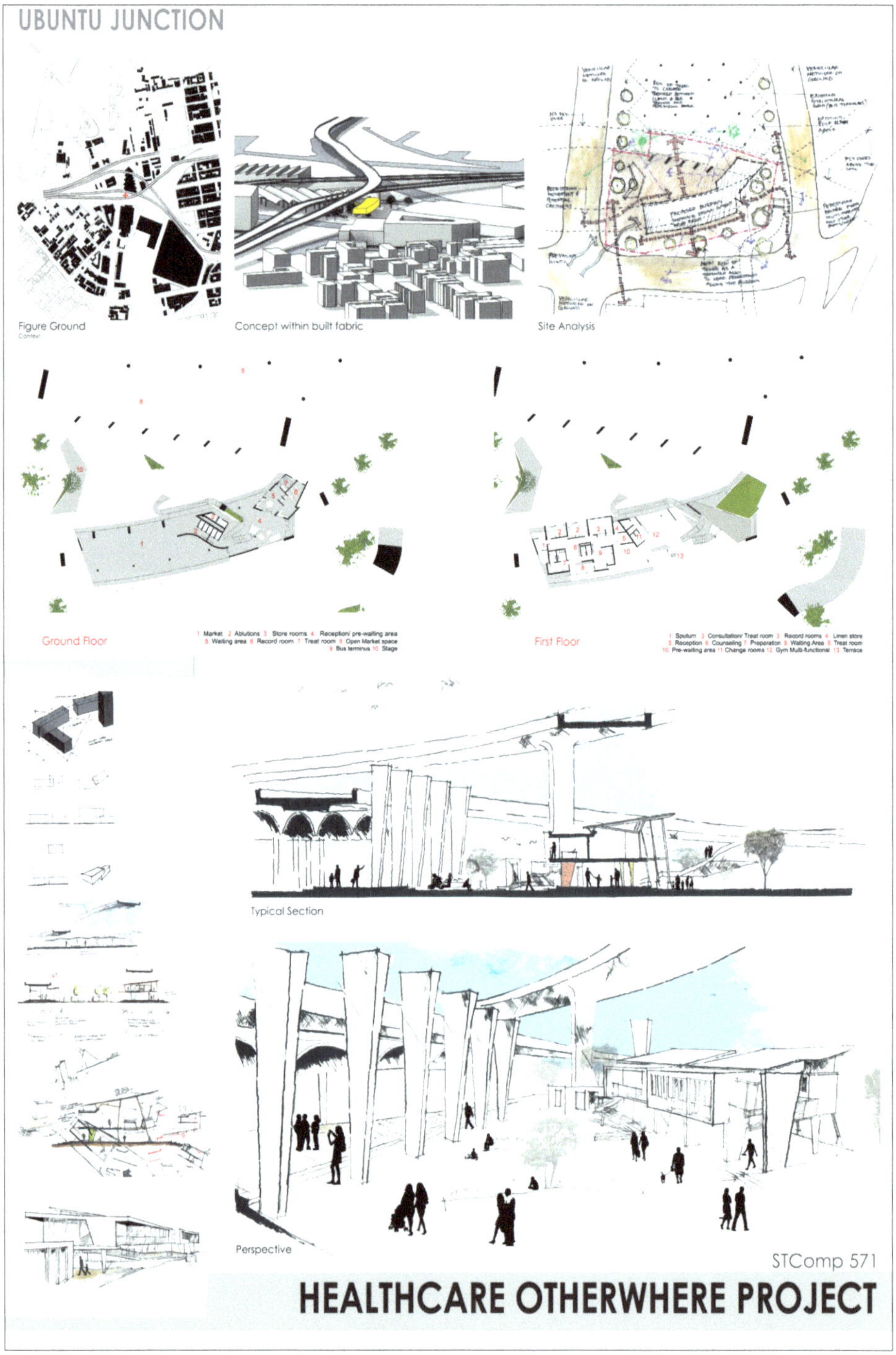

Figure 13. Top ten: Ayanda Ntsingana, Cape Peninsular University of Technology, South Africa.

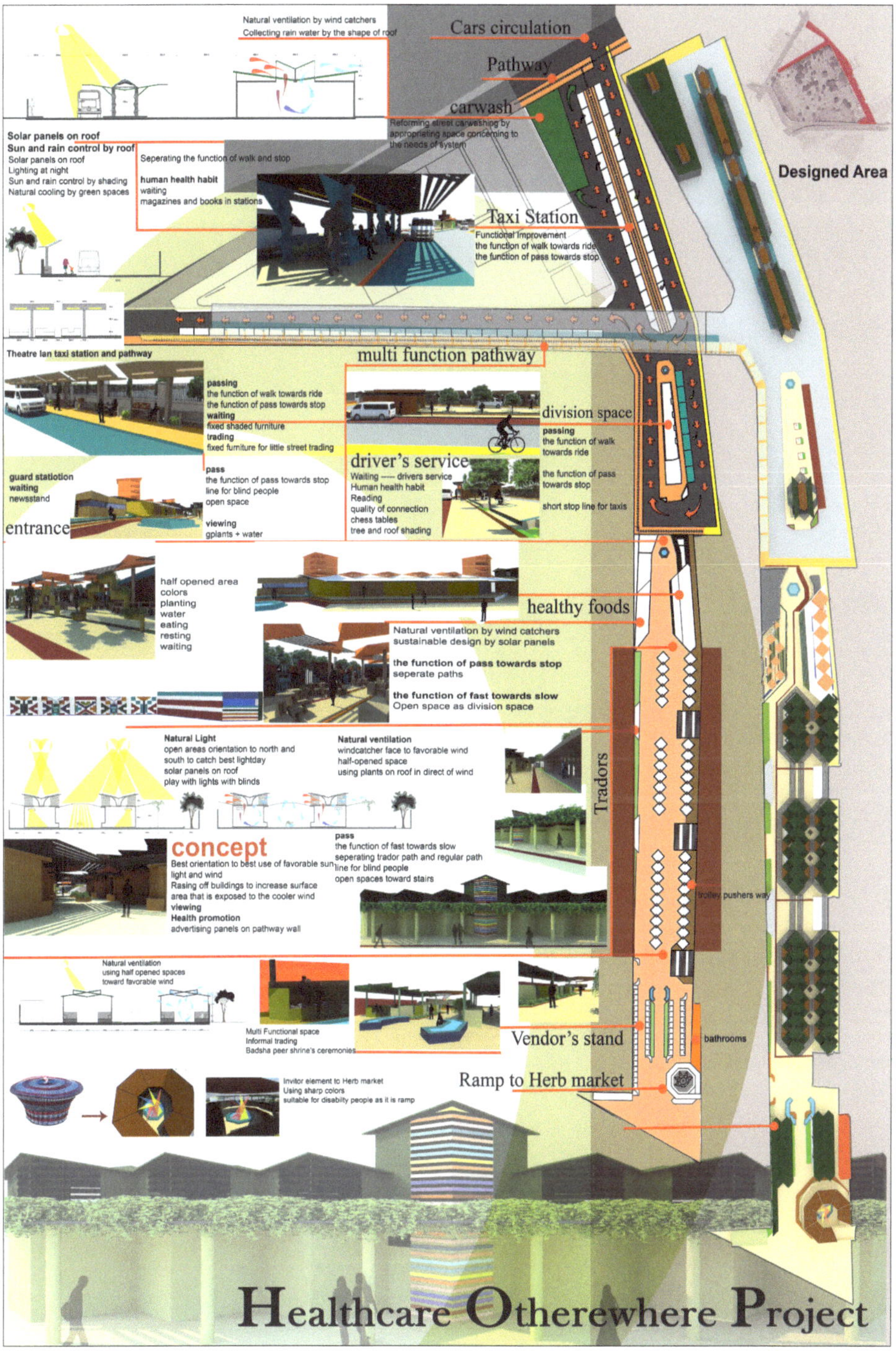

Figure 14. Top ten: Leili Mirzakhalili, Maziar Higher Educational Institute, Islamic Republic of Iran.

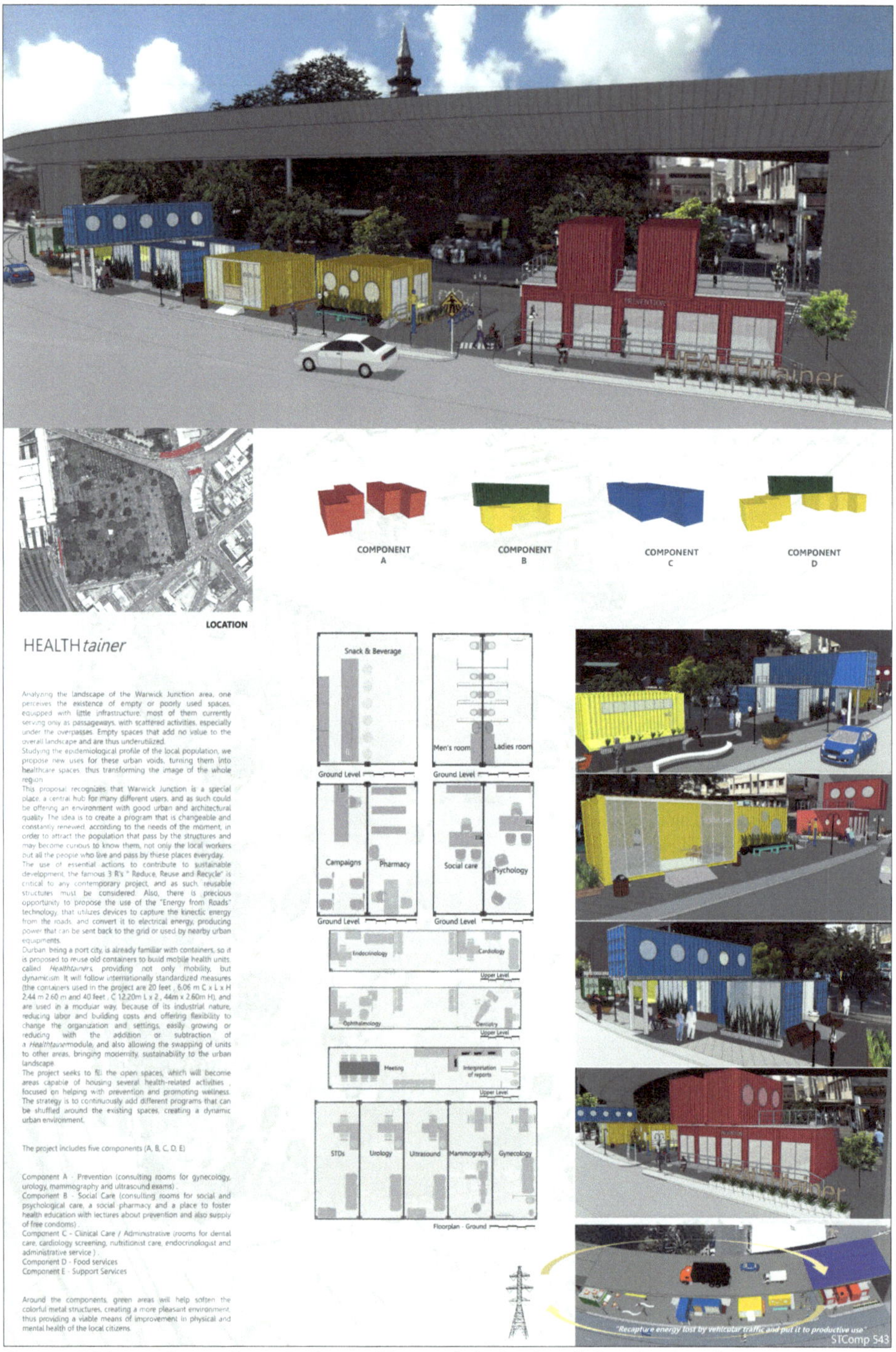

Figure 15. Top ten: Leticia Soares Rodrigues, Universidade Católica de Brasilia, Brazil.

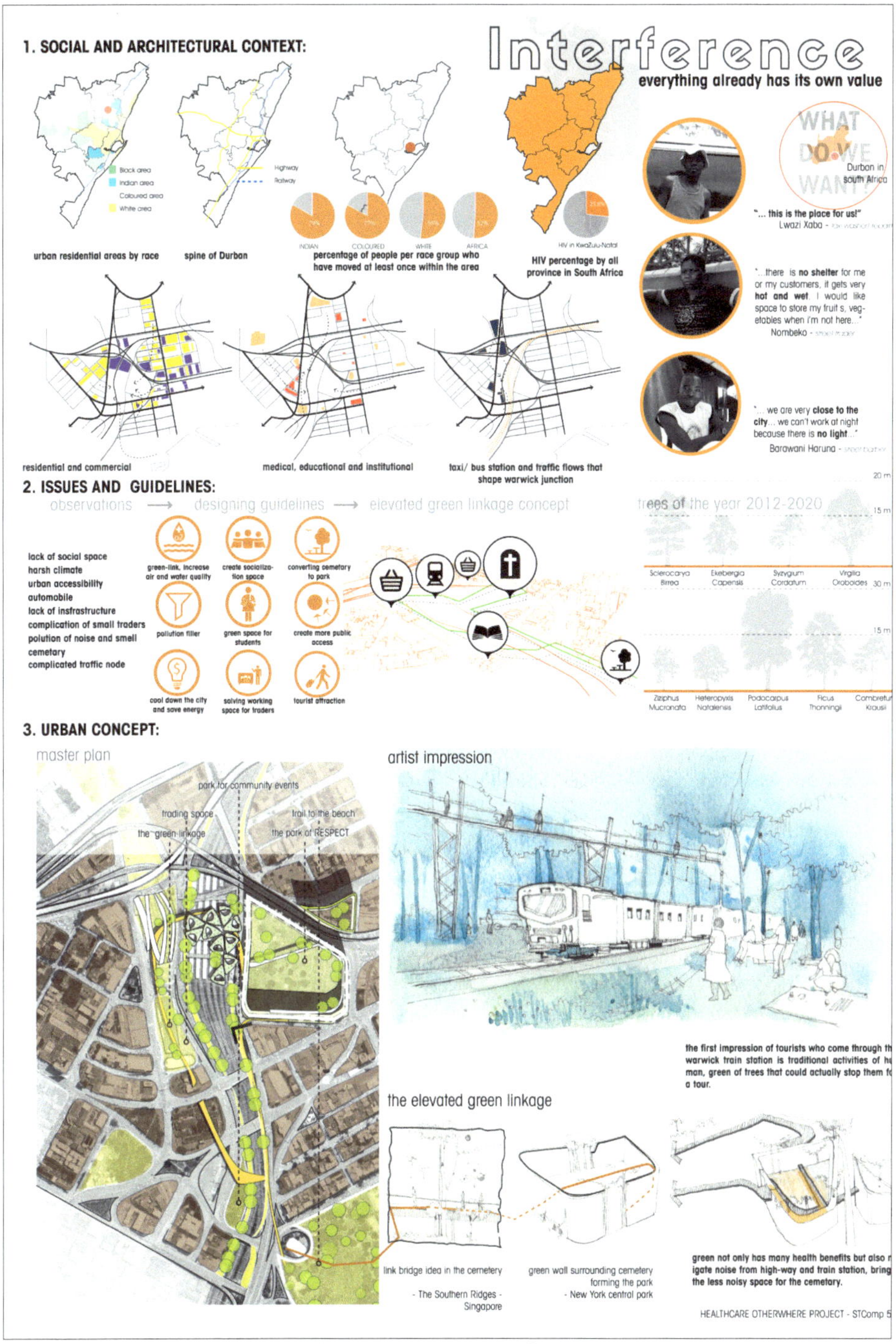

Figure 16. Third place: Chau Tran, Clemson University, United States.

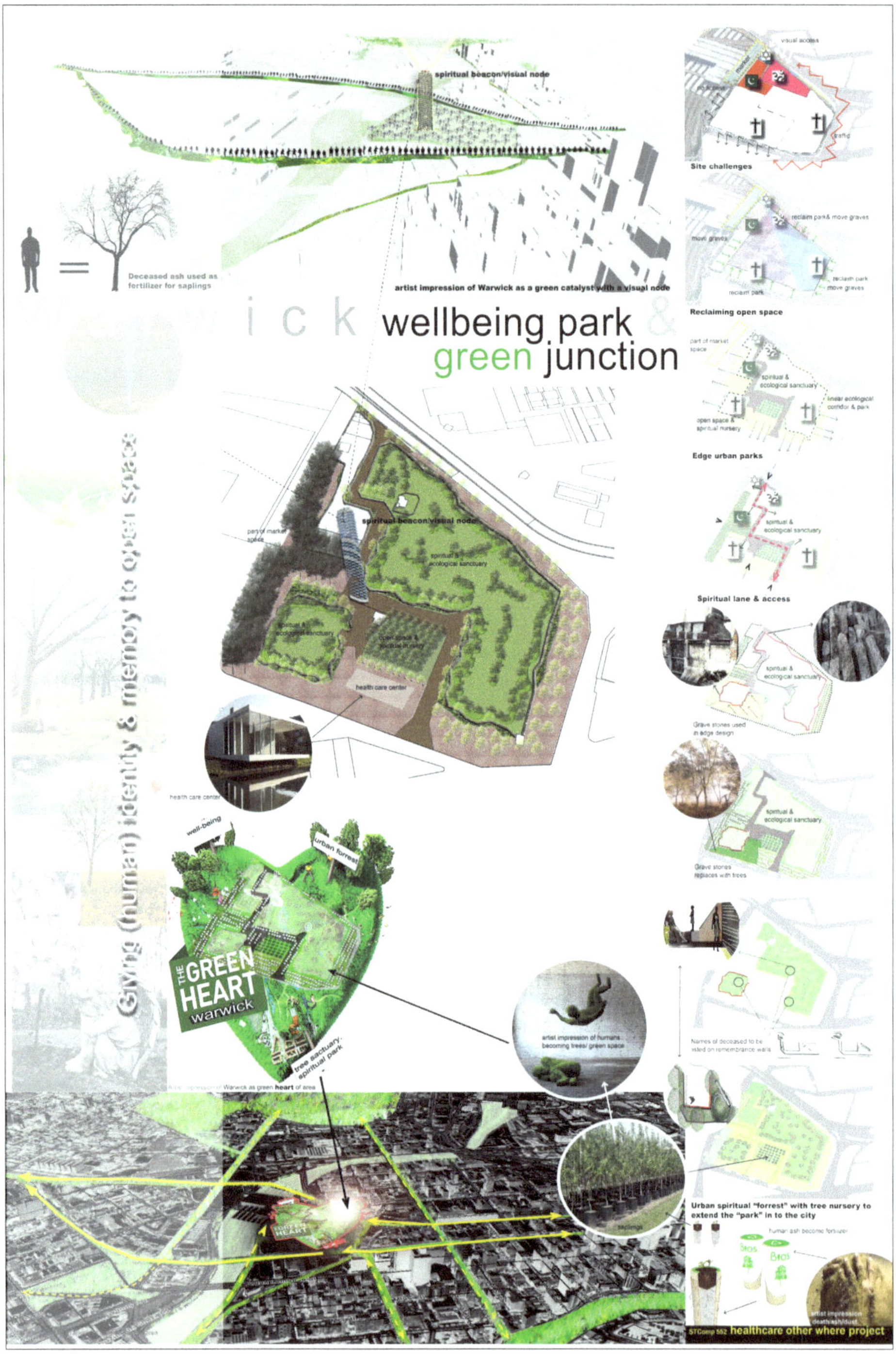

Figure 17. Second place: Henk Dippenaar, Tshwane University of Technology, South Africa.

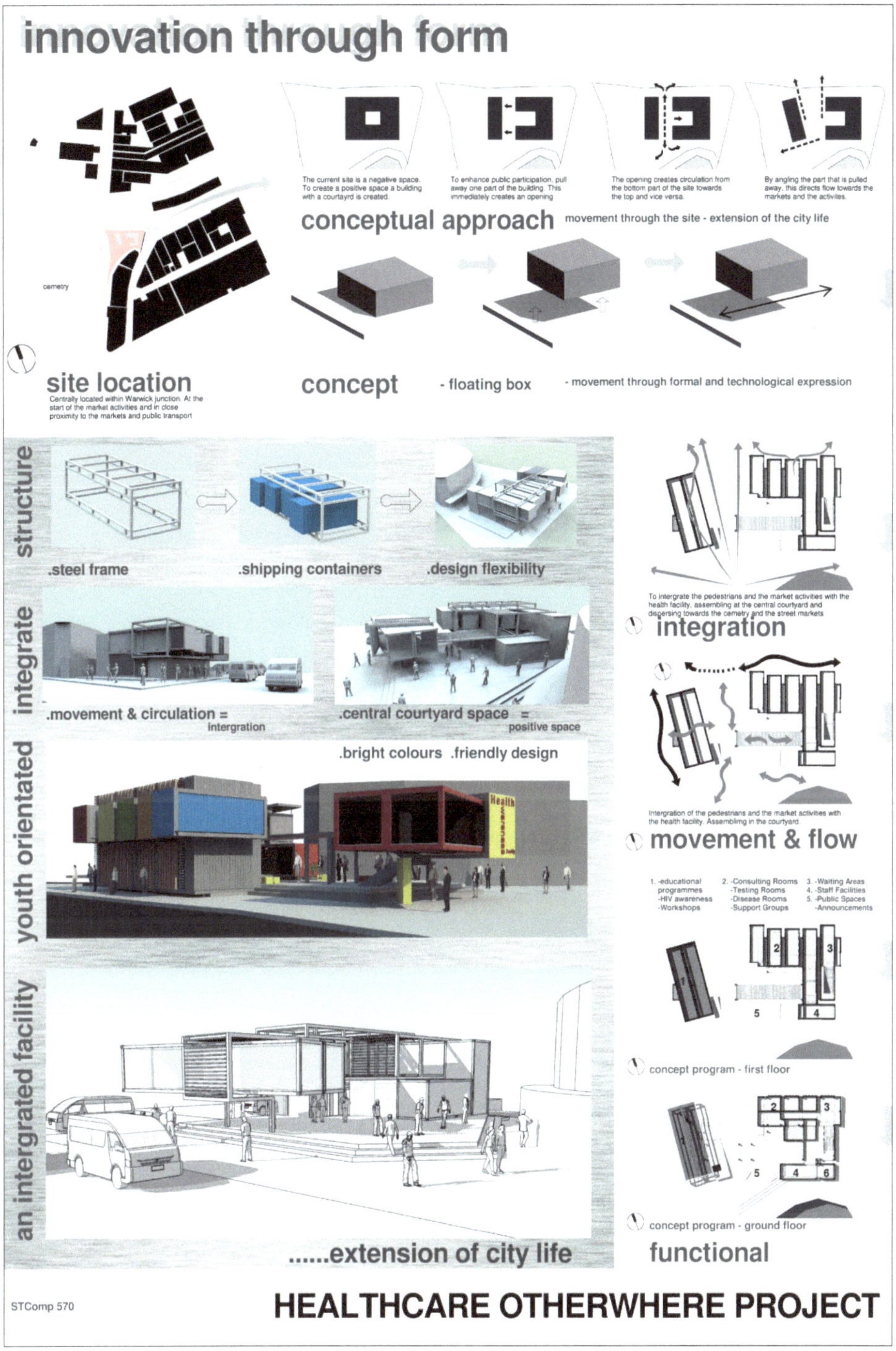

Figure 18. First place: Eugene Henning, Cape Peninsular University of Technology, South Africa.

211

AWARDS CEREMONY

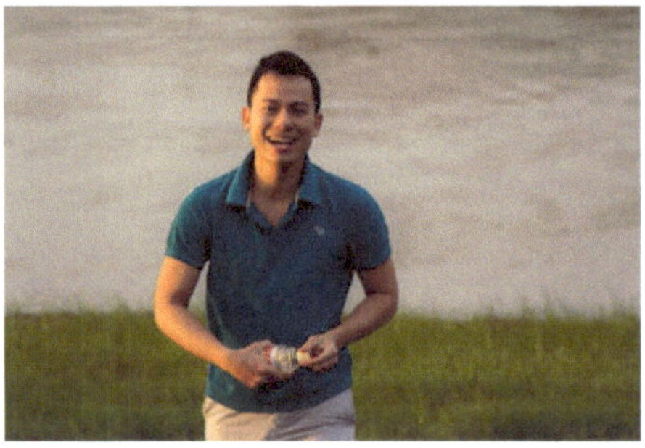

Figure 19. The international winner: Chau Tran, from Clemson University, USA was unfortunately not able to visit Durban.

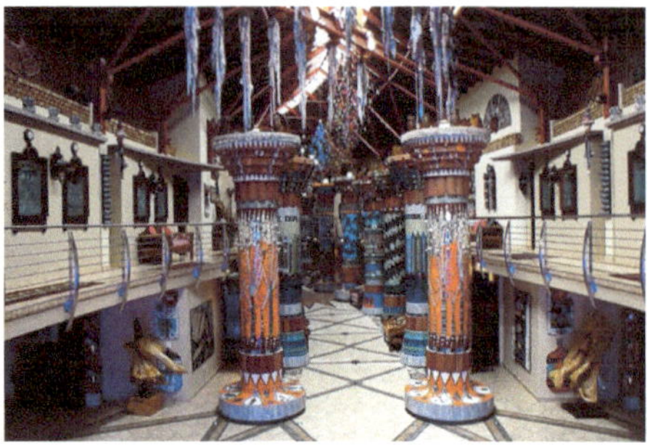

Figure 20. Gala dinner and awards were hosted at Ammazulu Palace on the 6th August 2014.

ACKNOWLEDGEMENTS

Generous sponsorship for the student competition exhibition was solicited by the local organising committee and was received from:
Copper Development Association, Frik Lange, A3, Gallagher Lourens, Consultium Project Planning and Management, John Staff, Revel Fox, Sharp Shop, John Royal, Harry Burger, Graceland, and Belgotex.
Exceedingly generous sponsorship was provided by Mike Nightingale Fellowship, Peter Pawlik and Saint Gobain South Africa for the prizes which were presented at an award ceremony at a gala dinner at Ammazulu African Palace.

SAINT-GOBAIN

MIKE NIGHTINGALE FELLOWSHIP Changing lives through sustainable development

TESIS Inter-University Research Centre "Systems and Technologies for Social and Healthcare Facilities"
University of Florence, Italy

www.ingramcontent.com/pod-product-compliance
Ingram Content Group UK Ltd.
Pitfield, Milton Keynes, MK11 3LW, UK
UKHW061541051026
15625UKWH00011B/560